National Jewish Center for Immunology and Respiratory Medicine
1400 Jackson Street
Denver, CO 80206
(303) 388-4461
800-222-5864

National Kidney Foundation
30 East 33rd Street
New York, NY 10016
(212) 889-2210

National Multiple Sclerosis Society
733 Third Avenue
New York, NY 10017

National Rehabilitation Information Center
8455 Colesville Road, Suite 935
Silver Spring, MD 20910
(301) 588-9284

Pediatric AIDS Foundation
1311 Colorado Avenue
Santa Monica, CA 90404
(310) 395-9051

Rehabilitation Services Administration
Department of Human Services,
Room 101M
605 G Street, NW
Washington, DC 20002
(202) 727-3211

Scleroderma Federation, Inc.
1182 Teaneck Road
Teaneck, NJ 07666

Sex Information and Education Council of the US
130 West 42nd Street, Suite 2500
New York, NY 10036
(212) 819-9770

United Network for Organ Sharing
National Organ Procurement and
Transplantation Network
1100 Boulders Parkway, Suite 500
P.O. Box 13770
Richmond, VA 23225
800-24-DONOR

United Scleroderma Foundation, Inc.
P.O. Box 399
Watsonville, CA 95077-0399
(408) 728-2202
1-800-HOPE

PROFESSIONAL ORGANIZATIONS

American Association of Neuroscience Nurses
224 N. Desplaines
Suite 601
Chicago, IL 60661
(312) 993-0043

American Congress of Rehabilitation Medicine
5700 Old Orchard Road, First Floor
Skokie, IL 60077-1024
(708) 966-0095

American Nephrology Nurses Association
ANNA National Office
North Woodbury Road
Box 56
Pitman, NJ 08071
(609) 589-2187

American Nurses Association
600 Maryland Avenue, SW
Suite 100 West
Washington, DC 20024
(202) 554-4444

Association of Rehabilitation Nurses
5700 Old Orchard Road, First Floor
Skokie, IL 60077-1024
(708) 966-3433

Joint Commission on Accreditation of Health Care Organizations
One Renaissance Boulevard
Oakbrook Terrace, IL 60181
(708) 916-5600

The Living Bank
4545 Post Oak Place, Suite 315
Houston, TX 77027
(713) 528-2971 or 800-528-2971

National Association of Orthopaedic Nurses
Box 56
North Woodbury Road
Pitman, NJ 08071
(609) 582-0111

North American Transplant Coordinators Association (NATCO)
P.O. Box 15384
Lenexa, KS 66215
913-492-3600

IMMUNOLOGIC DISORDERS

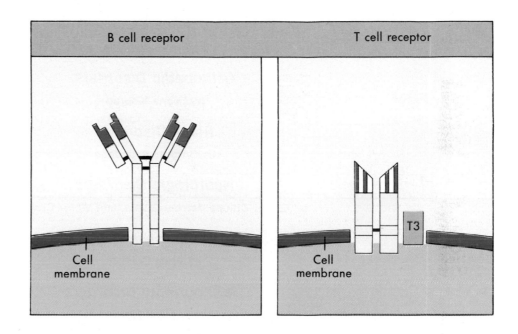

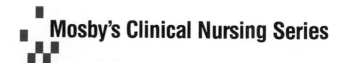

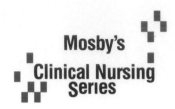

Mosby's Clinical Nursing Series

Cardiovascular Disorders
by Mary Canobbio

Respiratory Disorders
by Susan Wilson and June Thompson

Infectious Diseases
by Deanna Grimes

Orthopedic Disorders
by Leona Mourad

Renal Disorders
by Dorothy Brundage

Neurologic Disorders
by Esther Chipps, Norma Clanin, and Victor Campbell

Cancer Nursing
by Anne Belcher

Genitourinary Disorders
by Mikel Gray

Immunologic Disorders
by Christine Mudge-Grout

Gastrointestinal Disorders
by Dorothy Doughty and Debra Broadwell

IMMUNOLOGIC DISORDERS

CHRISTINE L. MUDGE-GROUT, R.N., M.S., C.C.R.N., C.N.N.

Clinical Nurse Specialist,
Assistant Clinical Professor,
University of California—San Francisco,
San Francisco, California

Original illustrations by

GEORGE J. WASSILCHENKO
Tulsa, Oklahoma

and

DONALD P. O'CONNOR
St. Peters, Missouri

Original photography by

PATRICK WATSON
Poughkeepsie, New York

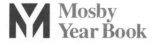 Mosby
Year Book

St. Louis Baltimore Boston Chicago London Philadelphia Sydney Toronto

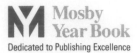
Mosby
Year Book
Dedicated to Publishing Excellence

Publisher: Alison Miller
Editor: Sally Schrefer
Developmental editor: Penny Rudolph
Project manager: Mark Spann
Production editors: Stephen Hetager, Christine O'Neil
Designer: Liz Fett
Layout: Doris Hallas

This book would not have been possible without the loving attention and patience of my family and friends. Most importantly, I would like to thank my husband, Jim Grout, for his invaluable support. I also wish to acknowledge the contributions of the University of California at San Francisco and the encouragement provided by Sally Schrefer.

Mosby–Year Book, Inc.
11830 Westline Industrial Drive
St. Louis, Missouri 63146

Library of Congress Cataloging-in-Publication Data

Immunologic disorders / Christine L. Mudge-Grout;
    original illustrations by George J. Wassilchenko and Donald P.
    O'Connor; original photography by Patrick Watson.
        p.   cm. — (Mosby's clinical nursing series)
    Includes bibliographical references and index.
    ISBN 0-8016-2775-3
    1. Immunologic diseases—Nursing.   2. Immunologic Diseases—
atlases.   3. Immunologic Diseases—nursing.   I. Mudge-Grout,
    Christine L. II. Series.
    [DNLM: WY 150 I325]
    RC582.I463   1992
    616.97—dc20
    DNLM/DLC
    for Library of Congress   92-49624
                                                     CIP

92 93 94 95 96 CL/CD/VH 9 8 7 6 5 4 3 2 1

Contributors

LINDA ABRAMOWITZ, R.N., M.S.
Clinical Nurse Specialist, Pediatric Bone Marrow
Transplant; Assistant Clinical Professor, University of
California at San Francisco, San Francisco, California
(*Severe combined immunodeficiency disease,
Wiskott-Aldrich syndrome*)

CYNTHIA RENO BALKSTRA, R.N.C., M.S.
Nursing Supervisor, Department of Nursing,
University of California at San Francisco, San
Francisco, California
(*Acquired immunodeficiency syndrome*)

JANA NIBBE HAGEN, R.N., M.S.
Independent Consultant, Pediatric Critical Care, St.
Paul, Minnesota
(*Autoimmune hemolytic anemia, Idiopathic
thrombocytopenic purpura, Idiopathic neutropenia,
Pernicious anemia*)

MARGIE STIRM, R.N., M.S., P.N.P., M.P.H.
Clinical Nurse Specialist, Pediatric Immunology/
Rheumatology, University of California at San
Francisco, San Francisco, California
(*X-linked agammaglobulinemia, Common variable
immunodeficiency*)

MARY ANN VAN DAM, R.N., M.S., P.N.P.
Clinical Nurse II, Pediatrics, University of California
at San Francisco; Clinical Pediatric Faculty, San
Francisco State University, San Francisco, California
(*Juvenile rheumatoid arthritis*)

CAROL S. VIELE, R.N., M.S.
Clinical Nurse Specialist, Department of Nursing,
Oncology/Hematology, Bone Marrow Transplant;
Assistant Clinical Professor, University of California at
San Francisco, San Francisco, California
(*Bone marrow transplantation*)

Consultants

DANIEL ADELMAN, M.D.
Assistant Professor of Clinical Medicine,
Allergy/Immunology Division, University of California
at San Francisco, San Francisco, California

LAURIE CARLSON, R.N., M.S.
Clinical Nurse Specialist, Department of Nursing,
Nephrology/Transplant, University of California at San
Francisco, San Francisco, California

MARVIN R. GAROVOY, M.D.
Director of Immunogenetics and Transplantation;
Professor in Residence, Surgery and Medicine,
University of California at San Francisco, San
Francisco, California

EDWARD J. GOETZL, M.D.
Robert L. Kroc Professor of Medicine, Director of
Division of Allergy and Immunology and
Microbiology/Immunology, University of California at
San Francisco, San Francisco, California

SUSAN JANSEN-BJERKLIE, R.N., D.N.Sc.
Associate Professor, Department of Physiological
Nursing, University of California at San Francisco, San
Francisco, California

SHARON LEWIS, R.N., Ph.D.
Associate Professor, College of Nursing; Research
Assistant Professor, Department of Pathology;
University of New Mexico, Albuquerque, New Mexico

OLIVIA MARTINEZ, Ph.D.
Assistant Research Immunologist, Liver Transplant
Division, Department of Surgery, University of
California at San Francisco, San Francisco, California

Preface

Immunologic Disorders is the ninth volume in *Mosby's Clinical Nursing Series*, a new kind of resource for practicing nurses. The *Series* is the result of the most elaborate market research ever undertaken by Mosby–Year Book, Inc. We first surveyed hundreds of working nurses to determine what kinds of resources practicing nurses want to meet their advanced information needs. We then approached clinical specialists, proven authors and experts, and asked them to develop a format that would meet the needs of nurses in practice. This format was presented to nine focus groups composed of working nurses and was refined among them. In the later stages we published a 32-page full-color sample so that detailed changes could be made to improve physical layout and appearance, section by section and page by page. The result is a new genre of professional books for nursing professionals.

Immunologic Disorders begins with a clear and concise Color Atlas of the Immune System. This is a complete and comprehensive review of the physiology of human defenses and immune responses. Every effort was made to explain the immune system in a way that rationalizes nursing interventions related to immunologic disorders.

Chapter 2 is a pictorial guide to the nurse's assessment of the immune system with reference to related disorders. Clear, full-color photographs show proper patient positioning and assessment techniques in sharp detail. All photos are accompanied by concise instructions in the text. Color manifestations of specific disorders complement this chapter.

Chapter 3 focuses on the laboratory tests used most frequently to diagnose or evaluate patients with immunoglic disorders. Biopsies and ophthalmologic tests are also presented. A consistent format for each procedure provides information about the purpose of the test, indications and contraindications, and nursing care, including patient teaching.

Chapters 4 to 12 present the nursing care of patients with immunologic disorders. Chapters 4 to 6 provide comprehensive overviews of acquired immunodeficiency syndrome (AIDS), common immunodeficiency disorders, and rheumatoid disorders. Chapters 7 to 11 discuss immune disorders focusing on a specific system—hemopoietic, vascular, renal, neurologic, and endocrine, respectively. Chapter 12 addresses medical interventions such as transplantation and plasmapheresis. Detailed charts and illustrations accompany the text. Each disease is presented in a format that you invented to meet your advanced practice needs. This format starts with the pathophysiology and clinical manifesta-

tions of each disease. Potential complications of each disorder are highlighted in a box for quick and easy reference. Definitive diagnostic tests with expected findings and the medical plan of treatment are briefly reviewed to promote collaboration among health care team members in an effort to provide optimum patient care. Patient teaching concerns are identified at the end of each disorder to enable the nurse to anticipate questions often asked by patient and family and to maximize teaching efforts and the use of time.

The nursing care for each disease represents the heart of the book and is presented according to the nursing process in easy-to-use tables. These pages have colored borders to make them easy to find and use on your unit. The nursing care is structured to integrate the five steps of the nursing process, centered around appropriate nursing diagnoses accepted by the North American Nursing Diagnosis Association (NANDA). The material can be used to develop individualized care plans quickly and accurately, and it meets the standards of nursing care required by the Joint Commission on the Accreditation of Healthcare Organizations (JCAHO). By facilitating the development of individualized and authoritative care plans, this book can actually allow you more time to spend on direct patient care.

In response to requests from scores of nurses participating in our research, a distinctive feature of this book is its use in patient teaching. Background information on diseases and medical interventions enables nurses to answer with authority questions patients often ask. The illustrations in the book, particularly those in the Color Atlas and in the chapter on diagnostic studies, are specifically designed to support patient teaching. In addition, the patient teaching section in each care plan provides nurses with a checklist of instructional concepts, promoting this vital aspect of care.

This book is intended for medical-surgical nurses, who invariably care for patients with immunologic disorders, practicing in both inpatient and outpatient settings. We expect it to be a helpful reference for nurses working primarily in hospital medical-surgical units, public health, home health, occupational health, and rehabilitation and long-term care facilities. We also anticipate that the book will be a valuable adjunct to medical-surgical nursing texts for nursing students. We hope that this book will contribute to the overall advancement of immunologic nursing and that it will promote the advancement of professional nursing by serving as a first step toward a body of professional nursing literature.

Contents

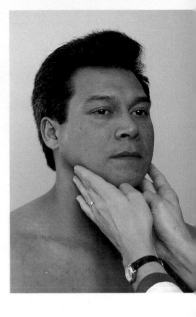

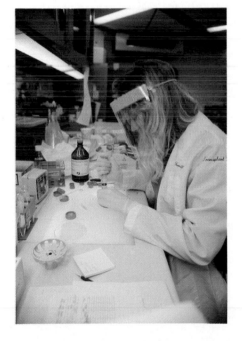

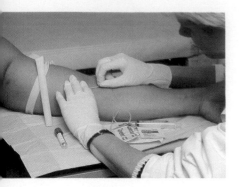

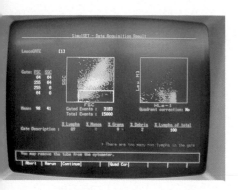

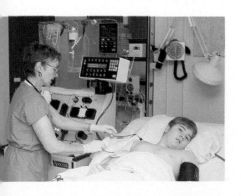

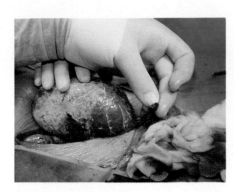

12 Transplantation and therapeutic procedures, 314

Appendix A   Complete blood count, 349

Appendix B   Examples of agglutination assays, 350

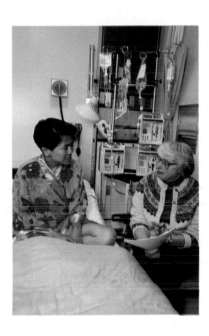

Color Plates

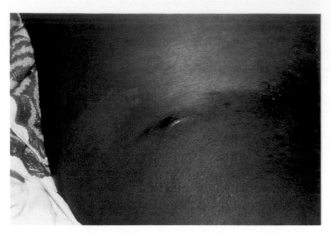

PLATE 1 Kaposi's sarcoma of the groin in patient with AIDS. (Courtesy The Centers for Disease Control, 1992.)

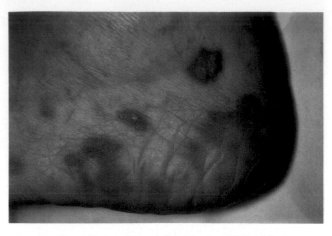

PLATE 2 Kaposi's sarcoma of distal heel and lateral foot. (Courtesy The Centers for Disease Control, 1992.)

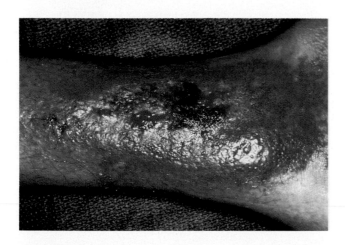

PLATE 3 Kaposi's sarcoma of distal leg and ankle. (Courtesy The Centers for Disease Control, 1992.)

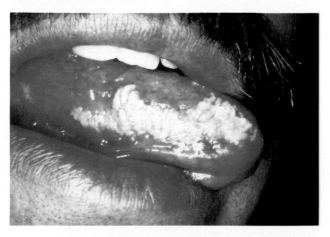

PLATE 4 Hairy leukoplakia on the tongue of a patient with AIDS. (Courtesy J.S. Greenspan, D.D.S., University of California—San Francisco; Courtesy The Centers for Disease Control, 1992.)

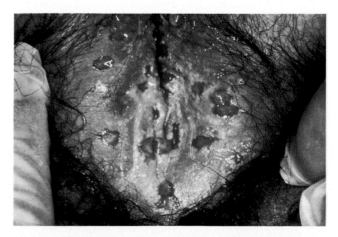

PLATE 5 Primary perineal herpes with methylene blue stain. (Courtesy The Centers for Disease Control, 1992.)

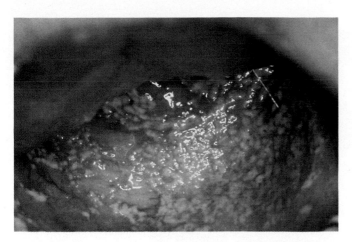

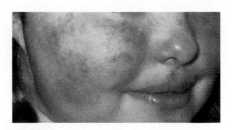

PLATE 7 Butterfly rash of systemic lupus erythematosus. (From Seidel et al.[157] Courtesy Walter Tunnessen, M.D., Johns Hopkins University School of Medicine, Baltimore, Md.)

PLATE 6 Soft palate showing extensive oral candidiasis in a patient with AIDS. (Courtesy Michael Glick, M.D., University of Pennsylvania, Philadelphia, Pa; Courtesy The Centers for Disease Control, 1992.)

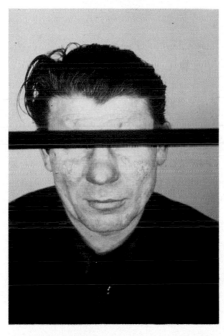

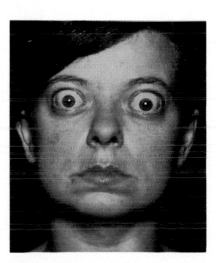

PLATE 9 Graves' disease. (From Seidel et al.[157] Courtesy Paul W. Ladenson, M.D., Johns Hopkins University and Hospital, Baltimore, Md.)

PLATE 8 Discoid lupus erythematosus. (Courtesy The Centers for Disease Control, 1992.)

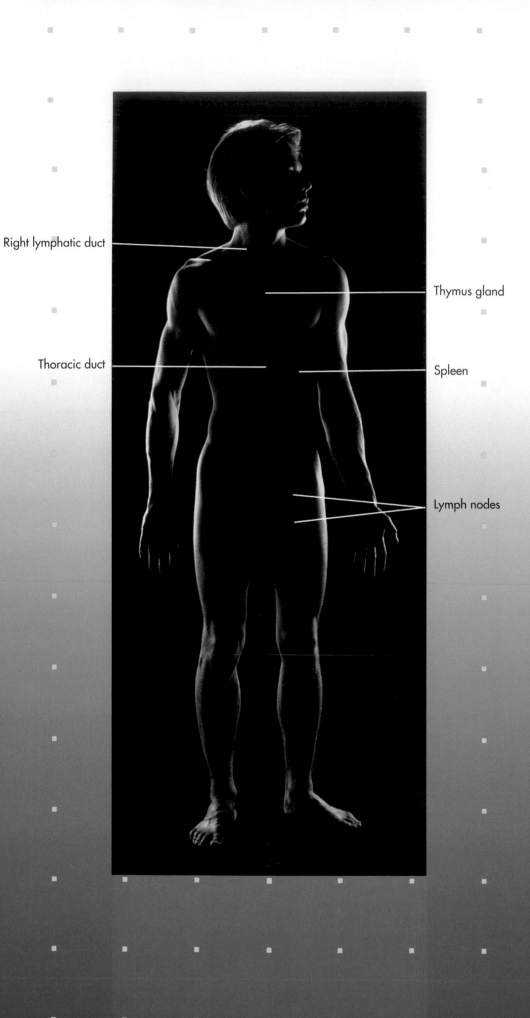

Right lymphatic duct

Thymus gland

Thoracic duct

Spleen

Lymph nodes

CHAPTER 1

Color Atlas of the Immune System

The word "immune" is derived from the Latin word *immunis*, meaning free from burden.

Immunology is an evolving science that essentially deals with the body's ability to distinguish *self* from *nonself*. This is accomplished through a complex network of highly specialized cells and tissues that collectively are called the *immune system*.

The immune system has three main functions: (1) to protect the body's internal milieu against invading organisms; (2) to maintain homeostasis by removing damaged cells from the circulation; and (3) to serve as a surveillance network for recognizing and guarding against the development, growth, and dissemination of abnormal cells. When the immune system responds appropriately to a foreign stimulus, the body's integrity is maintained; this is called *immunocompetence*. If the immune response is too weak or too vigorous, homeostasis is disrupted, causing a malfunction in the system, or *immunoincompetence*. Disruption of the homeostatic balance of the immune system can cause a number of diseases to manifest themselves. Inappropriate responses of the immune system have been classified into four categories: (1) hyperactive responses against environmental antigens (e.g., allergy); (2) inability to protect the body, as in immunodeficiency disorders (e.g., acquired immunodeficiency syndrome [AIDS]); (3) failure to recognize the body as self, as in autoimmune disorders (e.g., systemic lupus erythematosus); and (4) attacks on beneficial foreign tissue (e.g., organ transplantation rejection or transfusion reaction).

The advent of a number of molecular biologic techniques has greatly increased our knowledge of the immune system over the past decade. For example, immunomodulatory agents are widely used to augment immune function in cancer patients and people with immunodeficiency diseases. Histocompatibility matching and the development of pharmacologic agents that selectively depress immune reactivity have had a major impact on organ transplantation. The development of a variety of such techniques to treat and manage immunologic disorders, as well as our increasing knowledge of the immune system, will play an integral role in all clinical specialties in the future.

INNATE AND ADAPTIVE IMMUNITY

The immune system has two major defense mechanisms for protecting the body against foreign invasion: innate (nonspecific) immunity and adaptive (specific) immunity (Figure 1-1). **Innate** immunity is the first line of defense, providing physical and chemical barriers to invading pathogens. If these components fail to prevent invasion or to destroy a foreign pathogen, the adaptive immune response is summoned to assist in the battle. **Adaptive** immunity provides a specific reaction to each invading antigen and has the unique ability to remember the antigen that elicited the attack.

An **antigen** is a substance recognized by the body as foreign that can trigger an immune response. A characteristic known as memory enables the adaptive immune system to launch a quick response if reexposure to the antigen occurs. Certain diseases such as measles and chickenpox can produce lifelong immunity after the body has been exposed and infected.

Innate immunity is present from birth and is made up of a number of nonspecific defense systems. The body's exterior surface, including an intact skin and mucous membranes, provides an effective barrier and is the first line of defense against infectious and invasive organisms (Figure 1-2 diagrams the external defenses). Most infectious agents enter the body via the gastrointestinal tract, lungs, genitourinary tract, and nasopharynx. These structures not only serve as physical barriers to invasion, they also provide a milieu that is chemically unsuitable for microbial growth. Specific skin and mucosal secretions such as lysozyme, gastric acid, and lactic acid have bactericidal properties to protect the body. Lysozyme, for example, is a muco-

lytic, polysaccharide-specific enzyme found in nasal secretions, saliva, tears, and sweat that in the presence of complement can disrupt (lyse) the cell walls of many bacteria. The normal flora of the skin and mucous membranes also provides a defense against colonization of pathogenic bacteria. Resident microorganisms suppress the growth of infectious agents by competing for essential nutrients, producing growth-inhibiting substances, and altering the pH. Nonspecific mechanical factors, such as the ciliary action in the respiratory tract, also serve as protection.

When innate immunity fails to protect the body, the adaptive immune response comes into play. Adaptive immunity can be distinguished by its unique ability to mount a specific response to the invading microorganism and by its ability to remember the invader (memory). The primary components of adaptive immunity are the cellular immune response and the humoral immune response. These components ultimately are responsible for defending the body against a foreign invader by recognizing it as foreign, triggering a response against it, and remembering it in the event of future invasion. Innate and adapative immunity function interdependently, with the ultimate goal of protecting the body against foreign invasion.

THE BODY'S DEFENSE MECHANISMS

External physical and chemical defenses
Mononuclear phagocyte system
Inflammatory response
Immune response

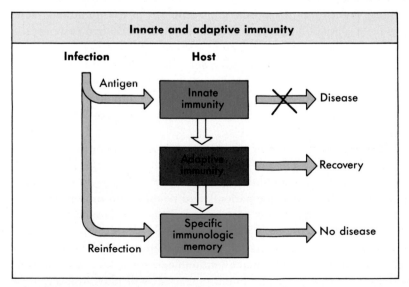

FIGURE 1-1
Innate and adaptive immunity.

INNATE AND ADAPTIVE IMMUNITY

Characteristics	Innate	Adaptive
Physical barriers	Physical defense: skin and mucous membranes	None
Response mechanisms	Nonspecific: mononuclear phagocytic system; inflammatory response	Specific immune response: humoral immunity, cellular immunity
Soluble factors	Chemical defense: lysozyme, complement, acute phase proteins, interferon	Antibodies, lymphokines
Cells	Phagocytes, natural killer (NK) cells	T lymphocytes, B lymphocytes
Specificity	None	Present
Memory	None	Present

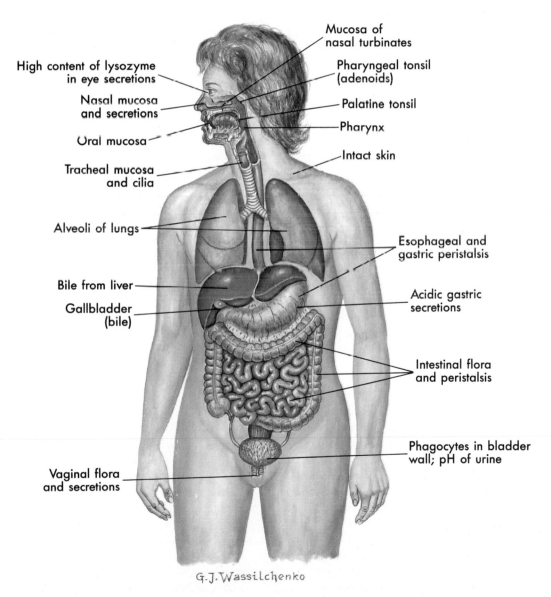

FIGURE 1-2
External defenses. (From Grimes D: *Infectious diseases,* St Louis, 1991, Mosby–Year Book.)

LEUKOCYTES

Through a process of differentiation, all blood cells are derived from precursor cells in the bone marrow, called **hematopoietic stem cells.** Some of these stem cells develop into leukocytes, whereas others become erythrocytes. Most leukocytes remain in the bone marrow until needed to combat an invading organism.

Leukocytes are white blood cells (WBCs) that are associated with the inflammatory and immune responses. These cells are the most important cellular components participating in the body's defense. They function collaboratively as a strong army to maintain the body's integrity by identifying, attacking, and killing unwanted invaders. (See Appendix A, p. 349.)

White blood cells are divided into three main groups: **granulocytes, monocytes,** and **lymphocytes.** All three types are derived from two main lines of differentiation, **lymphoid** lineage and **myeloid** lineage. The lymphoid lineage produces lymphocytes, and the myeloid lineage produces granulocytes and monocytes (Figure 1-3).

GRANULOCYTES

Cells of the granulocyte series are classified into three categories—**neutrophils, eosinophils,** and **basophils**—based on the histologic staining of their granules. These cells make up 60% to 80% of the total number of normal blood leukocytes. During an acute inflammation granulocytes, in conjunction with antibodies and complement, play a key role in protecting the body against microorganisms. Their main protective function is **phagocytosis,** a process in which a foreign object is engulfed and digested. Although considered front-line warriors against any invader, granulocytes lack two attributes typically associated with immunity: antigenic specificity and memory.

Phagocytosis

Phagocytosis is a multistep process through which granulocytes, monocytes, and macrophages remove foreign materials from the body. When a microorganism penetrates the epithelial surface, it comes in contact with these various cell types, which are strategically located throughout the body. The primary functions of the phagocytes are to engulf, internalize, and destroy invading organisms; this process is called **phagocytosis** (Figure 1-4).

Phagocytosis is initiated when a damaged or foreign substance attaches to the surface of a phagocytic cell. Particle recognition may occur at nonspecific membrane receptors or may be mediated by opsonic proteins. (**Opsonization** is a process whereby invading organisms or particles are coated with certain molecules

> **Granulocytes** and **monocytes** are the primary cells involved in the inflammatory response and are often referred to as phagocytes.
>
> **Lymphocytes** are predominantly involved in the immune response; they produce antibodies and mediate immunologic responses.

[e.g., IgG antibody or complement fragment C3b] that make them more attractive to phagocytes and thus readily phagocytized.) After particle attachment is complete, the cell membrane of the phagocyte's surface invaginates, encloses the particle, pinches it off, and internalizes it. The phagocytic vacuole subsequently fuses with lysosomal granules, which are the vacuoles within the cell that contain potent hydrolytic enzymes. During phagocytosis a number of metabolic changes occur within the cell, resulting in the release of toxic oxidative products, an event called the **respiratory burst;** also, under certain conditions, lysosomal enzymes and toxic oxygen products are released from the phagocytic cell. These events are responsible for much of the tissue damage that occurs during an ongoing inflammation.

LYMPHOCYTES

The maturation of lymphocytes depends on lymphoid tissue. The process begins during fetal development and continues throughout life. The two major classes of lymphocytes are T lymphocytes (T cells) and B lymphocytes (B cells). These cells are responsible for the immune response and play a key role in the development of adaptive immunity (Figure 1-5).

T lymphocytes, which represent 70% to 80% of the lymphocytes produced, are responsible for cell-mediated immunity. During fetal life the immature T cells (pre-T lymphocytes) migrate through the blood to the thymus. There, under the influence of thymic hormones (thymosin and thymopoietin), T cells proliferate and form mature T lymphocytes. In the environment provided by the thymus, each T cell develops the ability to recognize and attach to a specific antigen. The process of T-cell differentiation begins a couple of months before birth and continues through the first few months of life. If the thymus is removed after this time, T-cell immunity will not be impaired, because T cells have the ability to expand by cloning throughout life. (Refer to Nature of Clonal Selection, p. 23.)

B lymphocytes, which make up the remaining 10% to 20% of lymphocytes, are responsible for antibody production and humoral immunity. It is thought that

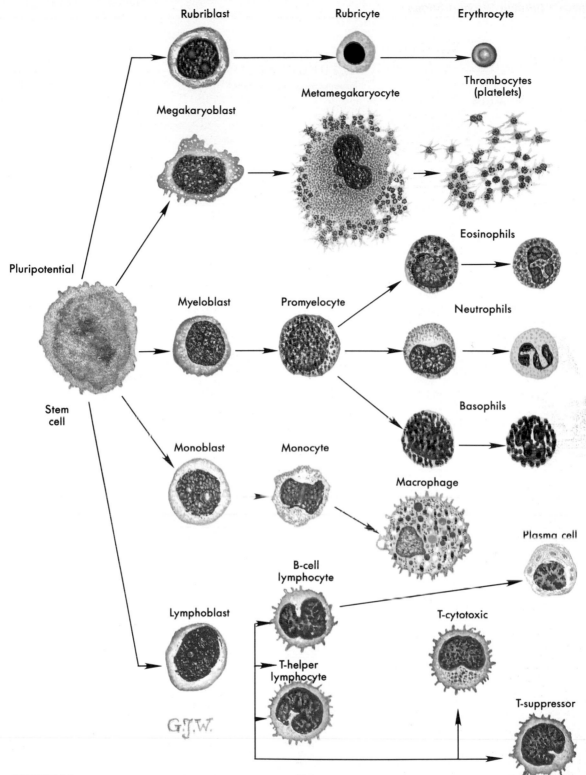

Rubriblast Rubricyte Erythrocyte

Thrombocytes
(platelets)

Metamegakaryocyte

Megakaryoblast

Eosinophils

Pluripotential

Myeloblast Promyelocyte Neutrophils

Stem
cell Basophils

Monoblast Monocyte

Macrophage

Plasma cell

B-cell
lymphocyte

T-cytotoxic

Lymphoblast

T-helper
lymphocyte

T-suppressor

G.J.W.

FIGURE 1-3
Differentiation of blood cells from a single stem cell. (From Belcher A: *Cancer nursing*, St Louis, 1992,
Mosby–Year Book.)

B-cell maturation and immunocompetence probably occur in the bone marrow, in lymphoid tissues lining the gastrointestinal tract (gut-associated lymphatic tissue [GALT]), or in the liver during the prenatal and neonatal periods. As with T cells, B cells are renewed throughout life by cell division.

After maturation T and B cells circulate in the blood and migrate into the lymphoid tissues, lymph nodes, and spleen. Lymphatic tissue is positioned strategically near the body's portals of entry, providing the lymphocytes with the advantage of being able to intercept antigens upon invasion. Most T and B cells circulate in the blood and lymphatic system, and the remainder are found primarily in lymph tissue.

LEUKOCYTES*

WHITE BLOOD CELLS (WBCs)

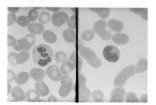

Participates in host defense; cytoplasmic granules contain enzymes that kill organisms after phagocytosis has occurred

MAST CELLS

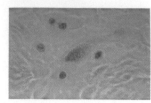

Releases heparin, histamine, and other potent mediators from granules into target tissue; defends against parasites

GRANULOCYTES NEUTROPHILS (POLYMORPHONU-CLEAR)

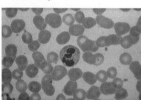

First to arrive at site of injury; releases antibacterial substances and digestive enzymes; remains active in the blood for at least 7 h and in the tissue for 48-72 h

MONONUCLEAR PHAGOCYTES MONOCYTES, MACROPHAGES

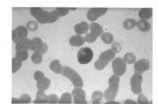

Has single, large nucleus that may be round or horseshoe shaped; cytoplasm contains few or no granules; stimulates T-cell maturation by secreting interleukin-1 (IL-1), which activates T-cell response; participates in antigen processing and presentation

EOSINOPHILS

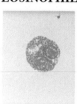

Defends against parasites; involved in allergic reactions

LYMPHOCYTES T LYMPHOCYTES

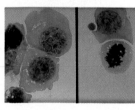

Plays a role in cellular immunity; active for months

BASOPHILS

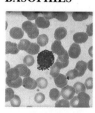

Has weakly phagocytic action; participates in allergic responses; releases heparin and histamine into surrounding tissue

B LYMPHOCYTES

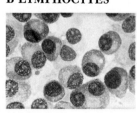

On contact with a specific antigen, will differentiate into antibody-producing plasma cells; plasma cells are active for 3-5 days; participates in antigen processing and presentation

*Color illustrations reprinted with permission from Sandoz Pharmaceuticals Corporation.

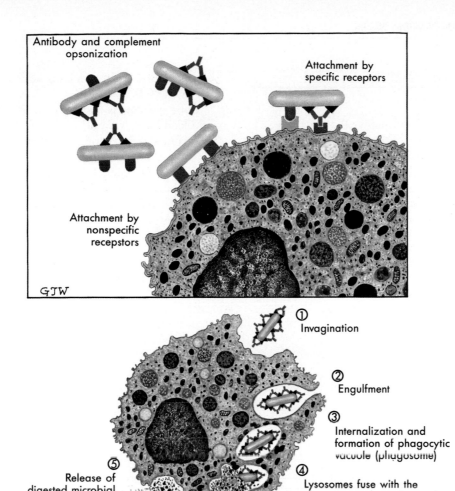

Antibody and complement opsonization

Attachment by specific receptors

Attachment by nonspecific recepstors

GJW

① Invagination

② Engulfment

③ Internalization and formation of phagocytic vacuole (phagosome)

④ Lysosomes fuse with the phagosome, damaging and digesting the phagocytosed material

⑤ Release of digested microbial products

FIGURE 1-4
Phagocytosis.

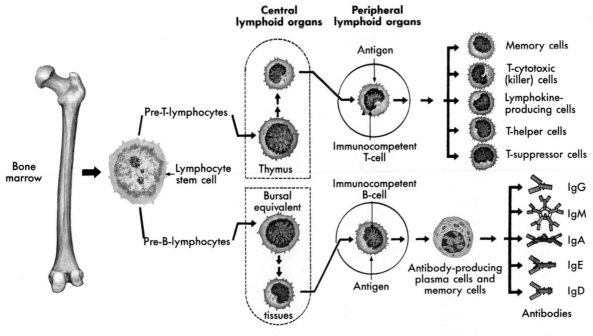

Central lymphoid organs

Peripheral lymphoid organs

Bone marrow

Lymphocyte stem cell

Pre-T-lymphocytes

Pre-B-lymphocytes

Thymus

Bursal equivalent

tissues

Antigen

Immunocompetent T-cell

Immunocompetent B-cell

Antigen

Antibody-producing plasma cells and memory cells

Memory cells

T-cytotoxic (killer) cells

Lymphokine-producing cells

T-helper cells

T-suppressor cells

IgG

IgM

IgA

IgE

IgD

Antibodies

FIGURE 1-5
Maturation, differentiation, and activation of lymphocytes. (From Grimes D: *Infectious diseases,* St Louis, 1991, Mosby−Year Book.)

ORGANS OF THE IMMUNE SYSTEM

To enable them to perform optimally, the cells involved in the immune system are organized into tissues and organs (Figure 1-6). These structures are classified as either primary or secondary lymphoid tissue and together are referred to as the lymphoid system. The **primary** lymphoid organs are the **bone marrow** and **thymus gland;** the **secondary** lymphoid organs, which house mature T and B cells, comprise the **spleen, lymph nodes, tonsils,** and other lymphoid tissue referred to as the **mucosa-associated lymphoid tissue,** or **MALT.**

Bone marrow is a spongy matrix of reticular cells and blood vessels found in the cavities of most bones. The average volume of bone marrow in an adult is 2 to 3 L, with the largest percentage located in the long bones. Functionally the bone marrow is responsible for producing all cellular components of the blood, including erythroid, lymphoid, and myeloid cells. It also serves as a storage place for the hematopoietic stem cells.

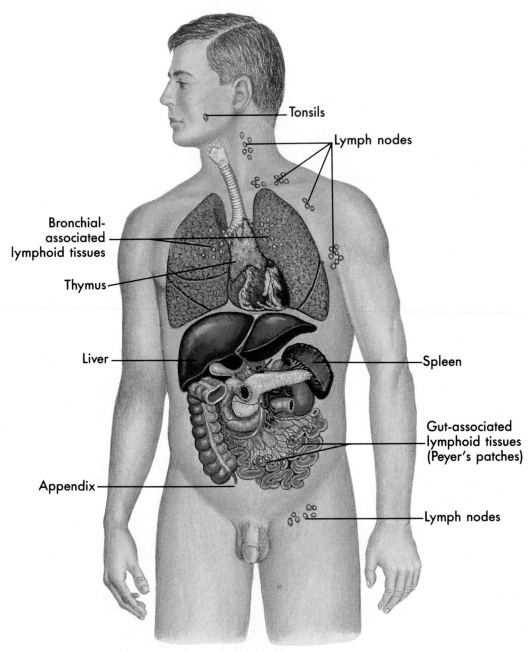

FIGURE 1-6
Components of the lymphatic system. (From Grimes D: *Infectious Diseases*, St Louis, 1991, Mosby–Year Book.)

The **thymus gland** is so named because of its resemblance to the leaf of a thyme plant (Figure 1-7). It is the first fetal organ to become lymphoid in character and functionally is considered the major site of T-cell maturation. It tends to be large during childhood and shrinks with age. In the elderly the thymus gland is composed mainly of fibrotic connective tissue. The cortex of the thymus contains most of the immature proliferating T cells, whereas the medulla houses the more developed and mature T cells. The rapidly dividing T cells in the cortex slowly migrate to the medulla, where they enter the bloodstream via the medullary veins to seek out foreign invaders.

The **spleen** is particularly important because its sinuses are lined with macrophages, allowing it to function as a major site of filtration of foreign particles from the blood (Figure 1-8). Two types of tissue are found in the spleen: red pulp and white pulp. The red pulp houses the reticular network and participates primarily in the removal and degradation of erythrocytes. The white pulp contains the majority of lymphoid tissue and is thought to participate in the maturation of B lymphocytes into antibody-producing plasma cells.

Lymph nodes are responsible for filtering foreign particles from the blood and for circulating lymphocytes throughout the body. When foreign substances enter the body, they are carried to regional lymph nodes for processing by lymphocytes and macrophages in the node.

Lymph nodes are small (1 to 25 mm in diameter), bean-shaped structures that are distributed throughout the body, generally at the junction of major lymphatics (Figure 1-9). Their principal function is to filter foreign antigens from the lymph circulation and to act as a site for antigen-specific lymphocyte maturation. The afferent lymphatics enter the node at the subcapsulary sinus, which is lined with phagocytic cells capable of engulfing and destroying foreign antigens. Lymphatic flow moves toward the efferent lymphatic duct, located at the hilus. Lymphocytes leave the lymphatic circulation and enter the node at the paracortex, migrate toward the medulla, and reenter the circulation via the efferent lymphatic. Lymph nodes have three principal regions: the outer cortex, which contains primarily B cells; the paracortex, populated mainly by T cells and macrophages; and the medulla. With antigen stimulation, lymphocyte production increases in the lymph nodes. Areas of the outer cortex that are particularly dense with B lymphocyte aggregates, called lymphoid follicles, become the focus of intense proliferative mitotic activity; these areas are known as germinal centers.

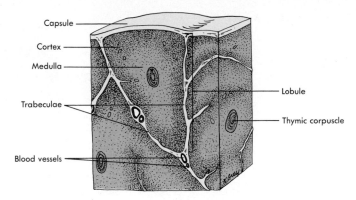

FIGURE 1-7
Cross section of the thymus gland. (From Seeley R et al: *Anatomy and physiology*, ed 2, St Louis, 1992, Mosby–Year Book.)

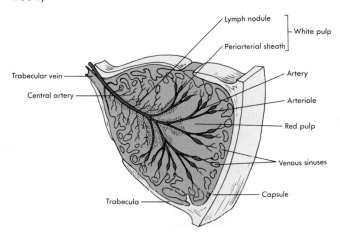

FIGURE 1-8
Cross section of the spleen. (From Seeley R et al: *Anatomy and physiology*, ed 2, St Louis, 1992, Mosby–Year Book.)

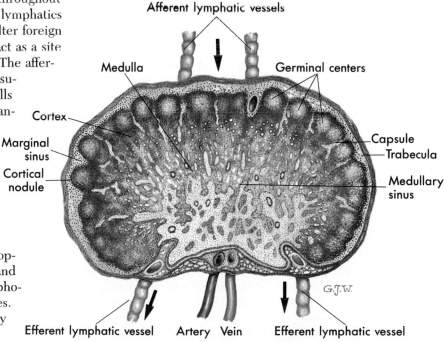

FIGURE 1-9
Structures of a lymph node. (From Belcher A: *Cancer nursing*, St Louis, 1992, Mosby–Year Book.)

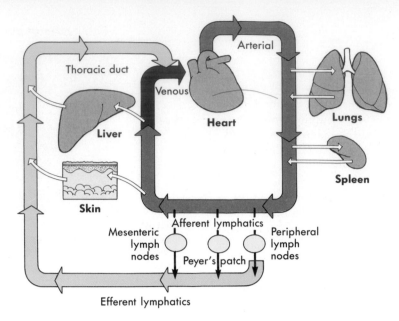

FIGURE 1-10
Lymphocyte traffic.

Proliferation occurs when B lymphocytes within the lymphoid follicles are specific for an antigen that has invaded the body; when such an invasion occurs, the B lymphocytes begin to proliferate and mature into specific antibody-producing plasma cells. The paracortex hypertrophies and contains large lymphocytes that come in direct contact with the antigen as it enters the node. During states of antigenic stimulation, such as with an infection, lymph nodes significantly enlarge because of the extensive hypertrophy of both the cortex and paracortex.

The acronym **MALT** (mucosa-associated lymphoid tissue) is used to identify encapsulated lymphoid tissue that is strategically located to protect the body from invading microorganisms. This tissue generally is well organized and is arranged either as diffuse aggregates of lymphocytes or as nodules with germinal centers for the development of mature lymphocytes. MALT acts as a sentinel at various entry sites where microorganisms might invade, particularly in the submucosal areas of the skin, respiratory, gastrointestinal, and genitourinary systems. These tissues are characterized as **gut-associated lymphoid tissue (GALT), bronchus-associated lymphoid tissue (BALT),** and **skin-associated lymphoid tissue (SALT).**

GALT comprises significant concentrations of lymphoid tissue that ranges from loose clusters of cells through the lamina propria to complex collections of lymphoid tissue such as the tonsils, Peyer's patches, or the appendix. The strategic location of the **tonsils** gives them direct exposure to airborne and alimentary antigens. Their structure and function are similar to those of the lymph nodes, and they act by trapping and removing invading antigens. **Peyer's patches** are pale nodules of lymphoid tissue that appear macroscopically on the outer wall of the intestines. Similar to the tonsils and the appendix, Peyer's patches are histologi-

cally well organized, with dependent T- and B-cell areas and germinal centers. Peyer's patches also harbor plasma cells (mature B cells) that produce the immunoglobulin IgA. These particular IgA-producing plasma cells protect the body by migrating to vulnerable areas exposed to the external environment (gastrointestinal tract, tear ducts, salivary glands, and upper respiratory tract). IgA is an important immunoglobulin in the defense against bacterial penetration of epithelial surfaces.

BALT structure and function closely resemble those of GALT. This type of tissue is composed of lymphocytes found primarily at the bifurcations of the bronchi and bronchioles. Most lymphocytes in BALT are B cells.

SALT consists of lymphocytes and specific cells, called Langerhans' cells, found in the epidermis of the skin. These cells can identify foreign antigens and transport them to regional lymph nodes for processing.

LYMPHOCYTE TRAFFIC

Mature lymphocytes circulate through various organs via the blood and lymphatic pathways (Figure 1-10). Lymphocytes leave the blood by traversing specialized endothelial venules of specific lymphoid tissue. The lymphocytes circulate through the lymphatic system, which coalesces into larger lymphatic vessels and eventually terminates in two major lymphatics, the thoracic duct and the right lymphatic duct. These two ducts empty the lymphocytes into the blood circulation at the great veins in the neck. T cells are highly mobile, whereas B cells tend to move more slowly and lodge for longer periods of time in the lymphatic organs. The recycling of lymphocytes through the blood and lymph circulation provides the body with a surveillance mechanism that allows recognition and removal of foreign antigens before they create a threat.

MONONUCLEAR PHAGOCYTE SYSTEM

The mononuclear phagocyte system (MPS) originally was called the reticuloendothelial system. It is made up of precursor cells derived from the bone marrow that develop into **monocytes** and **macrophages,** which are phagocytes. Monocytes circulate in the blood and, in only a few days, migrate into the tissue to become macrophages. Tissue macrophages tend to be larger in size and have a greater phagocytic capacity than do monocytes. Macrophages are located throughout the body in a variety of tissues (Table 1-1).

The mononuclear phagocyte system has three primary functions: (1) to protect the body from invading organisms through recognition and phagocytosis; (2) to clear tissue debris from sites of injury and possibly to serve as surveillance cells in antitumor defense; and (3) to participate in the immune response. Macrophages function as antigen-presenting cells (APCs), which process and present antigen to specific antigen-sensitive lymphocytes. The presentation of antigen initiates the immune response (see Immune Response, page 16). As secretory cells, macrophages release a number of very powerful chemicals, enzymes, complement proteins, and regulatory factors (e.g., interleukin-1). The functions of macrophages are augmented by a number of factors released from T cells (e.g., gamma-interferon).

Table 1-1

MONOCYTES AND MACROPHAGES OF THE MONONUCLEAR PHAGOCYTE SYSTEM

Name	Location
Blood monocytes	Blood
Kupffer cells	Liver
Intraglomerular mesangial cells	Kidneys
Alveolar macrophages	Lungs
Pleural macrophages	Pleural cavity
Serosal macrophages	Serosal space
Type A cells	Synovium
Microglial cells	Central nervous system
Spleen sinus macrophages	Spleen
Lymph node sinus macrophages	Lymph node
Histiocytes	Connective tissue
Bone marrow macrophages	Bone marrow
Osteoclasts	Bone tissue
Peritoneal macrophages	Peritoneal cavity
Langerhans' cells	Skin

INFLAMMATORY RESPONSE

The inflammatory response is a biochemical and cellular process that is launched immediately and aggressively by the body in response to cell injury and tissue damage. It may be triggered by immunologic or non-immunologic factors, including injury related to mechanical disruption (e.g., cuts); physical or chemical injury (e.g., burns, toxins); invasion of microorganisms (e.g., bacteria, fungi, or viruses); and immunologic injury (e.g., hypersensitivity reactions). The resultant cell damage initiates the inflammatory process by prompting the release of chemicals that in turn lead to a cascade of physiologic events. In response to cellular injury, inflammation is aimed at protecting the body and preventing further invasion by walling off and destroying or neutralizing the invading antigen. Repair and healing are also integral components of the inflammatory process.

The inflammatory response is important to both innate and adaptive immunity. However, in contrast to the immune response, which is antigen specific and has memory, the inflammatory response is nonspecific and lacks memory. It acts in the same manner each time, regardless of the stimulus or number of exposures to the same stimulus.

> The hallmarks of inflammation are swelling, heat, redness, pain, and loss of function.

The inflammatory response can be generated by cells (e.g., neutrophils, macrophages, mast cells, platelets, and endothelium) and by potent circulating proteins (e.g., complement components, coagulation factors, fibrinolysis, and kinin). However, the response is limited to vascularized tissues, because the molecular components of inflammation travel and are delivered to the site of injury via the blood vessels.

The cellular response to injury is the same regardless of the cause. When a cell has been injured, it undergoes a number of metabolic changes that cause it to swell. As the cell becomes further incapacitated, cellular atrophy results, reducing the cell's metabolic demands. Cell death eventually occurs if cellular metabolism cannot be maintained. When cell death occurs, lysosomal and digestive enzymes are released into the cell, dissolving cellular contents and stimulating the inflammatory process in surrounding tissues. Inflammation may remain local or become systemic. The **hallmarks** of inflammation, which were described more than 2,000 years ago, include **swelling** (tumor), **heat** (calor), **redness** (rubor), **pain** (dolor), and **loss of function** of the inflamed area.

> **IMMUNOLOGIC INDUCTION OF THE INFLAMMATORY RESPONSE**
>
> 1. Production of cytokines by macrophages and monocytes
> 2. Antigen-antibody (immune complex)-mediated generation of complement factors
> 3. IgE-mediated mast cell release of active and potent chemicals

STAGES OF THE ACUTE INFLAMMATORY RESPONSE

The process of inflammation occurs in a series of interrelated steps that involve blood vessels, fluid, and cellular components in the blood, lymphatics, and adjacent connective tissue. The complex mechanism of the inflammatory response has three stages: **vascular response, cellular response,** and **healing and repair.**

Vascular Response

The **vascular response** stage occurs immediately after cell injury. There is a very brief period of vasoconstriction, followed by the release of histamine and other chemical mediators from the injured cells (see box). In response to these mediators the vessels dilate in the surrounding area, causing local hyperemia (increased blood supply). As a result, filtration pressure in the blood vessels increases, which in turn increases capillary permeability. Fluid leaks from the blood vessels into the interstitial spaces. This fluid, known as **inflammatory exudate,** contains plasma proteins, en-

> **MEDIATORS OF INFLAMMATION**
>
> **Histamine:** Stored in granules of basophils, mast cells, and platelets; causes vasodilation, increased vascular permeability, and smooth muscle contraction
>
> **Serotonin:** Stored in platelets; causes vasodilation, increased vascular permeability, and smooth muscle contraction
>
> **Eosinophil chemotactic factor of anaphylaxis (ECF-A):** Located in mast cells; chemotactic for eosinophils
>
> **Neutrophil chemotactic factor of anaphylaxis (NCF-A):** Located in mast cells; chemotactic for neutrophils
>
> **Complement components (C3a, C5a):** Proteins derived from activation of the complement system; cause mast cell degranulation and histamine release, neutrophil and macrophage chemotaxis, smooth contraction, and increased capillary permeability
>
> **Kinins (e.g., bradykinin):** Substances produced by the kinin system; increase vascular permeability, cause vasodilation, and enhance chemotaxis for neutrophils and macrophages; pain
>
> **Prostaglandins (PGs):** Produced from arachidonic acid metabolism; PGI and PGE are potent vasodilators that react with histamine and kinins to increase vascular permeability; PGs promote platelet aggregation, stimulate the hypothalamus to regulate temperature, trigger pain receptors, may have antiinflammatory actions, and may modify immune function
>
> **Leukotrienes (LTB4, LTC4, and LTD4):** Produced from arachidonic acid metabolism; found predominantly as products of mucosal mast cells; promote inflammatory and hypersensitivity reactions; increase vascular permeability and smooth muscle constriction; LTB4 has chemotactic potency, promotes adherence of leukocytes to endothelial cells, and activates neutrophilic enzymes
>
> **Platelet activating factor (PAF):** Located in basophil, neutrophil, and macrophage cell membranes; when released activates platelet aggregation and neutrophils; causes increased vascular permeability and smooth muscle contraction; potent chemotactic stimuli for eosinophils
>
> **Proteinases (lysosomal enzymes):** Enzymes stored in lysosomes of leukocytes; produced in response to inflammation; able to break down bacteria and proteins generated by the inflammatory response
>
> **Clotting system:** Interacts with complement system to produce a number of products essential to the inflammatory response, tissue healing, and repair.
>
> **Lymphokines:** See Table 1-6

zymes, and other chemical components. The proteins tend to exert an oncotic pressure gradient, attracting more fluid into the interstitial spaces, which results in edema. As more fluid is mobilized from the vessels into the interstitial spaces, the inflammatory exudate is able to facilitate transportation of phagocytic cells into the site of injury.

Fibrinogen, a plasma protein, is activated into fibrin as it leaves the blood and migrates to the site of injury. Fibrin is deposited in collaboration with platelets to form a strong clot. The clot forms a web that can trap invading microorganisms and provide a framework for healing.

Cellular Response

The **cellular response** is first demonstrated by the migration of tissue macrophages through the extracellular space to the site of injury. The macrophages are drawn to the area by chemotactic factors released by damaged cells or invading organisms. Since there are few local tissue macrophages, other phagocytes are recruited (through chemotaxis) to the injured area when damage is extensive. Initially these phagocytes are primarily neutrophils, which soon become the prominent cellular components at the injured site. However, because of their short life span (approximately 10 to 15 hours) dead neutrophils begin to accumulate in the area. As a result, pus is formed from the combination of dead neutrophils, digested microorganisms, and cellular debris. To maintain the increased demand for more neutrophils, the bone marrow augments production and releases more neutrophils into the circulation. Occasionally the demand is so great that immature neutrophils (bands) are released from the bone marrow into the circulation, causing what is known as a **shift to the left.**

Within 24 hours monocytes are attracted to the site of injury; they are the second type of phagocyte to leave the peripheral blood and migrate to the site. Upon arriving at the inflamed tissue area, the monocytes differentiate and transform into macrophages; these macrophages are called inflammatory or exudative macrophages. They act as phagocytes to facilitate the digestion of cell debris, dying neutrophils, and microorganisms. They also participate in mediating leukocyte proliferation and capillary bud formation. Macrophages can stay in the inflamed areas for 2 to 12 months. They play a key role in cleaning the inflamed area of debris in preparation for repair and healing. Exudate ultimately is formed from the fluid and cellular debris in the surrounding inflamed area. Several forms of exudate can be produced locally, depending on the type and severity of the injury (Table 1-2).

Other cells that may be involved during an inflammation are (1) lymphocytes, which arrive at the site of injury much later and whose role primarily is related to cell-mediated immunity and antibody production (see the section on cell-mediated immunity, page 20); (2) eosinophils, which are present mainly during allergic reactions and which participate in the phagocytosis of IgE immune complexes; and (3) mast cells and basophils, which secrete from their granules inflammatory mediators (e.g., histamine and heparin) that augment the effects of the phagocytic cells.

Healing and Repair

Healing and repair of tissues is the final stage of the inflammatory response and involves both the process

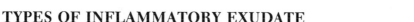

Table 1-2

TYPES OF INFLAMMATORY EXUDATE

Type	Characteristics	Example
Serous	Clear fluid; contains plasma proteins	Blisters, pleural effusion
Mucinous (catarrhal)	Clear mucous membrane secretions; may contain live or dead microorganisms	Postnasal drip with respiratory infections
Fibrinous	Contains excessive amounts of fibrinogen that has extravasated into tissues	Adhesions
Purulent (pus)	Cloudy, contains dead and live leukocytes, live and dead microorganisms, serous exudate, and liquified necrotic tissue	Abscess, empyema
Fibropurulent	Combination of fibrinous and purulent exudate	Granuloma
Hemorrhagic	Contains erythrocytes	Necrosis and rupture of a vessel wall

of regeneration and the process of repair. Regeneration is the body's ability to replace cells and tissues with the same type of cells that were destroyed from injury and/or infection. Repair is the replacement of damaged cells and tissues with connective tissue; this process generally results in the formation of a scar.

> Inflammation is always present in infection; however, infection is *not* always present in inflammation.

SUBACUTE INFLAMMATORY RESPONSE

A **subacute inflammatory response** is defined as a delayed phase of the acute inflammatory response. It is characterized by the neutrophils' inability to neutralize the inflamed area within a few hours and further accumulation of monocytes and lymphocytes at the site of tissue injury. These cells also attempt to localize the inflammatory response by creating a cellular barrier against the migration of the infectious organism into the lymphatic compartments or blood vessels. This is followed by proliferation of endothelial cells, induced primarily by factors from activated T cells and macrophages (e.g., fibroblast growth factors). These factors also encourage proliferation of cells and increase collagen synthesis. After the fine fibers of the fibroblasts have been laid down in the inflamed area, a bridge of connective tissue begins to form. When neutrophils, lymphocytes, and monocytes neutralize the inflamed area, epithelial cells and granulation tissue are laid down and inflammation subsides. An example of this type of inflammation would be subacute endocarditis.

ACUTE PHASE PROTEINS

The cellular response that occurs during inflammation is accompanied by a dramatic elevation in the levels of certain serum proteins. These proteins are collectively called **acute phase proteins;** they include C-reactive protein (CRP), serum amyloid A protein, alpha-1-antitrypsin, alpha-2-macroglobulin, fibrinogen, ceruloplasmin, and factor B. These proteins are used clinically to detect an infection or inflammation. The increased level of these serum proteins is manifested in the laboratory as an elevation in the **erythrocyte sedimentation rate (ESR),** a nonspecific indicator of an ongoing inflammation.

CHRONIC INFLAMMATION

Chronic inflammation may result if the inflammatory response is unsuccessful in eliciting an acute response. Chronic inflammation generally is caused by antigen substances that persist at the site of inflammation, provoking a continued reaction. Several factors, including age, nutritional status, and general health, influence an individual's ability to mount an effective inflammatory response and determine the outcome of the process. The antigens most often responsible for chronic inflammation are infectious, such as in tuberculosis or chronic active hepatitis. However, inadequate activation of the immune response or a hyperimmune response also can lead to chronic inflammation such as in autoimmune disorders or chronic inflammatory disorders.

Chronic inflammation is characterized by marked tissue infiltration by monocytes/macrophages, lymphocytes, and plasma cells that persist at the site of injury. Exudates usually are not formed. However, certain types of chronic disorders may have specific types of exudate. For example, the synovial effusions of rheumatoid arthritis are a specific type of exudate formed in the joints of patients with this disorder. Occasionally, chronic inflammation results in granuloma formation and potential functional loss of an area. **Granulomas** are 1- to 2-mm lesions that can be the result of prolonged inflammation characterized by the accumulation of lymphocytes and macrophages surrounding a central core of an infectious or foreign material. Fibrotic tissue is laid down on the periphery of the granuloma and acts as a physical barrier that separates the lesion from surrounding normal tissues, as in tuberculosis. The eventual outcome of this type of inflammatory response may be extensive tissue and organ destruction with severe cavitation and necrosis and/or fibrotic scarring.

PLATELETS

Platelets arise from the myeloid series and are derived from the large megakaryocytes in the bone marrow. They have an average life span of 8 to 11 days, and normal values are 150,000 to 400,000/µl. Containing many special factors and enzymes, platelets play an active role in blood clotting and in the immune response, particularly during inflammation. After an inflammatory response involving endothelial injury, platelets will aggregate and adhere to the affected endothelial surfaces. This is followed by the release of substances that increase permeability and factors that activate complement, which in turn attract leukocytes to the area. Platelets also participate in allergic reactions and, like basophils and mast cells, contain vasoactive substances and enzymes that can lead to tissue damage if released.

COMPLEMENT

The word "complement" came into use at the turn of the century when researchers recognized that blood plasma contained a substance necessary to complete the destruction of bacteria. It is now known that complement is a collective term used to identify a complex of at least 25 serum enzymatic proteins that mediate the inflammatory reaction and augment the immune response. Most of these proteins circulate in the blood in an inactive state until they are activated by either **immunologic stimuli (classic pathway)** or **nonimmuno-logic stimuli (alternate pathway)**. Once activated, the complement proteins produce a cascade of reactions through the interaction of proteins called **components**. The complement system has three primary functions: (1) lysis of cells and microorganisms; (2) facilitation of particle opsonization and clearance, which involves coating of foreign substances with a specific complement fragment to promote phagocytosis; and (3) gener-

ation of peptide fragments that mediate the inflammatory and immune responses. The proteins of the complement system cause vasodilation at the site of inflammation, provide chemotactic stimuli to encourage migration of phagocytes to the area, and directly participate in clearing infectious agents (Figure 1-11).

The two major pathways of complement activation, classic and alternative, both progress by sequential activation through a series of proteins that lead to the development of a complex enzyme capable of binding and cleaving complement component C3, which is common to both pathways. The two pathways then proceed together to form what is called the **membrane attack complex** (C5-9 on the surface of a target cell), which can cause cell lysis. This systematic reaction is called the **complement cascade.** Activation of the complement cascade results in activation of mast cells and basophils to release histamine, opsonization of antigen, and enhanced chemotaxis, which promotes phagocytosis by neutrophils and macrophages, cell lysis, agglutination of some microorganisms, and neutralization of viruses.

COMPLEMENT CASCADE

The components (C) of the classic and alternative pathways are identified by numbers following the letter "C." The early-acting components are numbered according to the order of their discovery, and the later-acting components according to their order of reaction. Thus the sequence of action of these components is C1, C4, C2, C3, C5, C6, C7, C8, and C9. C1 activates the classic pathway and is made up of three distinct proteins, C1q, C1r, and C1s. The alternative pathway is activated at C3 and involves properdin. The proteins of the alternative pathway are designated by letters such as Factor B or D. The proteins of each pathway react to each other in a precise and accurate sequence. The initial steps in the sequence are related to the grouping of complement cleavage fragments to form enzymes that subsequently bind to the next protein to continue the reaction cascade. Active enzymes in the cascade are identified by a bar over the character identifying the component. Although the complement system protects the body against infectious organisms and may play a role in destruction of tumor cells, the uncontrolled activation of this system would result in inflammatory changes and lytic destruction of body tissues. In addition, if a protein is missing, as in some genetic deficiencies, the sequence cannot continue and is interrupted at that point.

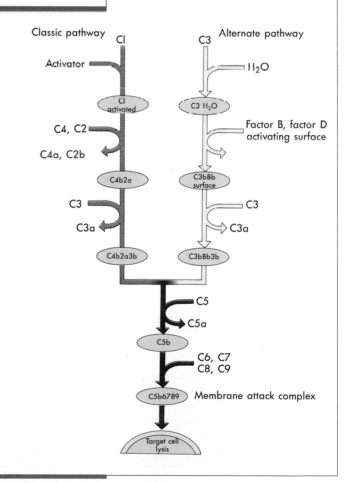

The **classic pathway** is activated by the formation of antigen-antibody immune complexes. IgG and IgM are complement-fixing antibodies that bind to antigen, forming the initial connector molecule to which one of the complement proteins (C1 [Clq, C1r, or Cls]) can attach. This triggers the complement cascade, which is subsequently lethal to the invading antigen.

The **alternative pathway** can be activated before the generation of a specific antibody or when antibody for a specific antigen is not available. Known activators of the alternative pathway include bacterial lipopolysaccharide, virus-infected cells, yeast, fungi, and certain bacterial cell walls. Aggregations of IgA and IgE also can activate the alternative pathway.

IMMUNE RESPONSE

The immune response, which represents adaptive immunity, is a highly complex sequence of events triggered by an antigenic stimulus. Three major cell types are involved in the immune response: macrophages, T lymphocytes (involved in cell-mediated immunity), and B lymphocytes (involved in humoral immunity). These cells interact with each other directly and under the supervision of cytokines (Table 1-3). The immune response is also integrally associated with complement, kinins, and the clotting and fibrocytic systems. Although much progress has been made in understanding the interaction of all these components, the exact mechanisms are not completely understood.

ANTIGENICITY

An **antigen** is a substance that the body recognizes as foreign and that can evoke an immune response. Examples of antigens are bacteria, viruses, grafted tissue, and pollen. Antigens are identified by characteristic shapes on their cell surface, called **epitopes.** All antigens carry a number (some carry hundreds) of different types of epitopes on their cell surface. **Autologous antigens** are self-antigens that under normal conditions do not evoke an immune response. However, when these "self"-antigens are changed by an infection or inflammation, the immune system recognizes its own tissues as foreign and produces an autoimmune response. The result of such an attack is an autoimmune disorder (e.g., systemic lupus erythematosus).

ANTIGEN PROCESSING AND PRESENTATION

Antigen processing and presentation are thought to be primarily the responsibility of macrophages. However, other cells such as B lymphocytes also have been shown to participate in this process (Table 1-4). When an antigen is identified by the body as foreign, the macrophages ingest the antigen and modify it chemically through an enzyme-mediated reaction; this is called **antigen processing** (Figure 1-11). Processed an-

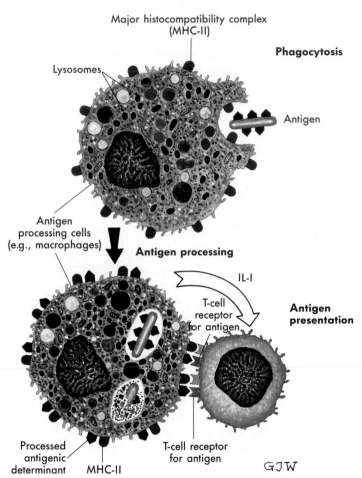

FIGURE 1-11
Antigen processing and presentation. Antigen-presenting cells (APC) (e.g., macrophages) identify, internalize, and degrade foreign antigens. The processed antigens are reexpressed on the APC surface in a highly immunogenic form for presentation to lymphocytes. Recognition of an antigen by specific receptors on the lymphocyte cell surface results in their stimulation and sequestration within the tissue.

tigen is reexpressed in association with HLA antigen on the macrophage cell surface in a highly immunogenetic form and presented to lymphocytes (T and B cells). This is called **antigen presentation,** lending the name **antigen-presenting cell (APC)** to macrophages. Recognition of the antigen as nonself by receptors on

Table 1-3

TYPES OF ADAPTIVE (ACQUIRED) IMMUNITY

Natural Immunity

Active	Acquired by natural infection with antigen (e.g., chickenpox)	Provides slow antigen-specific development of antibody
Passive	Acquired by natural contact with antibody transplacentally or through colostrum and breast milk (e.g., neonatal IgG and IgA from mother)	Provides immediate and temporary immunity to antigens that mother has immunity to

Artificial Immunity

Active	Acquired by inoculation with a variant of antigen, usually not the entire antigen (e.g., immunization, attenuated virus)	Provides permanent immunity to a specific antigen
Passive	Acquired by administration of antibody or antitoxin (e.g., gamma globulin, tetanus)	Provides immediate and temporary immunity

Table 1-4

ANTIGEN-PRESENTING CELLS (APC)

Type of Cell	Location
Macrophages	Lymphoid tissue (medulla of lymph nodes; red pulp of spleen) and circulation
Marginal zone macrophages	Spleen and lymph nodes
Langerhans' cells	Skin and regional lymph nodes; called veiled cells in afferent lymph and dendritic cells in lymph nodes
Dendritic leukocytes	Most tissues of the body
Follicular dendritic cells	Spleen and lymph node follicles
B cells	Lymphoid tissue

lymphocytes in blood, lymph, or tissue exudate sets up a chain of responses in an effort to destroy or neutralize the invading antigen.

The immune response is triggered by the processing and presentation of antigen. Two types of **antigen-specific** immune responses occur, cell-mediated immunity and humoral immunity. These responses are initiated by the activation and differentiation of lymphocytes after they have been presented with antigen by the macrophages. **Humoral immunity** is mediated by B lymphocytes that ultimately synthesize and secrete immunoglobulins in response to an antigenic challenge. **Cell-mediated immune** mechanisms involve T lymphocytes and macrophages. Although these two response are interdependent, it is helpful to consider them separately in understanding the immune response.

THE FOUR R'S OF THE IMMUNE RESPONSE

RECOGNIZE self from nonself. Normally the body recognizes its own cells as nonantigenic; therefore, an immune response generally is triggered only in response to agents that the body identifies as foreign. In autoimmune disorders the ability to differentiate self from nonself is disrupted, and the immune system attacks the body's own cells as if they were foreign antigens.

RESPOND to nonself invaders. The immune system responds in part by producing antibodies that target specific antigens for destruction. New antibodies are produced in response to new antigens. Deficits in the ability to respond can result in immunodeficiency disorders.

REMEMBER the invader. The ability to remember antigens that have invaded the body in the past is the immune system's memory. This characteristic allows for a quicker response if subsequent invasion by the *same* antigen occurs.

REGULATE its action. Self-regulation allows the immune system to monitor itself by "turning on" when an antigen invades and "turning off" when the invasion has been eradicated. Regulation prevents the destruction of healthy or host tissue. The inability to regulate could result in a chronic inflammation and damage to the host tissue.

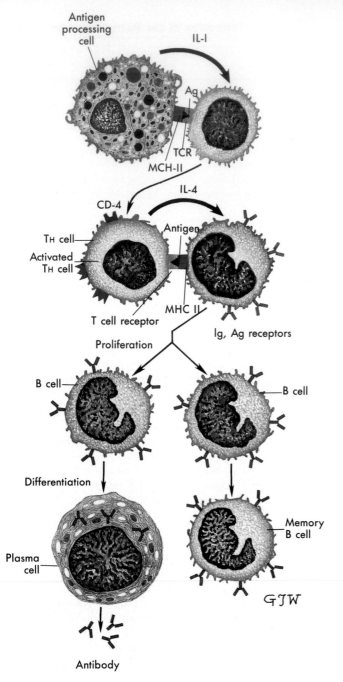

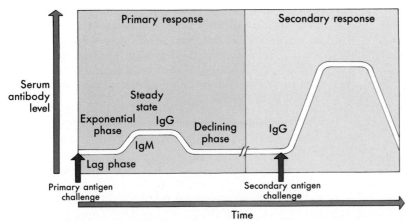

FIGURE 1-12
B-cell activation.

FIGURE 1-13
Primary and secondary immune responses.

HUMORAL IMMUNE RESPONSE

B lymphocytes differentiate into plasma cells, which produce antibodies that are responsible for humoral immunity. The production of antibodies protects the body against certain bacteria, aids in the neutralization of viruses, enhances phagocytosis, and activates the complement system.

Activation of B cells and humoral immunity may occur when antigen combines directly with antigen-binding receptors on B cells (Figure 1-12). This is called a **T cell–independent antigen response** and stimulates B-cell activation directly. However, more often B-cell activation is triggered by T cells binding to antigen, with appropriate help from regulatory T cells. This is called a **T cell–dependent antigen response.** In either case, stimulated B cells differentiate and proliferate into antibody-producing plasma cells and memory cells. Plasma cells secrete antibody into the circulation at a rate of approximately 2,000 molecules per second. Antibodies appear on the surface of plasma cells and bind antigen in a way similar to a key in a lock. Each plasma cell can produce only one specific type of antibody.

The initial contact with antigen that causes antibody production is called the **primary response** (Figure 1-13). Antibody production occurs approximately 2 to 8 days after first exposure to a particular antigen. Depending on the nature of the antigen and the efficacy of antibody production, the response peaks in 1 to 3 weeks. IgM is the first antibody formed, followed by IgG. Antibody titers usually can be detected within 10 days of exposure.

A **secondary response** occurs with subsequent exposure to the same antigen. Memory cells, which are quiescent until a subsequent exposure occurs, generate a rapid (1 or 2 days), prolific, and sustained response to the familiar invader. Antibody production, primarily IgG, produces much higher titers in a shorter time in a secondary response.

When an antibody-mediated response is generated against a soluble antigen, small antigen-antibody complexes form. These immune complexes may be rapidly cleared from the circulation by macrophages or deposited in tissues. Tissue-bound immune complexes can activate the complement system and provoke inflammatory destruction of normal, healthy cells. This is what occurs in some types of autoimmune diseases (e.g., rheumatoid arthritis, glomerulonephritis).

IMMUNOGLOBULINS (Ig)

Immunoglobulins (antibodies) are glycoproteins produced by plasma cells in response to

Table 1-5

CLASSES OF IMMUNOGLOBULINS

Class	Location, characteristics, and function	Class	Location, characteristics, and function
IgG	Most abundant in blood; also found in lymph, cerebrospinal, pleural, synovial, and peritoneal fluid, and breast milk Develops slowly during primary response, appears approximately 1 wk after IgM and peaks in 1-3 wk or longer after IgM peaks; may persist for years; highest concentration during secondary response; activates complement by alternative and classic pathways; facilitates phagocytosis through opsonization; attracts antigens directly; only immunoglobulin to cross the placenta and provide temporary immunity to neonate	IgA	Found in serum, secretions (bronchial, vaginal, prostatic, tears, saliva, colostrum), and mucosa (e.g., intestine, respiratory tract) Secretory antibody, primary defense against local invasion; by interfering with bacterial attachment to mucosal surfaces and impeding colonization, prevents entry of antigen into the circulation; may have specific antiviral properties; increases in chronic infection and inflammation; provides protection to neonate via maternal milk
IgM	Intravascular Predominant in primary immune response; first antibody to form in response to bacterial or viral infections; peaks in 1-2 wk after symptoms, is increased in chronic infections; in respiratory and gastrointestinal exposure to antigen, it increases in external secretions, is a potent activator of complement; is expressed on the surface of B cells; participates in blood transfusion reactions against blood types A and B antigens	IgE	Found in serum Triggers release of histamine and other mediators from mast cells and basophils upon binding with an allergen, in certain allergic disorders; high-affinity binding on surface membrane of mast cells and basophils; major mediator of allergic response; involved in type I hypersensitivity reactions; important defense against parasitic infections
		IgD	Found in serum Predominant antibody on the cell surface of B cells; may participate in the differentiation of these cells; increases with chronic infection

an invading antigen. Immunoglobulins make up a heterogeneous group of plasma proteins that constitute approximately 20% of total plasma proteins. Varying numbers of immunoglobulins are also found in the extravascular fluids and exocrine secretions and on the membrane surface of some lymphocytes.

Production of immunoglobulins is initiated in response to invasion by an antigen. The antibody gene is assembled from different parts of intracellular deoxyribonucleic acid (DNA) that are woven throughout the genetic material. The maturing B cells select and rearrange the genetic material from the DNA segments, formulate the material, and assemble it into antibody regions.

The new gene encoded antibody is absolutely unique. With B-cell proliferation, all offspring will manufacture this new antibody. As cells continue to proliferate, the natural selection of antigen-specific antibodies is formulated. The result of this process is that there appears to be a limited number of genetically unique B cells that can react to an endless array of invading antigens.

Immunoglobulins are considered bifunctional because they can bind to specific antigens that prompted their formation, and they also can interact with the body by initiating a number of immune regulatory activities (Table 1-5). The primary functions of immunoglobulins are to (1) directly attack antigens through the process of agglutination, precipitating neutralization, and lysis; (2) activate the complement system; (3) activate anaphylaxis by releasing histamine into the tissues and blood; and (4) stimulate antibody-mediated hypersensitivity.

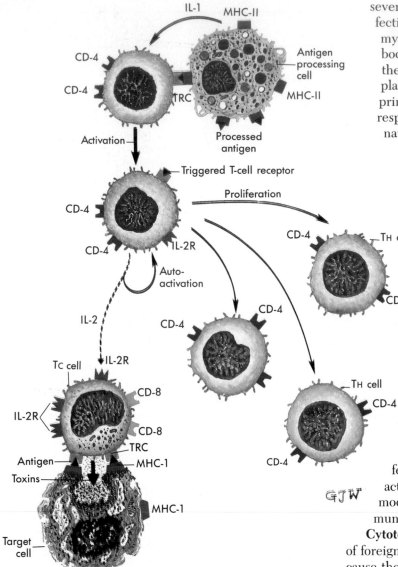

FIGURE 1-14
T-cell activation.

several ways: (1) It provides immunity against infections (including viral, fungal, protozoal, and mycobacterial types); (2) it plays a role in the body's response to tumors; (3) it participates in the rejection of transplanted tissues; and (4) it plays a role in hypersensitivity reactions. The primary cell types involved in the cell-mediated response are macrophages, T lymphocytes, and natural killer (NK) cells.

Cell-mediated immunity is directed primarily by T lymphocytes as the result of their interaction with antigen expressed on macrophages (APC). T-lymphocyte activation occurs when T cell antigen–binding receptors bind to antigen and class I or II proteins expressed on the surface of antigen-presenting cells (see Major Histocompatibility Complex in this chapter). With activation, **T-cell subsets,** which have previously been determined in the thymus, differentiate and proliferate. Functional T-cell subsets are classified as either **effector cells** (cytotoxic T cells and delayed hypersensitivity T cells) or **regulatory cells** (helper T cells and suppressor T cells). Although structurally these cells are very similar, they express different receptors on their cell surface and have different functions (Figure 1-14). Effector T cells act directly on antigen, whereas regulatory cells modulate the activity of other cells in the immune system. Some T cells become memory cells.

Cytotoxic T cells directly attack the cell membrane of foreign antigens by releasing toxic chemicals that cause the target cell to rupture and die. Cytotoxic T cells become sensitized when exposed to antigen and have antigen specificity. These cells are responsible for (1) protecting and ridding the body of cells infected with viruses and/or bacteria; (2) attacking cells that have been transformed by cancer; and (3) eliciting a rejection episode in grafted tissues or organs (e.g., a liver or kidney transplant).

Helper T cells and **suppressor T cells** are considered regulatory cells and participate in both cell-mediated and humoral immunity. When an antigen has been identified, **helper T cells** circulate and recruit help by interacting directly with B cells. Helper T cells interact with B cells that have identified the antigen, and they release lymphokines that stimulate clonal production of plasma cells and antibody formation. **Lymphokines** produced by helper T cells and other T cells also function indirectly to remove antigens from the body by (1) promoting the development

When a humoral immune response is triggered, one or more classes of immunoglobulins may be elaborated. The nature of the antibody response depends on the chemical and physical nature of the antigen, the route of antigen entry, and the individual's immunization history.

Five major classes of immunoglobulins have been identified: IgG, IgA, IgM, IgD, and IgE. The normal concentration of total immunoglobulin in the serum is 300 to 1,800 mg/dl in adults.

CELL-MEDIATED IMMUNE RESPONSE

The interaction of immune system cells with antigen is called cell-mediated immunity, which is important in

and proliferation of cytotoxic T and B lymphocytes; (2) attracting other leukocytes into the area; and (3) enhancing phagocytosis of macrophages. As the lymphokines attract more cells to the site, the antigen becomes overwhelmed and is subsequently eliminated (Table 1-7).

Suppressor T cells release chemicals that inhibit the activity of helper T cells and other immune cells. These chemicals indirectly suppress B-cell antibody formation and cytotoxic T-cell functions. Suppressor T cells are responsible for "turning off" the helper T lymphocytes. Without the suppressor cells, the helper T cells, in conjunction with other cells, would continue their activities even after the antigen had been destroyed. Together, helper T and suppressor T cells keep the immune system in check and balance.

The relative numbers of functional helper T (Th) and suppressor T (Ts) cells contribute to determining the strength and persistence of an immune response. When the delicate balance between Th and Ts cells is disrupted, autoimmune or immunodeficiency diseases may result. Since T lymphocytes have distinct surface markers and can be readily discriminated in the laboratory, immune function can be estimated by measuring the Th:Ts ratio. Normally there are twice as many Th cells as Ts cells. In contrast, individuals with AIDS frequently demonstrate a decrease in Th cells, with a ratio of 1:1 or less, whereas people with autoimmune disorders may have a decrease in Ts cells in proportion to Th cells, indicating an exaggerated or hyperactive immune response.

Natural killer (NK) cells are part of the third group of lymphocytes, referred to as **null cells.** They are not T or B lymphocytes, but they do participate in cell-mediated immunity. They often are referred to as large, granular lymphocytes because, unlike T or B lymphocytes, they have granules in their cytoplasm. Although NK cells lack memory, they are available to kill antigen without prior sensitization and are thought to play an important role in innate immunity. NK cells are thought to participate in the immune response by the nonspecific killing of virally infected cells, tumor cells, and transplanted tissues before cell-mediated effector cells have been sensitized. They may also be involved in protecting the body by functioning as a component of immune surveillance.

> **Cluster of differentiation (CD)** is a characteristic cell surface marker found on human leukocytes. For example, all T cells (T3) express the marker known as CD3, whereas helper T cells express a CD4 marker, and suppressor T cells express the CD8 marker. (See Chapter 3.)

MECHANISMS OF ANTIGEN-ANTIBODY INTERACTIONS

Agglutination: Antigen combines with antibody to form clumps in the serum or tissues (agglutination usually refers to cells).

Precipitation: Antigen and antibody combine to make an insoluble lattice formation that precipitates.

Opsonization: The process by which a molecule (opsonin) coats an antigen, increasing its attractiveness to neutrophils and macrophages, thereby enhancing phagocytosis; examples of opsonins: IgG, C3b.

Neutralization: Antibodies provide toxic and viral neutralization; antibodies specific for a certain antigenic toxin bind and render them inactive, promoting their removal by the mononuclear phagocyte system. Antibodies specific for epitopes on certain viruses will attach to them, blocking viral binding to host cells.

Complement: Certain antibodies, when bound to antigen, can activate complement, causing cell lysis.

Lymphocytes become immunocompetent when they are capable of generating an immune response. The presence of specific proteins on their surface membranes indicates immunocompetence and enables them to identify specific antigens, bind to them, and render them inactive.

Lymphokine-activated killer (LAK) cells are lymphocytes that have been exposed to and activated by interleukin-2 (IL-2). They differ from NK cells in that they manifest nonspecific antigen cytotoxicity against a much wider range of target antigens. Clinically LAK cells have proved effective in combating a number of metastatic malignancies.

T-CELL SUBSETS

Effector Cells

Cytotoxic T cells: Mediate antigen-specific cytotoxicity by binding to the surface of the cell, disrupting its membrane, and killing it directly with lymphokines; cytotoxic T cells kill microorganisms that are perceived as foreign (e.g., virus-infected cells, cancer cells, or allogenic cells introduced by transplantation); they release lymphokines and promote phagocytosis.

Delayed hypersensitivity T cells: Trigger allergic reactions, anaphylaxis, and autoimmune reactions

Regulatory Cells

Helper T cells: Amplify the cell-mediated immune response through production of lymphokines; augment the response of B cells and cytotoxic T cells to antigens, and stimulate the activity of all other T cells, monocytes, and macrophages

Suppressor T cells: Modulate the immune response by "turning off" or "on" the action of helper and cytotoxic T cells, to prevent them from causing excessive damage and potentially harmful immune reactions

The basic unit of the immunoglobulin molecule consists of four polypeptide chains linked together by disulfide bonds. There are two **variable** regions (V) and two **constant** regions (C). The variable region on all immunoglobulins is the area that binds to antigen; it is also the area of difference between immunoglobulins, which allows for greater flexibility and assistance with antigen binding.

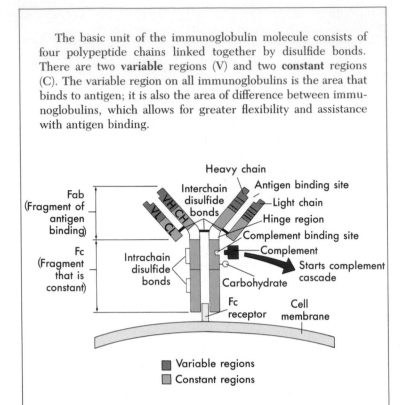

CYTOKINES

The immune response is extremely complex and requires constant interaction by the involved cells. Communication between cells is facilitated by the secretion of extremely potent chemical messengers, called **cytokines.** They act in part by enhancing cell growth, promoting cell activation, directing cellular traffic, stimulating macrophage function, and destroying antigens (Table 1-6). Cytokines can be classified as **lymphokines,** secreted by lymphocytes, or **monokines,** secreted by monocytes or macrophages.

Interferon (**IFN**) is a type of lymphokine that has been shown to defend the body against tumor cell growth and viruses. Interferons can also activate NK cells and increase their cytotoxic abilities. Three types of interferons have been identified, based on their function and cell origin: alpha-interferon, beta-interferon, and gamma-interferon. Interferons currently are undergoing human trials to determine their effectiveness in treating malignancies.

CELL COOPERATION IN THE IMMUNE RESPONSE

Macrophages are antigen-presenting cells (APC) that process and present antigen to helper T cells (CD4) and release interleukin-1 (IL-1). Helper T cells are activated when T cell antigen–binding receptors bind to antigen and to class II proteins expressed on the cell surface of macrophages simultaneously. Activated helper T cells release interleukin-2 (IL-2) and other cytokines, which stimulate the activation of (1) B cells into antibody-secreting plasma cells, and (2) cytotoxic T cells (CD8), which release cytotoxins, causing subsequent target cell (antigen) death. The generation of memory cells after initial exposure to antigen prepares the immune system to provide an augmented response upon subsequent encounters with the same antigen. Regulation of the immune response involves a complex network of interactions between helper T cells, suppressor T cells, and antibody feedback mechanisms (Figure 1-15).

Table 1-6

CYTOKINES

Type	Source	Main Functions
Interleukins (IL)		
IL-1 (endogenous pyrogen)	Predominantly macrophages	Augments the immune response; inflammatory mediator; activates T cells; activates phagocytes; promotes prostaglandin production; induces a fever
IL-2 (T-cell growth factor [TCGF])	Predominantly helper T lymphocytes	Activates T lymphocytes and NK cells; promotes growth and proliferation of T cells
IL-3 (multi-CSF)	T lymphocytes, mast cells	Hematopoietic growth factor for immature hematopoietic precursor cells
IL-4 (B-cell growth factor [BCGF])	T lymphocytes	Growth factor for T cells, activated B cells, and mast cells; macrophage-activating factor, enhances IgE reactions
IL-5	T lymphocytes, macrophages	Promotes growth and proliferation of activated B cells
IL-6	Monocytes, T and B lymphocytes, fibroblasts	B-cell stimulatory and differentiation factor; promotes hematopoiesis, enhances the inflammatory response
IL-7	Bone marrow, thymus	Promotes growth of lymphoid cells
IL-8 (monocyte-derived neutrophil chemotactic factor)	Macrophages, monocytes	Triggers chemotactic activity of neutrophils and lymphocytes
IL-9	Helper T cells	T-cell and mast-cell growth factor; supports maturation of erythroid progenitors
IL-10	Helper T cells	Inhibits proliferation of helper T cells; induces MHC antigen expression
Interferons		
Alpha-interferon	Leukocytes	Provides antiviral protection; inhibits cell proliferation; stimulates production of IL-2 immunomodulator
Beta-interferon	Fibroblasts, macrophages, epithelial cells	Provides antiviral protection
Gamma-interferon	T lymphocytes, NK cells	Activates macrophages, promotes B cell differentiation and NK cell activity; inhibits neoplastic cell proliferation
Tumor necrosis factor (TNF)	Macrophages, lymphocytes, fibroblasts, endothelial cells	Promotes the immune and inflammatory responses; kills tumor cells
Colony-stimulating factors (CSF)		
G-CSF	Monocytes, fibroblasts	Myeloid growth factor
GM-CSF	T cells, fibroblasts, monocytes, endothelial cells	Myelocytic growth factor
M-CSF	Monocytes, lymphocytes, fibroblasts, endothelial and epithelial cells	Macrophage growth factor
Transforming growth factor (TGF)	Lymphocytes, macrophages, platelets, bone	Stimulates fibroblasts for wound healing; inhibits the immune response

NATURE OF CLONAL SELECTION

Adaptive immunity is based on the specificity of lymphocytes. The manner in which lymphocytes can identify specific antigens and proliferate is a process called clonal selection. When an antigen invades the body, it binds to a few cells that recognize it as foreign. Recognition and binding cause the specific clones of the antigen-binding cells to proliferate, enabling them to mount a satisfactory immune response. Both B and T cells participate in clonal selection. B cells develop into antibody-producing plasma cells at a rapid rate on initial exposure and then begin to die. T cells have an-

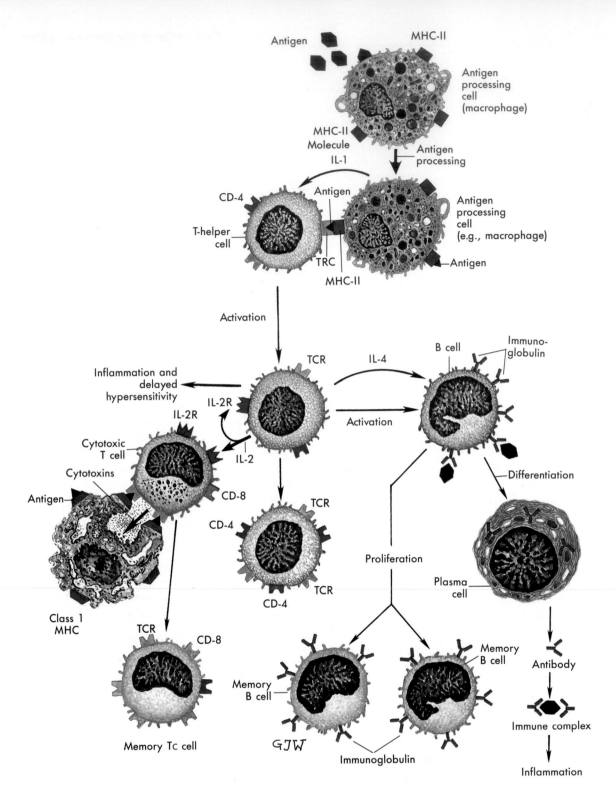

FIGURE 1-15
The immune response.

tigen receptors that recognize specific antigens in association with HLA antigens. When an antigen stimulates the right T-cell clone, that clone becomes activated, proliferates, and destroys the antigen through cell-mediated immunity. Primary exposure to every antigen that enters the body stimulates the development of memory B- and T-cell clones for that specific antigen. Their primary responsibility is to maintain specific immunologic memory for antigens that have been encountered. Memory for each antigen that has been previously identified enables the body to mount a rapid and more aggressive response to subsequent exposures to the same antigen.

MAJOR HISTOCOMPATIBILITY COMPLEX

The **major histocompatibility complex** (MHC) is a chromosomal region consisting of a group of genes found in every mammalian species studied. This gene complex is important for cell-cell interaction, immune recognition, and the coding of cell-surface histocompatibility antigens that are essential for evoking an immune response, particularly in transplanted tissue rejection. In mice, where much of the research has been conducted, the complex is referred to as H-2 and is located on the mouse chromosome 17. In humans the complex is called the **human leukocyte antigen (HLA)** system and is located on chromosome 6 (Figure 1-16). Every individual inherits two haplotypes for chromosome 6, one from each parent. A haplotype is a set of genes located on a single chromosome with specific characteristics. One maternal HLA haploid genotype (haplotype) and one paternal haploid genotype make up the genetic composition of every individual. Computerized technology, specific HLA antigen testing, and recombinant DNA technology have allowed the identification of hundreds of individual genes and many possible patterns of the HLA complex.

The antigens located on the HLA complex are divided into three groups, called class I, class II, and class III antigens. Each genetic region of the HLA complex is called a **locus. Class I antigens** (loci: HLA-A, HLA-B, and HLA-C) of the major histocompatibility complex are found on the surface of all nucleated cells and platelets (with the exception of sperm). These antigens are mainly involved in immune recognition, tissue graft rejection (class I antigens are the target antigens recognized by the cytotoxic T lymphocytes), and elimination of virally infected cells. **Class II** MHC antigens (loci: HLA-D, HLA-DR, HLA-DQ, and HLA-DP) are found expressed primarily on immunocompetent cells, including B cells, resting and activated T cells, macrophages, and monocytes. Class II molecules provide regulatory communication between various T cells. The presentation of antigens to T cells by the antigen-presenting cells is important in

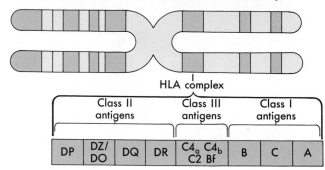

Chromosome 6: Site of genes that encode HLA antigens

FIGURE 1-16
The human leukocyte antigen (HLA) is located on chromosome 6.

enhancing the cooperation of T and B cells for the production of antibodies. **Class III** MHC antigens (complement) are located between class I and class II antigens on chromosome 6 of the HLA complex. These antigens are involved in both the alternative and classic pathways of the complement system.

Each locus has an allele and there are many different alleles that could be located at a given locus. An **allele** is a variant form of the gene and is recognized by a numerical indicator. For example, in HLA-A1, the 1 is the allele of the A loci on the HLA complex. Alleles that have been identified at a specific locus but that have not been officially recognized by the International HLA Nomenclature Committee are coded with a "w" to be placed in front of the allele number to signify "workshop" or working (e.g., HLA-DRw4). When official recognition has been confirmed, the "w" is eliminated and replaced with the appropriate number.

Identifying individual cellular specificities on the major histocompatibility complex is a process called tissue typing; it is used in transplantation and paternity testing and in association with various diseases, particularly autoimmune disorders. For example, HLA-DR3 often is seen in association with systemic lupus erythematosus (SLE) and myasthenia gravis, whereas HLA-DR4 is more commonly seen in rheumatoid arthritis. Once an individual has been tissue typed for HLA, it is not necessary to repeat this test, since genetic identity does not change.

HYPERSENSITIVITY REACTIONS

Hypersensitivity reactions are altered immunologic responses to a specific antigen that result in an exaggerated or inappropriate immune response. The classification of hypersensitivity reactions, derived from a schema developed by Gell and Coombs, defines four types based on the speed of the reaction and the im-

mune mechanisms involved: (1) type I: immediate reaction (IgE mediated), (2) type II: cytotoxic reaction (antibody mediated), (3) type III: immune complex–mediated reaction, and (4) type IV: cell-mediated reaction. The first three types are antibody-mediated responses, and the last is a cell-mediated response. These four reactions often are interrelated and may occur simultaneously. They may be secondary to a disease process or the primary cause of tissue destruc-

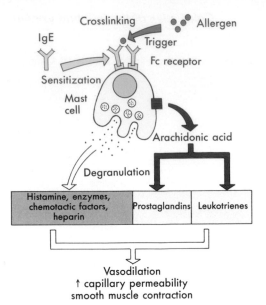

FIGURE 1-17
Type I (immediate hypersensitivity) reaction.

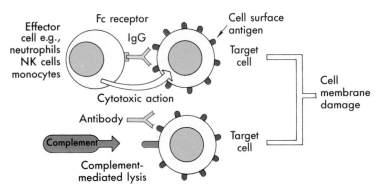

FIGURE 1-18
Type II (cytotoxic hypersensitivity) reaction.

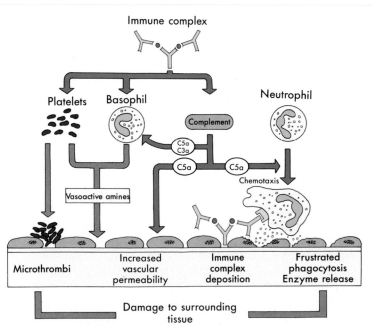

FIGURE 1-19
Type III (immune complex–mediated) reaction.

tion. The response time for clinical symptoms may be immediate or delayed. Anaphylaxis is an example of an immediate hypersensitivity reaction, and contact dermatitis is a type of delayed hypersensitivity reaction.

TYPE I REACTIONS

Type I (immediate hypersensitivity) reactions are IgE antibody mediated; they are initiated by antigen that usually is an environmental protein (e.g., animal dander, bee sting, or pollen) (Figure 1-17). The reaction occurs within minutes of exposure to the antigen and depends on the activation of mast cells and the release of their potent mediators. The stimulus for mast cells to release their potent substances requires that at least two of the receptors on the Fc region of the IgE antibody be bridged together with the antigen; this is called **cross-linking.** Once cross-linking has occurred, the mast cell undergoes degranulation, releasing its potent mediators and causing acute inflammation. Products of arachidonic acid metabolism (e.g., prostaglandins and leukotrienes) are generated and contribute to the delayed component of the reaction that often evolves hours after the initial exposure. Clinical manifestations are the result of the action of the inflammatory mediators on the surrounding tissue and blood vessels (i.e., smooth muscle constriction, increased vascular permeability, and vasodilation). Common type I hypersensitivity reactions include allergic rhinitis (hay fever), urticaria (hives), and anaphylaxis.

TYPE II REACTIONS

Type II (cytotoxic hypersensitivity) reactions are antibody mediated and occur when antibodies (IgA and IgM) are directed against antigen on host cells (Figure 1-18). The antibodies sensitize host cells, resulting in cytotoxic action by effector cells or cell lysis mediated by complement.

Most cells have a number of antigens on their surface membranes. Histocompatibility antigens (HLA) are one type of antigen. Generally the others are identified as tissue-specific antigens, which are selectively expressed on the membranes of specific cells. Because of the specificity of such antigens, antibody reactions are limited to cells (tissues) that express the "specific" antigen. Type II hypersensitivity reactions are commonly observed in the erythrocyte destruction of ABO-incompatible blood transfusions, and in some immune disorders such as myasthenia gravis and Goodpasture's syndrome.

TYPE III REACTIONS

Type III (immune complex–mediated) reactions are the result of antigen-antibody complexes deposited in tissues and blood vessels (Figure 1-19). Deposition of immune complexes causes the activation of complement and attracts phagocytes into the area, resulting in local inflammation and tissue damage. The difference between type III and type II reactions is that cell destruction caused by type II reactions is localized to a certain cell type, whereas type III reactions destroy tissue or organs where the immune complexes are most likely to be deposited. Frequent sites of immune complex deposition are the kidneys, resulting in glomerulonephritis, and the skin and joints, as seen in systemic lupus erythematosus and arthritis. Immune complex–mediated reactions are associated with a large amount of antigen and an ineffective antibody response.

TYPE IV REACTIONS

Type IV (delayed hypersensitivity) reactions develop 12 to 24 hours after the initial antigen exposure (Figure 1-20). This reaction is mediated by antigen-sensitized helper T cells after a second exposure to the same antigen. Helper T cells release cytokines that promote the recruitment and activation of macrophages, which release inflammatory mediators. If the antigen persists,

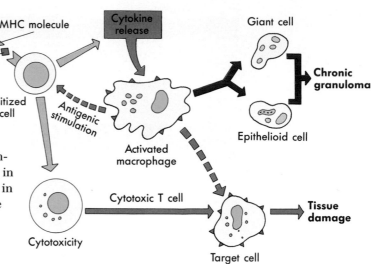

FIGURE 1-20
Type IV (delayed hypersensitivity) reaction.

tissue damage caused by macrophages may develop into a chronic granulomatous reaction. Examples of type IV reactions include a tuberculin reaction, contact dermatitis, and patch testing.

Table 1-7

MEDIATORS OF IMMEDIATE HYPERSENSITIVITY

Mediator	Function	Reaction
Histamine released from mast cells and basophil granules	Increases vascular permeability and vasodilation; causes smooth muscle contraction	Edema of airways, bronchoconstriction, bronchospasms, urticaria, pruritus, nausea, vomiting, diarrhea, hypotension, shock
Eosinophilic chemotactic factor of anaphylaxis (ECF-A) released from mast cells	Attracts eosinophils to target area	Increase in eosinophils; release of histamine
Serotonin released from platelets	Constricts smooth muscle; increases vascular permeability	Bronchoconstriction, bronchospasm, mucosal edema
Leukotrienes (metabolites of arachidonic acid)	Constrict airway smooth muscle; increase vascular permeability	Bronchial constriction; promotes histamine effect on smooth muscle
Prostaglandins (metabolites of arachidonic acid)	Constrict smooth muscle; stimulate vasodilation	Bronchospasm, hypotension, skin wheal and flare reaction
Platelet activating factor (PAF) released from mast cells	Aggregates platelets; stimulates vasodilation; chemotactic for eosinophils	Systemic hypotension, eosinophilic infiltrate
Kinins (e.g., bradykinin)	Contract smooth muscle; increase capillary permeability; cause vasodilation, hypotension, and pain; facilitate arachidonic acid metabolism	Angioedema, painful swelling, bronchial constriction
Anaphylatoxins (C3a, C4a, C5a derived from complement activation)	Stimulate histamine release	Same as histamine

CHAPTER 2

Assessment

An immunologic nursing assessment starts with the evaluation of the patient's medical-surgical, family, psychosocial, cultural, and occupational history and proceeds with a close, systematic physical examination. The immune system is evaluated primarily by laboratory data, but because a variety of immune disorders can affect many organ systems, a detailed history and complete physical examination are important.

HEALTH HISTORY

Demographic data

Age, sex, race, place of birth, occupation

Chief complaint

Guides the interview and should be stated in the patient's own words, reflecting why he is seeking medical attention. The following are examples of possible chief complaints related to immunologic disorders.

Fatigue and weakness

Extreme fatigue and weakness may result from anemia or neuropathy secondary to an autoimmune or immunodeficiency disorder.

Altered ability to perform activities of daily living (ADLs)

Changes in activity level

Sleep patterns: (e.g., difficulty sleeping; when, where, and number of hours; number of naps during the day)

Greater fatigue or weakness in the morning or at night

Greater weakness on one side or the other

Persistent or intermittent fatigue or weakness

Aggravating or precipitating factors for fatigue and weakness (e.g., physical activity, climbing stairs, gardening, overexposure to the sun)

Factors that relieve fatigue or weakness (e.g., minimizing physical activity, medication to enhance a full night's sleep)

Does weakness affect the joints

Fever

Fever may indicate an inflammation, an impaired immune system, or rapid proliferation of white blood cells (WBCs).

High fevers of 39.4°-40° C (103°-104° F) may demonstrate serum sickness, whereas low-grade fevers of 37.2°-37.7° C (99°-100° F) may indicate an allergy. Fever may also be a sign of organ or tissue transplant rejection.

How long has fever been present

How high has it been

Does fever fluctuate

Periods of being afebrile (does the fever occur only at night)

Intermittent or persistent fevers

Does perspiration or night sweats accompany fever

Does a flushed appearance accompany fever

Joint pain

Pain in the knees, hands, wrists, or elbows may indicate an autoimmune disorder (e.g., systemic lupus erythematosus, rheumatoid arthritis). Aching in the bones can be caused by expanding bone marrow; heat and salicylates decrease joint pain from inflammation.

What joints are affected

Is pain bilateral or unilateral

When does joint pain occur

Is pain intermittent or continuous

Rate pain on a scale of 1-10

What are the aggravating or precipitating factors (e.g., increased physical activity)

What are the relieving factors (e.g., medication, ice or heat, or minimizing physical activity)

Do redness, swelling, and warmth accompany pain

Does pain alter activity

Is there pain at rest

HEALTH HISTORY—cont'd

Is there early morning stiffness
Bone pain or aching

Abnormal bleeding

Abnormal bleeding may indicate a platelet or clotting factor abnormality, which can be seen with certain immunodeficiency disorders, some immune disorders, antineoplastic drug therapy, immunosuppressive therapy in organ transplantation, and malignancies involving the bone marrow (e.g., leukemias, lymphomas). Excessive blood loss often results in anemia.
Presence and site of unusual bleeding
    Frequent nose bleeds
    Bleeding from gums (during flossing) or mouth
    Easy and frequent bruising from an unidentified cause
    Hematemesis
    Black, tarry stools
    Bloody urine
    Heavy menstrual periods
Character of bleeding (onset, frequency, duration, amount, color [bright red, coffee colored, black])
Is bleeding prolonged after a minor cut or dental work
Does bleeding start for no apparent reason

Lymphadenopathy

Swollen lymph nodes typically signal inflammation or infection, which may be associated with immunodeficiency disorders. Increased lymphocyte production is commonly seen in certain leukemias. Enlarged lymph nodes accompany Hodgkin's disease, non-Hodgkin's lymphoma, and lymphoproliferative disorder seen as a complication of organ or tissue transplantation.
Swelling in neck, armpits, or groin
Are areas of swelling erythematous, painful/tender, warm
Are nodes firm, mobile, red, warm, tender
Recent surgery or trauma
Organ or bone marrow transplant (when)
When was swelling first noticed
Is swelling constant, intermittent, or transient
Is swelling bilateral or unilateral
Is edema pitting in nature
Recent insect sting
Interventions used to decrease or inhibit swelling
Has a lymph node biopsy been performed
Efforts to treat (e.g., support stockings, elevation)

Skin rash

A skin rash may be present with allergic disorders (e.g., urticaria) and some autoimmune diseases (e.g., butterfly facial pattern in systemic lupus erythematosus).
Location of rash
Itching
Type of lesion
Is rash constant, intermittent, or transient
Is rash related to a specific activity or substance (e.g., sun exposure, soap, food, animals)
Is there dermal sensitivity
Interventions used to decrease or avoid rash
Is rash associated with redness, warmth, tender or sensitive areas, or pruritus
Any recent insect sting
Any recent environmental exposure (e.g., chemicals)

Chronic or recurrent infections

Persistent infections may indicate an impaired immune system secondary to an immunodeficiency disorder, an autoimmune disease, or organ or tissue transplantation.
Organ system typically affected
What organism is usually involved
How does the infection present itself
Is there a fever
Human immunodeficiency virus (HIV) status
Previous infections

Patient's perception of the problem

To what degree are the patient and family concerned about the symptoms?
What does the patient feel has caused or will alleviate the symptoms?
In general, does the patient feel in "good health"?

Patient history: factors relating to immunologic disorders

Concurrent disorders

Autoimmune disorders
Immunodeficiency disorders
HIV status
Infections (chronic, recurrent)
Malignancies
Chronic systemic disorders (diabetes, renal failure)
Asthma
Organ or tissue transplant

HEALTH HISTORY—cont'd

Allergies/hypersensitivity

Allergic to:
  Inhalants (e.g., pollens, mold, spores, animal dander)
  Contactants (e.g., metals, plants, fibers, chemicals)
  Injectables (e.g., drugs, blood transfusions, venoms, vaccines)
  Ingestants (e.g., foods, food additives, drugs)
Symptoms accompanying allergic reaction
  Weeping eyes
  Coughing, nasal congestion
  Edema, erythema
  Shortness of breath
  Rash/urticaria
  Itching

Family history

Family members with:
  Allergies
  Autoimmune diseases
  Immunodeficiency diseases
  Chronic or recurrent infections
  Arthritis
  Anemia
  Asthma
  Malignancy
  Any symptoms similar to the patient's

Medications

Prescription
  Chemotherapy
  Antibiotics
  Immunosuppressive agents
  Antihistamines
  Nonsteroidal antiinflammatory agents
Nonprescription
  Cold and flu preparations
  Aspirin or ibuprofen
  Allergy preparations
  Sleep agents
  Herbal remedies
  Vitamin, mineral, or iron supplements
  Illicit drug use (cocaine, heroin, marijuana)

Radiation

Total body irradiation
Localized body irradiation

Immunizations/previous tests

Immunizations
  Tetanus, pertussis, diphtheria
  Polio
  Mumps
  Rubella
  Rubeola (measles)
  Tuberculosis skin test

Influenza
Haemophilus influenzae type B
Previous tests
  Allergy testing
  Antibody testing
  Skin testing

Surgery

Organ or tissue transplantation
Thymectomy
Splenectomy
Surgery, with trauma to regional lymph nodes
Breast implants

Diet and nutrition

Weight
  Actual and ideal
  Recent loss or gain; deliberate or unintentional
Dietary restrictions
  Prescribed by physician, nutritionist, or self-prescribed
  Tolerance
Routine dietary intake
Food intolerances or allergies

Activity history

Level of daily activity
Indoor or outdoor activity, sun exposure
Response to activity (urticaria, nausea, itching, unusual shortness of breath)

Psychosocial

Stresses or life-change events
Relationship with others
  Support systems
  Marital status, children, siblings, friends
  Significant others
Response to stress
Methods of coping
Response to pain or discomfort
Adjustment to the current problem
Self-image
Loss of interest in work or play; lethargic
Sexual preference

Social-cultural history

Cultural and spiritual values
Educational level
Occupation: determine type, hours worked per week, indoors or outdoors, physical or sedentary, contact with chemicals, retired, job history
Military service (exposure to Agent Orange)
Leisure activities and hobbies
Economic resources: insurance and other
Tobacco and alcohol use
Recent travel

ASSESS BEHAVIOR, MENTAL STATUS, AND FACIAL FEATURES

Assess the patient's **behavior** and **mental status** to determine mood, **emotional stability,** and **cognition.** It is not uncommon for patients with chronic diseases to be depressed or angry regardless of the nature of the disorder. However, irritability, confusion, memory loss, and paranoid thinking (or other symptoms of psychosis) may develop with an immune disorder, particularly in autoimmune diseases such as systemic lupus erythematosus (SLE). Other problems of cognition, such as forgetfulness, short-term memory loss, and impaired ability to solve complex, abstract problems, may occur with multiple sclerosis (MS) or progressive acquired immunodeficiency syndrome (AIDS). AIDS patients with progressive dementia may have HIV encephalopathy.

Observe the patient for facial expression, weakness, and edema. Changes in facial expression may be seen in myasthenia gravis (MG), reflecting a snarl that replaces a smile or a "flat" expression, demonstrating facial weakness. Facial weakness may also be seen with other autoimmune disorders such as MS. Facial edema may indicate Hashimoto's disease or a renal abnormality, such as glomerulonephritis, which accompanies certain autoimmune disorders such as SLE.

ASSESS THE SKIN

Assess the skin for **color** and **integrity.** Check for **lesions, rashes, nodules,** and any signs or symptoms of infection or inflammation.

Inspect the patient's skin **color** for pallor, **cyanosis, jaundice, erythema,** or **petechiae.** Pallor reflects decreased oxyhemoglobin concentration. A generalized pallor can occur as the result of pernicious or hemolytic anemia or may be present with a number of autoimmune or immunodeficiency disorders. **Cyanosis** is caused by an increased amount of deoxygenated hemoglobin, which appears with some anemias. Cyanosis or pallor in the patient's fingertips, toes, nose, or tongue can be seen in Raynaud's phenomenon, which may appear independently or may accompany some autoimmune disorders such as scleroderma or SLE. Jaundice is the result of an elevated bilirubin level. It is most easily seen in the patient's sclerae, mucous membranes, and skin. Jaundice may be secondary to increased erythrocyte hemolysis (hereditary or acquired) or to autoimmune chronic active hepatitis. Jaundice and pallor found simultaneously may indicate hemolytic anemia. Check for areas of erythema that may be caused by local inflammation or infection. Examine the skin for petechiae or purpuric lesions, which are classic signs of autoimmune thrombocytopenic purpura.

The **integrity** of the skin is evaluated by palpation and is based on turgor, texture, temperature, and moisture. **Turgor** reflects skin elasticity and the water content of the skin and subcutaneous tissues. It is assessed by lifting up a fold of skin, usually on the abdomen or over the radius at the wrist, and observing how quickly it returns to its normal shape. Normally the skin will return to its normal shape very quickly. Loss of normal skin turgor is often due to dehydration, large weight loss, normal aging, or chronic illness.

Skin **texture** varies considerably between individuals and on different parts of the body. The descriptive terms usually used are thick, thin, coarse, tight, and smooth. Patients with scleroderma have taut, thickening skin, whereas patients with Hashimoto's disease often have very dry, coarse skin.

Palpate the skin to determine **temperature** and **moisture.** Moisture on the skin may be thin and watery or thick and oily. Fluid from any observed lesion must be described as to color, amount, thickness, and odor. Abnormally dry skin may indicate dehydration or an autoimmune disorder such as Sjögren's syndrome. Skin that is typically pink, warm, smooth, and sweaty may indicate Graves' disease. An increase in local or systemic temperature generally indicates inflammation or infection, whereas a decrease in peripheral temperature indicates arterial insufficiency, as in Raynaud's disease.

Inspect the skin for any type of **lesion,** noting the type and characteristics (size, shape, color, texture, and elevation or depression), location, distribution, and any exudate (amount, color, and consistency). Lesions may indicate an immune disorder or may be the result of an acute or chronic infection, as is frequently seen in immunodeficiency diseases.

Inspect the skin for **rashes** and their distribution. Gentle palpation of the skin with the fingertips is the best method of detecting a rash that may not be visible. Ask the patient if the skin itches, and observe for signs of scratching. Certain immune disorders have characteristic rashes. For example, a rash across the bridge of the nose and on the cheeks in a butterfly pattern is indicative of SLE. Hivelike plaques on the knees, elbows, buttocks, upper back, and posterior neck may indicate dermatitis herpetiformis. Rashes around the anterior and posterior neck may suggest an atopic dermatitis. A rash in the axilla may represent an atopic allergic reaction to the patient's deodorant.

Check for allergic skin reactions such as eczema, rashes, wheals, or angioneurotic edema.

Palpate for **nodules,** particularly around the joints of the elbows, wrists, hands, fingers, knees, ankles, and feet. Nodules generally are easily palpable, elevated, firm, and approximately 1 to 2 cm in diameter. Subcutaneous nodules often are palpable in rheumatoid arthritis. Nodules in rheumatoid arthritis are frequently accompanied by joint swelling, heat, and pain.

ASSESS THE HAIR AND NAILS

Hair

Inspect and palpate hair for **growth, texture, distribution, color,** and **amount.**

Inspect hair growth patterns, and note patches of alopecia on the head, arms, and legs. Check for short, broken hairs above the hairline on the forehead, a common finding in SLE. Palpate the hair to assess texture and amount.

Hair that is thin, dry, brittle, or nonresilient or that shows signs of broken hair shafts may indicate a chronic illness (e.g., Graves' disease), medication (e.g., prednisone), and/or malnutrition (e.g., related to dysphagia).

Nails

Inspect the nails for **color, symmetry, cleanliness, length, configuration,** and **adherence** of the nail to the nail bed.

Check the nails for koilonychia (spoon nail), which is associated with Raynaud's phenomena, anemia, and other systemic disorders. Observe for onycholysis (loosening of the nail from the nail bed) and brittleness, often seen in Hashimoto's disease. Depressions that can be palpated on all nail surfaces generally occur in response to a systemic disease. Longitudinal white streaks may indicate a systemic disorder or anemia. Evaluate nails for signs of infection.

ASSESS THE EYES

Stand in front of the patient and inspect the **eyebrows** and **external eye.** Eyebrows that are short and coarse may suggest hypothyroidism associated with Hashimoto's thyroiditis late in the disease trajectory. Periorbital puffiness may reflect the loss of elasticity that develops with aging. Periorbital edema is abnormal and may indicate allergies, renal disease, or thyroid hypoactivity. Abnormal protrusion of the eyeballs, presenting a wideeyed, staring appearance, is called exophthalmos. Bilateral exophthalmos is characteristic of Graves' disease. Check for lid lag, as demonstrated by the edge of the sclera appearing between the upper lid and the iris, also a sign of Graves' disease. Note any fasciculations or tremors of the lids, suggesting MS or hyperthyroidism. Observe for ptosis, a drooping of the eyelids, which is a common finding in myasthenia gravis.

Check the **conjunctivae** for erythema or pallor. Erythema may suggest conjunctivitis, seen in allergies or immunodeficiency disorders (e.g., AIDS). Pallor of the conjunctivae may indicate hemolytic anemia or the anemia that accompanies SLE or rheumatoid arthritis. Engorged or enlarged vessels in the conjunctivae may suggest keratoconjunctivitis or the scleritis may accompany rheumatoid arthritis.

Palpate the eye. An eye that feels firm and resists palpation may suggest hyperthyroidism, as in Hashimoto's disease. Palpate the upper and lower lid margins. If the lid feels full, evert the lid and inspect the lacrimal gland. These glands may become enlarged in Sjögren's syndrome and sarcoid disease. Despite lacrimal gland enlargement, these patients often complain of "dry eyes" because of inadequate tear production.

The six cardinal fields of gaze are used to assess ocular muscle strength and determine muscle weakness that may be seen in certain immunologic disorders (e.g., MS, Graves' disease).

ASSESS THE SUPERFICIAL LYMPH NODES

Lymph nodes are located along the lymphatic vessels; they can be identified as superficial nodes in the subcutaneous connective tissue or as deep nodes under the muscular fascia. They rarely are found isolated, but rather are grouped in chains or clusters. The exact number of lymph nodes varies from one individual to another, but smaller lymph nodes appear to be more proliferative.

Physical assessment of the superficial lymph nodes enables the nurse to detect enlarged, tender, or mobile lymph nodes, providing functional information about the immune system.

Lymph node assessment includes inspection and palpation. Using a centimeter ruler may be helpful in measuring the exact size of the lymph node being examined. When a node has been identified, it must be evaluated according to location, size, surface characteristics, consistency, symmetry, fixation and mobility, tenderness and pain, erythema, heat, and increased vascularity (see box). *Assessment of the lymph nodes begins with the neck nodes and proceeds to other nodal areas as each related area of the body is examined.*

Inspect the body for prominent lymph nodes, erythema, and red streaks that follow lymphatic drainage patterns. Palpate the lymph nodes using the pads of the second, third, and fourth fingers. Start by pressing very lightly, using a rotary motion; gradually increase the pressure. Heavier pressure can move the node before it can be felt. Concern is warranted when the node

---

INFECTION

Local inflammation is manifested by redness, heat, pain, swelling, and loss of function. Systemic inflammation is manifested by fever, increased heart rate and respirations, leukocytosis with a shift to the left, and weight loss. Subjective findings that often accompany infection include malaise, nausea, anorexia, fatigue, and apathy.

ASSESSMENT CHARACTERISTICS OF LYMPH NODES OR MASSES

Location: Be specific in describing the site; use imaginary body lines or bony prominences to relate findings; draw pictures when appropriate.

Size: Define the volume in centimeters, using a tape measure, from the three dimensions of length, width, and thickness; state the total volume; accurately describe the shape (round, cylindric); if irregular, draw pictures.

Surface characteristics: Describe accurately as smooth, nodular, or irregular.

Consistency: Describe as hard, firm, soft, resilient, spongy, cystic (cysts usually are transluminal; nodes are not).

Symmetry: Describe symmetry, and compare with other structures; clearly define the edges.

Fixation and mobility: Describe the exact mobile parameters in centimeters; if the mass is fixed in position, identify whether fixation is to underlying or overlying tissue by trying to move it with your fingers; matted nodes are enlarged nodes that feel like a mass.

Tenderness and pain: Describe whether present without stimulation or elicited by palpation or movement; indicate whether direct, referred, or rebound; malignant nodes generally are nontender; inflamed and infected nodes generally are painful.

Erythema: Describe the extent of color change, if present, and the area of distribution.

Heat: Describe the extent if present.

Increased vascularity: Describe the prominence of overlying veins or cyanosis of the area.

---

is firm and fixed. When enlarged nodes are identified, evaluate the adjacent areas and those regions drained by the involved nodes for infection or malignancy (Figure 2-1).

Normal Findings

Generally lymph nodes are not palpable in a healthy, well-developed adult. In a child, thin adult, or someone who has had a viral infection, they will be easier to feel. When lymph nodes are palpable, they should be smooth, symmetric, slightly soft, and mobile and have clearly defined edges. The node should have no pain, tenderness, erythema, or warmth to touch.

Normal lymph nodes vary considerably in size, from next to unidentifiable to the size of a coffee bean or even as large as an olive. They usually are round or oval in shape. However, they have also been observed as flat and elongated or cylindric. Generally lymph nodes closer to the middle of the body are smaller than those that are more superficial. For example, the axillary and inguinal lymph nodes typically are larger than the supraclavicular or iliac lymph nodes. Small, movable nodes less than 1 cm in size are of minimal concern. For example, an occasional small, firm node found in the cervical or inguinal regions is called a "shotty" node; these shotty nodes usually are clinically insignificant.

Infants and children under 2 years of age often have widespread lymph node enlargement, which usually decreases with age. Fibrosis and fatty degeneration typically are found on pathologic examination of nodes in the elderly.

Abnormal Findings

Inflamed, tender, fixed, or matted nodes indicate a problem and require further evaluation. Infected nodes usually are warm and tender to the touch and may be matted. Red streaks covering a node usually indicate lymphadenitis, and there generally is an obvious site of infection. Enlarged and tender nodes often suggest an acute inflammatory response to a viral, fungal, or bacterial infection. The source of infection can be identified from the pattern of lymph node enlargement and the drainage route. For example, ear infections drain to the preauricular, retropharyngeal, and deep cervical nodes, which may also be tender and enlarged. This may be in response to the ear infection (otitis media) or the cause of the ear infection. Matted nodes are enlarged nodes that feel like a mass. If a mass is transluminal with a flashlight, it probably is not a node but a cyst. Hard, firm, immobile, irregularly shaped, and nontender nodes often involve a malignancy.

Generalized lymphadenopathy involving three or more nodal regions may indicate an inflammation, infection, autoimmune disorder, or neoplastic process. In some autoimmune disorders, such as SLE, the nodal enlargement may be either diffuse or local. Any node that is enlarged, tender, painful, immobile, matted, or inflamed requires further investigation.

ASSESS THE HEAD AND NECK LYMPH NODES

A systematic approach to assessing the lymph nodes of the head and neck is mandatory. If a meticulous method is not used during the assessment, portions of

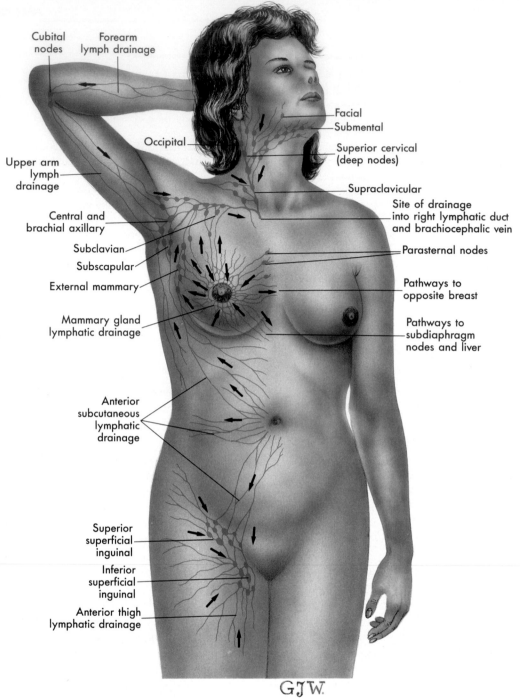

Cubital nodes
Forearm lymph drainage
Occipital
Facial
Submental
Superior cervical (deep nodes)
Upper arm lymph drainage
Supraclavicular
Site of drainage into right lymphatic duct and brachiocephalic vein
Central and brachial axillary
Parasternal nodes
Subclavian
Subscapular
Pathways to opposite breast
External mammary
Mammary gland lymphatic drainage
Pathways to subdiaphragm nodes and liver
Anterior subcutaneous lymphatic drainage
Superior superficial inguinal
Inferior superficial inguinal
Anterior thigh lymphatic drainage

GJW

FIGURE 2-1
Lymphatic drainage.

the lymph node chain probably will be overlooked.

Inspect the regions where the lymph nodes are located. Have the patient slightly rotate his head to either side and tilt it backward. Look for any obvious swollen or reddened lymph nodes, asymmetry, masses, or lesions. Ask the patient if he has any tenderness in his head or neck.

Most of the nodes in the body that are palpable are located in the head and neck. Identifying the anterior and posterior triangles at the lateral side of the neck can assist the examiner in palpating the lymph nodes of the head and neck (Figure 2-2).

The lymph nodes of the head and neck are palpated with the patient in a sitting position. The patient's neck should be flexed slightly forward and toward the side being examined. Face the patient, and place the fingertips of your right hand at the location of the preauricular nodes, just anterior to the ear (Figure 2-3). Use your left hand to support the patient's head. By using the pads of the index finger and middle fingers of both hands, the skin is rolled in a gentle but firm circular motion (not pushed) over the underlying tissue. Gentle, firm, and consistent pressure should be applied

Table 2-1

REGIONAL LYMPH NODE ASSESSMENT

Lymph node region	Normal findings	Abnormal findings
Head and neck nodes	Small (<1 cm), smooth, nontender, possibly firm (as in a "shotty node"), and with well-defined edges	Tender or enlarged nodes: preauricular or postauricular (mastoid)—indicates ear infection; submental, submandibular, suprahyoid, thyrolingual, and internal jugular—indicates a mouth or tongue infection
Cervical nodes	Palpable in children and adolescents; gradually diminish with age, and by fifth decade are reduced by 50%	Deep nodes are enlarged with throat infections, rubella, infectious mononucleosis, and hepatitis; nodes with a diameter of ≥1 cm indicate a malignancy; enlarged nodes in children usually are due to an infection
Supraclavicular nodes	Should not be palpable	Enlarged, firm, fixed nodes in patients >35 yr indicate malignancy; tender nodes suggest infection or inflammation
Axillary nodes	Most are not palpable; of the central axillary nodes, one or two nontender, small nodes may be palpable	Enlarged or tender nodes may indicate a malignancy; this mandates reexamination of the supraclavicular and infraclavicular nodes
Upper extremity nodes: epitrochlear node	Not palpable or very small (<1 cm)	Enlargement may suggest secondary syphilis or inflammation
Lower extremity nodes: popliteal and inguinal nodes	Popliteal nodes generally are not palpable; inguinal nodes are larger than other nodes in the body (approximately 1 cm) and may be palpable; if so, they should be small, soft, and mobile.	Popliteal enlargement or tenderness indicates inflammation or lymphangitis; enlarged inguinal nodes (>1 cm) indicate a lesion or inflammation in the vulva, lower aspect of the vagina, penis, or scrotal surface; red streaks arising as the result of an infection generally follow the lymphatic drainage up the leg; this may indicate lymphangitis

(pushing too hard on the nodes will obliterate them in the deeper soft tissue). Next, sequentially palpate the postauricular nodes located behind the ear, the occipital nodes at the base of the skull, and the tonsillar nodes. Then, move your fingertips to the underside of the mandible on the side you are examining. Pull the skin and subcutaneous tissue laterally over the ramus of the mandible at the location of the submandibular nodes, between the chin and the angle of the mandible (Figure 2-4). Sequentially palpate the submandibular, sublingual, and submental nodes. Examine the other side. Assessment of the thyroid typically follows evaluation of the lymph nodes of the head and neck if Graves' disease or Hashimoto's disease is suspected.

The posterior **cervical nodes** (spinal nerve chain and posterior superficial cervical chain) are examined next (Figure 2-5). The patient should be in a sitting position.

Palpable lymph nodes of the head and neck should be examined in the following order:
  Preauricular nodes
  Postauricular (mastoid) nodes
  Occipital nodes
  Tonsillar (retropharyngeal) nodes
  Submaxillary (submandibular) nodes
  Sublingual nodes
  Submental nodes
  Posterior superficial cervical chain (transverse cervical artery chain)
  Posterior cervical chain
  Deep cervical chain
  Supraclavicular nodes

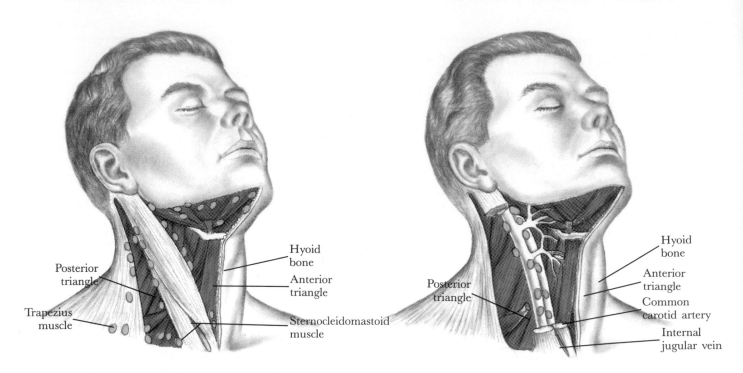

FIGURE 2-2
Anterior and posterior triangles of the neck. (From Seidel et al.[157])

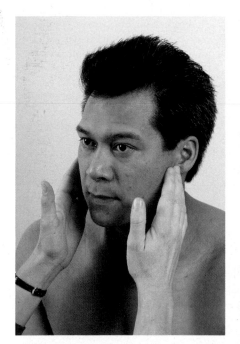

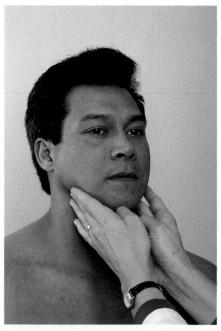

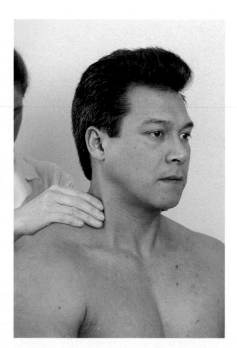

FIGURE 2-3
Palpation of the preauricular lymph nodes.

FIGURE 2-4
Palpation of the submandibular lymph nodes.

FIGURE 2-5
Palpation of the postcervical lymph nodes.

Inspection of the neck begins with having the patient raise his chin and tilt his head slightly backward. Look for asymmetry, swelling, obvious lymph nodes, or masses, and palpate these areas.

Palpation may be initiated from either in front or in back of the patient. To examine the posterior cervical nodes, support the patient's head with one hand and with the fingertips of the other hand palpate along the anterior surface of the trapezius muscle. Use a circular motion, moving toward the posterior surface of the sternocleidomastoid muscle. Examine the other side.

The anterior triangle, which harbors the deep cervical chain, is largely obstructed by the overlying sternomastoid muscle (Figure 2-2). However, it is possible to palpate the nodes at either end of this chain, the tonsillar and supraclavicular nodes, respectively. To examine the anterior triangle, hold the patient's chin in your left hand and gently palpate the nodes of this chain. Start with the tonsillar node and move the fingertips down the neck to the terminal node of this chain, the supraclavicular node. Then examine the other side.

For examination of the **supraclavicular nodes** (Virchow's nodes), the patient should be in a sitting position. Encourage the patient to relax the muscles of the upper body and allow the clavicles to drop. Bend the patient's head forward with your right hand (this promotes relaxation of the sternocleidomastoid muscle and the anterior neck, promoting exposure of the scalene triangle) (Figure 2-6). Inspect the area for nodal enlargement or erythema. To palpate these nodes, hook your left index finger over the clavicle lateral to the tendinous portion of the sternocleidomastoid muscle. The index finger should probe deeply in a rotary motion into the scalene triangle to allow the supraclavicular nodes to be palpated. At the completion of the examination, the entire neck is lightly palpated for nodes.

ASSESS THE AXILLARY NODES

Examination of the axillary nodes is approached by visualizing the area as a four-sided pyramid with its apex being the most superior point. The apex is located at the level between the first rib and clavicle in the axilla (the apex is the uppermost part of the armpit).

The axillary nodes are **inspected** with the patient in a sitting position. Observe for any obvious swollen or reddened lymph nodes. Inspect the skin of each axilla, and observe for evidence of a rash, erythema, or changes in pigmentation.

To palpate the axillary nodes, stand in front of the patient and ask him to relax his left arm down (Figure 2-7). Assist him by supporting his left wrist with your left hand. To palpate the patient's left axilla, cup the fingers of your right hand and reach high into the apex of the patient's axilla. Slowly bring your fingers down in

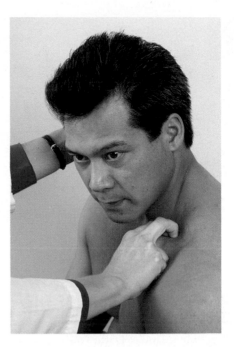

FIGURE 2-6
Palpation of the supraclavicular lymph nodes.

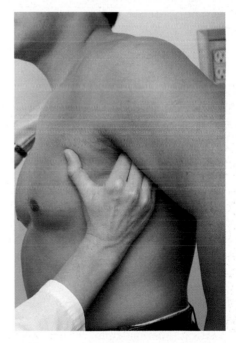

FIGURE 2-7
Palpation of the axillary lymph nodes.

a rotary motion over the surface of his ribs, milking the axillary contents downward. Feel for the central nodes by compressing them against the chest wall and muscles of the axilla. Continue to palpate in a rotary motion deep inside the anterior and posterior axillary folds and along the upper humerus to feel for the pectoral (anterior), subcapsular (posterior), and lateral axillary nodes. If these last nodes are difficult to palpate, they may be more easily palpated by standing behind the patient. Then examine the other side.

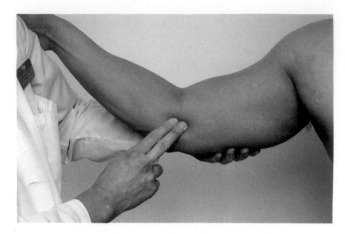

FIGURE 2-8
Palpation of the epitrochlear lymph nodes.

ASSESS THE LYMPH NODES OF THE EXTREMITIES

The **epitrochlear node** is the only peripheral lymph center in the upper extremities. It is located on the medial surface of the arm above the elbow in the depression above and posterior to the medial condyle of the humerus.

The epitrochlear nodes are **inspected** with the patient in a sitting position (Figure 2-8). Observe for any obvious swollen or reddened lymph nodes. Inspect the skin, and check for evidence of nodules, rash, erythema, or changes in pigmentation. To palpate the epitrochlear nodes, support the patient's elbow with one hand and assess the nodes with the other. Use the same rotary motion with the pads of the first three fingers. Examine the other side.

The lower extremities are made up of an extensive network of deep and superficial lymphatic ducts. Only the superficial ducts are palpable. They drain lymph from the legs primarily into the **popliteal** and **superficial inguinal lymph centers**. The popliteal lymph center comprises two or three nodes. It is located posterior to the knee close to the terminal end of the saphenous vein. There are two groups of superficial inguinal lymph centers, the horizontal (superior) group and the vertical (inferior) group (Figure 2-9).

The horizontal group comprises five or six nodes located just inferior and parallel to the inguinal ligament. The vertical group comprises four or five large lymph nodes located just inferior to the junction of the saphenous and femoral veins. Only the horizontal and vertical superficial inguinal lymph nodes are palpable. The nodes are examined with the patient in the supine position, legs slightly apart, with the examiner to one side. Maintain the patient's modesty by covering the genitalia during the examination.

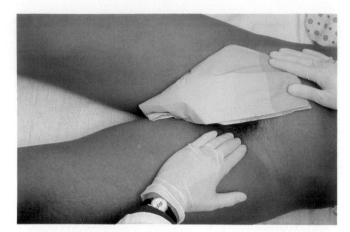

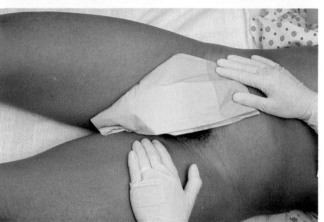

FIGURE 2-9
Palpation of the inguinal lymph nodes. **A,** Superior (horizontal). **B,** Inferior (vertical).

Inspect the nodal area for edema, redness, and changes in the skin. Observe for enlarged nodes. Palpate the vertical inguinal lymph nodes by placing your right thumb on top of the upper aspect of the patient's right thigh. Then use the pads of the first three fingers, which should cup right over to the medial aspect of the leg, to palpate these inguinal nodes. Continue to use a rotary motion when palpating for these nodes. To palpate for the horizontal nodes, move the fingers of the right hand to the area just below the inguinal ligament, using the same rotary motion. Examine the other side.

ASSESS THE NOSE, MOUTH, AND TONSILS AND ADENOIDS

Nose

The nasal cavity is inspected by pushing the tip of the patient's nose upward and shining a flashlight into the nostrils (Figure 2-10). Increased redness may suggest infection, whereas ulceration of the mucous membranes may indicate SLE. Turbinates that are boggy and swollen with a pale or bluish gray color suggest an allergic

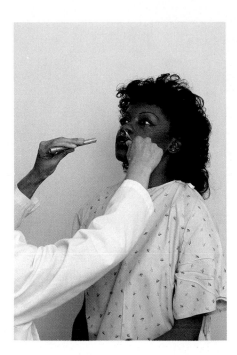

FIGURE 2-10
Inspection of the nasal cavity. (From Wilson S and Thompson J: *Respiratory disorders*, St Louis, 1991, Mosby–Year Book.)

disorder. The presence of polyps may indicate a chronic allergic condition.

Mouth

Inspect the **lips** and **mucous membranes** of the mouth using a penlight. Check for changes in color, ulcerations, lesions, and white patches of exudate. Patients with SLE can develop oral ulcerations. Patients with immunodeficiency disorders are at greater risk for developing herpes simplex, which is characterized as a recurrent, vesicular, crusting lesion generally located on the lip. The most common oral infection is candidiasis (thrush), which leaves a white exudate over the tongue and mucous membranes. This infection frequently is seen in infants and in patients receiving chemotherapy or immunosuppression drugs (organ or tissue transplant) or who have an immunodeficiency disorder (AIDS, common variable immunodeficiency).

Inspect all borders of the tongue. An infection or malignancy should be suspected with any ulceration, nodule, or thickened red or white patch. Check for white irregular lesions, usually on the lateral side of the tongue, called "oral hairy leukoplakia," an early manifestation of AIDS. These lesions may have prominent folds or "hairy" projections. Tongue enlargement may be seen with certain immunologic disorders such as Hashimoto's disease. Have the patient stick out his tongue as far as possible, and observe for a fine tremor, which may occur in Graves' disease.

Tonsils and Adenoids

Inspect the tonsils and adenoids. Tonsils or adenoids that are enlarged, reddened, or covered with white or yellow exudate may indicate an infection.

PULMONARY ASSESSMENT

Inspect the patient's breathing pattern. Observe for signs of respiratory distress, specifically dyspnea, persistent coughing, wheezing, and cyanosis. AIDS patients often have tachypnea with shallow, labored breathing patterns secondary to pneumonia and *Pneumocystis carinii* infection.

Assess the patient's cough. A productive cough may be a sign of infection, and a sputum specimen should be obtained. Sputum that is thin, white, and frothy may suggest an asthmatic attack or may be secondary to volume overload caused by the renal failure from glomerulonephritis seen in SLE. Sputum that is green or yellow and tenacious suggests an infection.

Palpate thoracic expansion from posterior and anterior positions. Limitation in chest expansion may indicate pain, inflammation, or restriction secondary to scleroderma. Percuss the chest wall systematically from side to side to compare tone. Dullness indicates consolidation, as with pneumonia, whereas hyperresonance may suggest trapped air, as with bronchial asthma.

Auscultate anterior and posterior breath sounds. In patients with pneumonia or *P. carinii* infection, crackles and bronchial breath sounds often are heard over the affected area. Wheezes are a more common finding in asthma and other allergic disorders. Pleural effusions may develop in patients with rheumatoid arthritis or SLE.

CARDIOVASCULAR ASSESSMENT

Auscultate for cardiac rate and rhythm and abnormal heart sounds. Listen for murmurs. Tachycardia and an irregular heart rate suggest atrial fibrillation or atrial flutter and may indicate Graves' disease, anemia, or infection. Apical systolic murmurs can result from severe anemia caused by an autoimmune disease or immunodeficiency disorder. Pericardial friction rubs are associated with endocarditis and pericarditis with effusion, as are seen in patients with SLE, rheumatoid arthritis, or scleroderma. Assess peripheral circulation for impairments.

ABDOMINAL ASSESSMENT

Inspect the skin of the abdomen for color changes. Check for surface characteristics, noting any unusual lesions, nodules, or scars. Auscultate all four quadrants to assess bowel sounds. Hyperactive bowel sounds may be heard as the result of diarrhea that may be found with certain autoimmune disorders such as ulcerative colitis

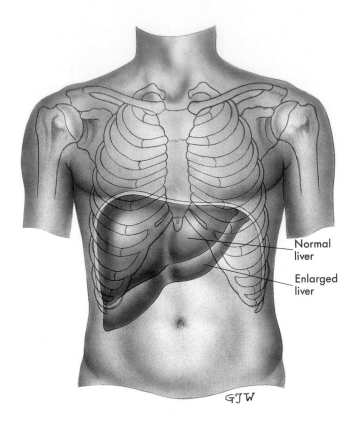

FIGURE 2-11
Size and location of normal liver and enlarged liver.

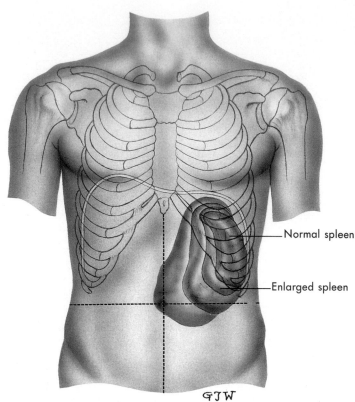

FIGURE 2-12
Size and location of normal spleen and enlarged spleen.

and Crohn's disease. Hypoactive bowel sounds may be heard secondary to constipation in other autoimmune disorders such as scleroderma. Percuss all quadrants to determine overall tympany and dullness. Then go back and percuss the liver and spleen independently. Dullness should be heard only over solid organs such as the liver and spleen (Figures 2-11 and 2-12). Palpate all four quadrants to determine areas of tenderness. Progress to a deeper palpation to assess abdominal organs. Dullness in areas not over a solid organ indicates a mass. Tenderness may suggest an infection, which is more common in individuals with immunodeficiency disorders. **Hepatosplenomegaly** is found with a number of immune disorders such as hemolytic anemia, immunodeficiency disorders, lymphomas, idiopathic thrombocytopenic purpura, and autoimmune hepatic diseases. Splenomegaly generally is a complication of portal hypertension, whereas splenic tenderness usually is the result of an inflammatory process seen in patients with immunodeficiency disorders.

NEUROMUSCULAR ASSESSMENT

Inspect all muscle groups and joints for swelling, erythema, asymmetry, or nodules suggestive of rheumatoid arthritis or an infection. With SLE joints may be erythematous, swollen, and painful with movement but not deformed as in rheumatoid arthritis. Palpate for muscle tone, warmth, and tenderness. Weakened muscle tone may be associated with multiple sclerosis or SLE. Heat and tenderness over a joint may suggest rheumatoid arthritis or an infection. Joint involvement in rheumatoid arthritis usually is symmetric, with red, deformed, and swollen joints, and subsequently results in limited mobility and muscle weakness.

Assess the patient's **gait, muscle strength, coordination,** and **range of joint motion.** A spastic gait pattern may suggest MS, whereas a shuffling gait pattern may be a sign of extreme weakness, as seen in myasthenia gravis. Gait ataxia similar to Parkinson's disease often occurs in the patient with advancing AIDS. Pain with mobility may suggest rheumatoid arthritis.

Patients with extreme muscle weakness will have difficulty standing up or holding their arms above their heads. Muscle weakness is common in patients with myasthenia gravis, SLE, rheumatoid arthritis, and progressive AIDS. It also may be seen in other immunodeficiency disorders as the result of anemia. In some cases muscle weakness can be observed in altered speech patterns. Changes in speech patterns and voice volume are most commonly seen in MS and myasthenia gravis.

Coordination can be determined by asking the seated patient to pat his knees with both hands, alter-

Table 2-2

ASSESSMENT OF THE CRANIAL NERVES

Cranial nerve/function	Examination procedure	Abnormalities found in immune disorders
I: olfactory (sense of smell)	Identification of familiar odors; testing one naris at a time	Allergies
II: optic (vision)	Use of the Snellen chart and Rosenbaum near vision chart	Diplopia with myasthenia gravis and MS; cytomegalovirus (CMV) blindness with AIDS; photophobia with SLE
III: oculomotor IV: trochlear VI: abducens (pupillary constriction, motor movement of eye and upper eyelid)	Inspect for drooping eyelids and pupil size, direction, consensual response to light, and accommodation	Ptosis with myasthenia gravis; lid lag with Graves' disease; fasciculation and tremors with MS or early Hashimoto's disease; nystagmus with MS
V: trigeminal (motor movement of temporal muscle and masseter muscle of jaw)	Inspect face for atrophy and tremors; palpate jaw muscles for tone and strength while patient clenches his teeth; check for touch and pain sensation; test corneal reflexes with cotton swab	Decreased muscle strength with MS and myasthenia gravis, as demonstrated by difficulty chewing; sensory loss may be due to conversion reaction in severe SLE, MS, or AIDS
VII: facial (motor affecting muscle around forehead, eyes, and mouth; sensory affecting anterior tongue)	Inspect facial symmetry with various facial expressions (e.g., smiling, frowning, puffed cheeks); check sweet and salty sensations	Snarling facial expression with myasthenia gravis; facial weakness with SLE and MS
VIII: acoustic (hearing and balance)	Test hearing with whisper screening; check bone (Rinne) and air (Weber) conduction	Impaired hearing with MS and with chronic otitis media stemming from immunodeficiency disorders
IX: glossopharyngeal (motor: pharynx; sensory: ear, pharynx, and posterior tongue, taste)	Check gag reflex and ability to swallow	Difficulty swallowing with myasthenia gravis, MS, and systemic sclerodema
X: vagus (motor: palate, pharynx, larynx; sensory: pharynx, larynx)	Inspect palate for symmetry with speech sound and gag reflex; check swallowing; assess speech	Dysarthric speech seen with myasthenia gravis; slurred speech with MS; hoarseness may result from chronic allergies
XI: spinal accessory (motor: sternomastoid, upper aspect of trapezius)	Check muscle strength; shrug shoulders against resistance	Extreme muscle weakness with myasthenia gravis; general muscle weakness with rheumatoid arthritis, SLE, MS, and AIDS
XII: hypoglossal (motor function of tongue)	Inspect tongue for symmetry, tremors, and atrophy; test for tongue strength with index finger when tongue is pressed against cheek; assess quality of speech sounds	Tremors may be seen in muscle weakness of MS or myasthenia gravis

nating turning up the palm and back of the hands and gradually increasing in speed. Patients with myasthenia gravis or MS may have difficulty performing this maneuver because of lack of coordination and muscle weakness. Patients with rheumatoid arthritis may find it too painful.

Evaluate the patient's **balance** using the Romberg test. Loss of balance is seen in disorders involving extreme weakness, as in Graves' disease or ataxia in advanced AIDS.

Evaluate **range of joint motion** and **muscle**

strength. Pay particular attention to the hands, wrists, and knees. Patients with rheumatoid arthritis or SLE may have a limited range of motion and decreased muscle strength.

Evaluation of primary **sensory** functions includes superficial touch, pain, temperature, and vibration. Alteration in sensation may occur in a variety of autoimmune disorders (e.g., SLE, multiple sclerosis, Raynaud's phenomenon) or allergic disorders (asthma, urticaria). Also, observe for neuropathies that may occur with SLE and rheumatoid arthritis.

CHAPTER 3

Diagnostic and Laboratory Procedures

OBTAINING A BLOOD SPECIMEN

PATIENT TEACHING

Tell the patient why and when the specimen will be obtained. Instruct her that blood specimens require a venipuncture, which usually takes about 3 minutes to perform, and that she may feel transient discomfort from the tourniquet or needle. A small amount of bleeding or a hematoma may result when the needle is removed. The patient can apply pressure to the site of the venipuncture until the bleeding has subsided (Figure 3-1).

Protect yourself and others during blood sampling. Before you draw blood, always wash your hands, and wear gloves while collecting or handling blood. If there is concern that the blood might "spray," wear goggles. Do not recap needles. Needles should be disposed of immediately in a sharps-only container. If some blood is spilled, it should be cleaned up with bleach or another comparable agent.

COLLECTING A BLOOD SPECIMEN

Instruct the patient in the procedure, and assemble the equipment: appropriate tubes for the tests being performed, 10- to 30-ml syringes (depending on the amount of blood needed for the test; often less blood is required for children), 21-gauge needle (butterfly), gloves, alcohol swabs, tourniquet, one 2 × 2 sterile gauze pad, plastic bandage strip (e.g., Band-Aid), and appropriate labels and forms. Wash your hands, and then clean the area with an alcohol swab in a circular

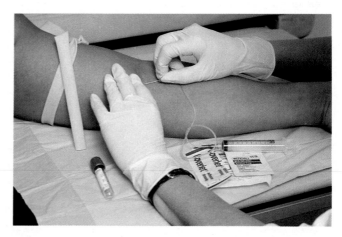

FIGURE 3-1
Performing a venipuncture to obtain a blood specimen.

motion from the inside out to remove superficial dirt and body oil. Allow the area to dry. Apply the tourniquet, and put on the gloves. Identify the vein, and perform the venipuncture, drawing up the appropriate amount of blood for the test.

Remove the tourniquet and then the needle, applying pressure to the site with the sterile gauze. Insert the needle with the syringe of blood into the appropriate tubes, and apply the plastic bandage strip to the venipuncture site.

Label the tubes, and complete the appropriate forms. The following information should be on all forms and tubes: patient's name, date, time the blood was drawn, and whether the blood was obtained peripherally or from a central line. Finally, send the specimen to the appropriate laboratory for testing. Many institutions have more than one laboratory for immunologic testing.

COMPLETE BLOOD COUNT (CBC) AND DIFFERENTIAL

A complete blood count (CBC) and differential provides information about general health through the quantitative values of hemoglobin (Hb), hematocrit (Hct), red blood cells (RBCs), and white blood cells (WBCs). Hemoglobin, hematocrit, and red blood cells help evaluate oxygen-carrying capacity, percentage of RBCs, and hydration status. The white count and differential is determined by the number of white cells in a cubic millimeter (mm^3) of blood. The differential is the determination of the specific value for neutrophils, lymphocytes, monocytes, eosinophils, and basophils in a sample of 100 white blood cells. The percentage of each cell type is reported in the total (Figure 3-2).

Anemia is demonstrated by a decreased hemoglobin and hematocrit, which is very common in patients with rheumatoid arthritis, systemic lupus erythematosus (SLE), and Goodpasture's syndrome. Alterations in the white cell count and differential vary considerably (see Appendix A, Complete Blood Count). Thrombocytopenia is associated with such disorders as SLE, infection with the human immunodeficiency virus (HIV), and idiopathic thrombocytopenic purpura.

INDICATIONS

Chronic infections	Autoimmune disorders
Immunodeficiency disorders	Allergic disorders

PATIENT TEACHING

Explain to the patient and family the reason for the test and that a blood sample will be drawn.

TESTS FOR NONSPECIFIC INFLAMMATION

The **erythrocyte sedimentation rate (ESR, sed rate)** is a very nonspecific and unreliable test that is greatly influenced by increased protein in the plasma and other factors. It measures the distance and rate at which RBCs fall in a specially marked tube over 1 hour. As the patient's RBCs fall in the tube, plasma is displaced upward, impeding the downward flow of the settling blood components. Factors that influence this test are

Note: Procedures for drawing blood from central or hemodialysis lines vary between institutions. Be sure you are familiar with the procedure in your facility before obtaining a blood sample from such a line.

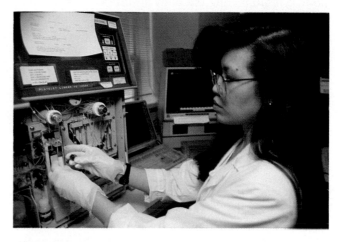

FIGURE 3-2
Medical technologist performing a complete blood count (CBC).

RBC density and volume, surface area, aggregation, and cell surface charge (Figure 3-3). Normal ESR values are reflected in mm/hr. RBCs normally fall at a rate of 10 to 15 mm/hr in men and 15 to 20 mm/hr in women. The ESR increases with age, but the upper limit of normal for patients over 60 years of age has not been clearly defined. An increased ESR is seen with rheumatoid arthritis, rheumatic fever, hemolytic anemia, thyroid disorders, autoimmune disorders, nephritis, and some malignancies. Decreased levels are seen with polycythemia vera, hypofibrinogenemia, sickle cell anemia, and congestive heart failure.

C-reactive protein (CRP) enhances the phagocytic activity of polymorphonuclear neutrophils directed toward invading antigens. It is produced by the liver and excreted into the blood during periods of acute inflammation. CRP can be detected by radioimmunoassay (RIA) or latex agglutination. The test is performed when an active inflammation is suspected; however, it is nonspecific for any one disorder. The normal value is less than 6 μg/ml.

INDICATIONS

Chronic or acute inflammation	Suspected infection
Autoimmune disorders	Rheumatoid arthritis

PATIENT TEACHING

Explain the purpose of the test and that a blood sample will need to be drawn.

PHAGOCYTIC CELL FUNCTION TESTS

Polymorphonuclear leukocytes (PMNs) and **monocyte-macrophage** cells are evaluated when determining phagocytic cell function. These cells are extremely important in protecting the body against antigen invasion. Disorders of phagocytic function include chronic granulomatous disease, Chédiak-Higashi syndrome, Job syndrome, myeloperoxidase deficiency, and glucose 6-phosphate dehydrogenase (G6PD) deficiency.

Two primary tests are used to determine phagocytic cell function: the relative and absolute number of cells, and the neutrophil functional assays.

The **absolute and relative numbers** of monocytes and PMNs are determined from the CBC (see Appendix A, p. 349). This type of testing generally excludes bone marrow dysfunction. If a high or low neutrophil count is identified, a bone marrow biopsy may be necessary to evaluate granulocytopoiesis.

Neutrophil functional assays evaluate five stages of phagocytosis: motility, recognition and adhesion, ingestion, degranulation, and killing. Neutrophil **motility** is determined by testing for chemotaxis using an immunodiffusion method. Tests for **recognition and adhesion** are performed by evaluating opsonins (antibodies and complement [C3 or C3b]) on the cell membrane surface. These tests generally are used in research and are not helpful in the clinical setting. **Ingestion** is assessed by exposing the neutrophils to various microorganisms or other labeled particles and counting how many of the particles were engulfed.

Testing for **degranulation,** called **frustrated phagocytosis,** allows for examination of degranulation separate from ingestion. Frustrated phagocytosis occurs when a phagocyte attaches to a particle that cannot be phagocytized because of factors added to the medium when the test is performed. The phagocyte releases lysosomal enzymes into the area, damaging the particle membrane. Measurement of this activity is accomplished by placing the neutrophils in a medium that is in contact with a foreign particle. As the neutrophils fail to phagocytize these particles, they discharge their contents into the medium. The rate of release of specific enzymes is calculated, providing an estimate of degranulation.

The last and most important function of neutrophils is to kill invading microorganisms. The neutrophils' ability to complete this last stage depends on the successful completion of the prior stages. **Killing** ability is examined by the **nitroblue tetrazolium test** (NBT) and by **chemiluminescence. NBT** is a clear, yellow substance that is converted into deep blue formazan that stains cells on reduction. When neutrophils ingest particles, a metabolic burst (respiratory burst) occurs; this increases oxygen consumption and glucose metabolism, reducing the NBT to deep blue formazan. The reduced dye is extracted and measured photometrically. The degree of reduction demonstrates phagocytic killing activity.

Neutrophil killing ability can also be measured by the emission of light, called chemiluminescence. Neutrophils emit a small amount of light after ingesting a microorganism as a result of the metabolic burst. Oxygen-containing substances that form within the vacuoles of the neutrophils emit light in proportion to the number of oxygen-containing substances that form. This provides a precise connection between light emission and killing activity of the neutrophil. The light is measured by photomultiplier tubes.

INDICATIONS

Chronic infections; congenital immunodeficiency disorders; diabetes; recurrent sinus, pulmonary, or skin infections; suspected neutrophil or phagocytic dysfunction

PATIENT TEACHING

Explain to the patient and family the purpose of the test and the procedure for collecting a blood sample.

METHODS OF DETECTING ANTIGENS AND ANTIBODIES

Antigens and antibodies are detected through a number of in vitro techniques, including immunodiffusion, agglutination, enzyme-linked immunosorbent assay (ELISA), radioimmunoassay (RIA), immunofluorescence, and monoclonal antibodies.

IMMUNODIFFUSION AND ELECTROPHORESIS

Immunodiffusion and electrophoresis are techniques used to detect antigen-antibody reactions by measuring **precipitation.**

Precipitation is the simplest and most direct qualitative method of detecting antigen-antibody reactions. It occurs when a soluble antibody and a soluble antigen migrate toward each other in a test medium and cross-link, forming a latticelike complex. This formation results from the numerous receptor sites on the antigen and antibody surfaces that promote cross-linking. As more and more complexes are formed, they precipitate in the solution or gel. Precipitation lines or bands form in the medium when the concentrations of antibody and antigen are equal, indicating that they have identified each other and formed complexes. These bands of precipitated antigen-antibody complexes generally are sharp with a very faint fuzziness at the edges.

This type of testing allows the distinction of separate antigen-antibody reactions that are produced by various antibodies in the serum. The amount of antibody and antigen in the medium determines the precipitation reaction. An excess of either antigen or antibody may produce a false negative result. These tests usually are performed on an agar or agarose gel medium and take approximately 2 to 4 days to complete.

Immunodiffusion reactions can be classified as single or double reactions. Single immunodiffusion reactions occur when the antigen or antibody remains fixed and the other reactant is left mobile in the medium to form the complex. An example of this would be an agar or gel disc containing a specific antibody to a specific antigen. A small well is made in the agar and filled with the specific antigen. When the complexes are formed, a single band precipitates around the well in the gel medium.

A double immunodiffusion reaction occurs when both the antigen and the antibody are freely mobile to migrate toward each other, precipitate, and form complexes within the medium. An example is seen with the use of a single agar dish with two small wells punctured in it, one containing antigen and the other antibody. After some time, precipitation lines will form where the optimum concentrations of antigen and antibody meet. The number of precipitating lines indicates the various antigen-antibody complexes.

Electrophoretic assays are used to augment immunodiffusion by adding an electrical field to the medium. Applying an electric voltage to a pH-specific agar medium causes the antigen and antibody to move toward each other and precipitate. Electrophoretic assays are performed to measure serum immunoglobulins and other proteins. They are more specific and generally much quicker than plain immunodiffusion, requiring approximately 1½ to 4 hours to complete. These tests include electroimmunodiffusion, immunoelectrophoresis, and countercurrent, rocket, and immunofixation electrophoresis.

Precipitation assays allow detection of a number of foreign antigens (e.g., microorganisms, allergens) and antibodies. They frequently are used to aid in the diagnosis of immunodeficiency diseases. For example, the Western blot test is an immunoelectrophoretic assay used to test for HIV.

AGGLUTINATION

Agglutination reactions involve the clumping of particulate matter such as cells or other material by antibodies called agglutinins (Figure 3-3). The reaction occurs

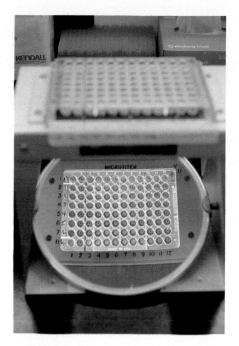

FIGURE 3-3
Agglutination assay.

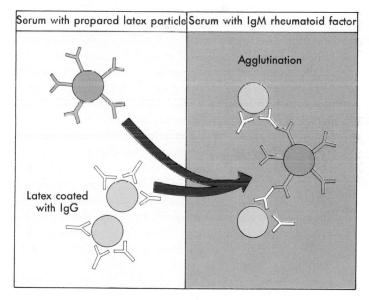

FIGURE 3-4
Example of rheumatoid factor test by agglutination.

on the surface of certain particles such as erythrocytes, microorganisms, or latex with antigens that subsequently bind to antibodies (Figure 3-4). It is a sensitive process that demonstrates the antibodies' ability to attach to insoluble antigens or antigen-coated particles and form a clumping reaction. This reaction may be observed in a test tube, slide, or other formulated medium. Agglutination is clinically useful for detecting a variety of antibodies.

Agglutination reactions are classified as direct or indirect. Direct agglutination occurs when antibodies attach directly to antigens. Indirect agglutination occurs when the antigen has been coated with a chemical or has coupled with erythrocytes or other inert particles that attract antibodies. Many antigens will couple with erythrocytes and form a stable complex that is attractive to antibodies, causing subsequent agglutination and antibody identification. Agglutination is used in ABO blood typing, to identify antibodies against a variety of microorganisms (syphilis, salmonellosis), and in autoimmune disorders. (See Appendix B, p. 350, for examples of agglutination assays).

An agglutination inhibition test is done to determine the specificity and titer of a specific antibody. This test is based on the competition between the particulate and soluble antigens for antibody receptor sites. The test is used most often to check for human chorionic gonadotropin, which is the confirming laboratory test for pregnancy. Agglutination inhibition has also been used to test for titers of antiviral antibodies.

ENZYME-LINKED IMMUNOSORBENT ASSAY (ELISA)

The enzyme-linked immunosorbent assay (ELISA) is extremely sensitive in detecting antigens and antibodies. Commercial kits are available with a specific antigen or antibody that is labeled with an enzyme to provide a standard of testing (Figure 3-5).

To measure a specific antibody, antigen is fixed to a solid plate medium and incubated with a serum sample. Excess antigen is washed away, and a test antibody that binds to the antigen is added. A ligand that is covalently coupled with an enzyme and able to recognize the antibody is added. Excess unbound enzyme is washed away, and a colorless substrate is added. This substrate acts by hydrolysis on the enzyme portion of the ligand, ultimately producing a color change. This is quantified on the developed plate, either visually or by a spectrophotometer. The amount of hydrolyzed substrate is precisely proportional to the quantity of antibody or antigen in the serum.

Clinically the ELISA is useful in detecting numerous antibodies (e.g., anti-DNA antibodies, as in SLE; antibody to HIV) and antigens.

RADIOIMMUNOASSAY (RIA)

RIA uses a radiolabeled ligand and is done mainly to detect small amounts of antigen, antibody, or antigen-antibody complexes in the serum. A known amount of a specific antigen (or antibody) is labeled with a radioactive ligand and added to the serum specimen, causing antigen-antibody complexes to precipitate. The radioactive ligand in the precipitate is counted on a gamma counter, and the result is converted into a titer.

A second RIA technique is based on the competition between radiolabeled antigen (or antibody) and unlabeled antigen (or antibody) for binding sites on limited amounts of antibody (or antigen). This technique deter-

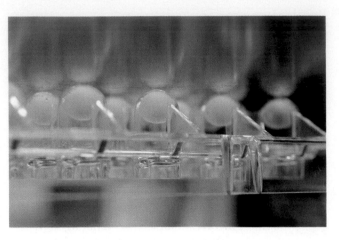

FIGURE 3-5
Enzyme-linked immunosorbent assay (ELISA) for detecting antigens and antibodies.

SCREENING FOR HIV ANTIBODIES

The ELISA method, which is both sensitive and specific, is the first screening test used to detect HIV antibodies. To perform the test, viral antigen is placed in a multiwell tray and test serum is added. If viral antibody is present in the serum, it will bind to the viral antigen at the bottom of the well. An enzyme-linked antihuman antibody is then added that will bind to the complex, which is detected colorimetrically. The ELISA method is not accurate all the time and may give false positive results. If a patient tests positive with this technique, the Western blot test should be done. This test takes the whole virus and reduces it to a number of protein fragments. The fragments are separated electophoretically, and the specimen is examined for specific antibodies directed against the various fragments. Antibodies to the protein fragments of HIV will bind to the specific viral protein, confirming the presence of the virus.

mines the *amount* of antigen (or antibody) in the serum specimen. The procedure is conducted by adding radiolabeled antigen to the specimen; this antigen binds with approximately 70% of the available antibody. Various amounts of unlabeled antibody are then added to the specimen to allow the serum antigen to bind with it. This creates competition between labeled and unlabeled antigen for binding sites on the antibody. The radioactivity of the plate is counted for the amount of radiolabeled antigen at various unlabeled antigen concentrations, and a titration curve is developed. The titration curve demonstrates the amount of antigen present in the serum sample. Clinically the RIA methods are used to detect allergens and antibodies associated with allergy, as well as antibodies in various diseases.

IMMUNOFLUORESCENCE

Fluorescence is the emission of light of one color based on the wavelength of the light. Immunofluorescence is used to detect antibodies and autoantibodies directed against tissue or cellular antigens. The antigen is detected by using fluorescence-labeled immunoglobulins that become fixed to antigens, forming a stable immune complex (Figure 3-6). The antigen-antibody complex can be seen with a fluorescence microscope or flow cytometer. Two methods use fluorescent antibodies: direct immunofluorescence and indirect immunofluorescence.

Direct immunofluorescence is used primarily to detect antigen. It involves fluorescence labeling with specific antibodies that will react with antigens. This test is clinically used to detect viruses and lymphocytic subsets and to check for protein deposition in particular tissues (e.g., renal immune complexes in SLE).

With **indirect immunofluorescence,** the antibody-specific antigen is not labeled. The unlabeled antibody is put in contact with the antigen and binds to it, forming an immune complex. The antigen is detected by adding a fluorescently labeled antiimmunoglobulin, which binds to the antibody on the antigen-antibody immune complex. This test is used to screen sera for antideoxyribonucleic acid (anti-DNA) antibodies, as in SLE.

MONOCLONAL ANTIBODIES

Monoclonal antibodies are large numbers of identical antibodies that are active against a specific antigenic target. They are exactly reproducible, and their clones are genetically identical. This technology has been available only since 1975, when Milstein and Kohler, who later shared in the Nobel Prize, discovered the technique for making monoclonal antibodies. Before that time it was impossible to produce large amounts of identical antibody to a single antigen, because B lymphocytes, which produce antigen-specific antibodies, could not be grown to produce single antibodies.

Monoclonal antibody technology provides antibody-producing B lymphocytes that are fused with nonsecreting antibody tumor cells (e.g., myeloma cells) that can replicate indefinitely in a culture medium. Clones derived from these cells can survive in cell culture and produce large quantities of identical monoclonal antibodies.

Clinical application of this technology is becoming increasingly more diversified. It currently is being used therapeutically in organ transplantation, autoimmune disorders, and antitumor therapy, as well as to treat graft-versus-host disease. Diagnostic application is progressing rapidly and includes detection of HLA antigens, microorganisms, lymphocyte subsets, and a variety of others.

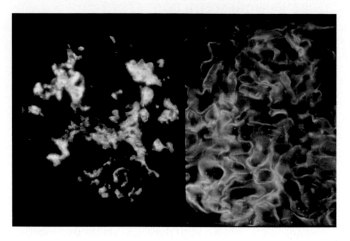

FIGURE 3-6
Immunofluorescence for detecting immune complexes.

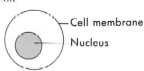

PATTERNS OF IMMUNOFLUORESCENT STAINING FOR ANTINUCLEAR ANTIBODIES

Homogeneous pattern (diffuse)
Associated with SLE, connective tissue disorders

Cell membrane
Nucleus

Outline pattern (peripheral)
Associated with SLE

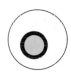

Speckled pattern
Associated with SLE, connective tissue disorders, Sjögren's syndrome, scleroderma, polymyositis, rheumatoid arthritis

Nucleolar pattern
Associated with scleroderma, polymyositis

IMMUNOHEMATOLOGIC TESTS

Immunohematologic tests are used to assess antigens on RBC surfaces. These tests are clinically indicated to monitor potential blood transfusion reactions, hemolytic anemia, blood type (ABO) compatibility and Rh typing, antibody screening (indirect Coombs' test), and antiglobulin testing (direct Coombs' test).

ABO blood typing is performed to decrease the risk of a blood transfusion reaction. Isohemagglutinins are naturally occurring antibodies to RBCs. They are present in all immunocompetent individuals by 2 years of age except for individuals with AB blood type. For example, individuals with type A blood have anti-B isoantibodies, those with type B have anti-A isoantibodies, and persons with type O have both anti-A and anti-B isoantibodies; individuals with type AB have neither. This allows individuals with type O blood to be universal donors and those with type AB to be universal recipients. To determine an individual's specific blood type, separate aliquots of the patient's RBCs are mixed with anti-A serum and anti-B serum. The results depend on the presence or absence of agglutination. For example, patients whose RBCs agglutinate in the presence of anti-A serum will have either A or AB blood type. Patients whose RBCs agglutinate with both anti-A and anti-B serum are AB blood type.

The **antiglobulin test (Coombs' test)** is used to detect any immunoglobulin that is bound to antigen by using antiimmunoglobulin.

The **indirect Coombs' test** is a type of *antibody screening* that detects specific serum antibodies to RBC antigens that are not attached to the cell. It is performed by adding antiimmunoglobulins to particles, usually RBCs, that are suspected of having antibodies bound to the antigens on their cell surface. This results in agglutination of the red blood cells, confirming the presence of antibody. This type of testing is performed before RBC transfusions and to detect Rh-positive antibody in maternal blood.

The **direct Coombs' test** is an *antiglobulin test* that detects serum antibodies that coat RBCs but do not result in agglutination. This test is performed by adding antiimmunoglobulin (anti-IgG or anticomplement) to saline-washed RBCs. If immunoglobulin or complement is present, agglutination will occur, indicating a positive reaction. A positive reaction may be useful in the diagnosis of newborn hemolytic disease or autoimmune disorders.

INDICATIONS FOR COOMBS' TESTING

To **determine** Rh factor
To **evaluate:** Suspected blood transfusion reaction; SLE; drug reactions; hemolytic anemia

COMPLEMENT ASSAYS

Complement is a group of serum proteins. These proteins function as one of the primary mechanisms of antigen-antibody reactions. One of these functions causes the lysis of cells and tissue damage. Complement testing currently involves the primary complement components of the classic pathway and a number from the alternative pathway, as well as several inhibitors. There are three primary tests to assess complement: the CH_{50} **test** (complement hemolytic 50%), measurement of the individual **complement components** (total or functional level), and **complement fixation** (CF).

The overall integrity of the complement system can be determined by the CH_{50} test. It provides an adequate screening of the complement cascade, since the entire system must be intact to reflect a normal value. This test uses a suspension of sheep red cells coated with anti−red cell antibody to measure the amount of

serum necessary for a 50% lysis. Normal results are between 100 and 200 U/ml. A low value may indicate a complement deficiency.

It is important to determine each **complement component** individually to evaluate both total level and function. The total level of a particular component may be normal, even though functionally it is inactive.

Antibody preparations against complement components are used to detect complement components and complement inhibitors by applying electroimmunodiffusion techniques. To test total levels of complement components, RIA or ELISA methods (see p. 46) are employed by using a specific antibody for every component being evaluated.

The reduction in serum complement may be due to a number of disorders, including complement consumption by antigen-antibody immune complexes, increased synthesis or catabolism of complement, or the development of an inhibitor to complement. Increased levels generally are due to complement overproduction.

Complement fixaton (use) occurs during antigen-antibody reactions. Therefore, the utilization or fixation of complement during these reactions can be used to detect antigens, antibodies, or both.

Complement fixation is a two-step process based on the principle that one or more of the complement components can be fixed (used) in an antigen-antibody reaction. The test is initiated by adding a known amount of complement to the patient's serum. The added complement is then fixed. The second step measures the hemolytic activity of complement. This step detects the amount of complement fixed and the proportion of antibody or antigen in the patient's serum. The second step is performed by adding antigenic sheep red blood cells (SRBCs) to the serum. The remaining unfixed complement will lyse the SRBCs. Therefore lysis occurs when complement is unfixed, indicating that the serum is deficient in either antigen or antibody. Lysis does not oc-

cur if all complement if fixed, indicating the presence of antigen and antibody in the serum.

The results of complement fixation are expressed in titers. Clinically, complement fixation is used to detect the presence af anti-DNA, immunoglobulins, and anti-platelet antibodies.

INDICATIONS

To evaluate:
Decreased complement activity: SLE, myasthenia gravis, severe combined immunodeficiency and immune-complex disorders, chronic infection, angioedema, chronic infections
Increased serum complement: rheumatoid arthritis, periarteritis nodosa, and diabetes

PATIENT TEACHING

Explain that this test reveals complement component and activity, which may be indicators in infection or autoimmune disorders. Instruct the patient that the test requires a blood sample.

CRYOGLOBULINS

Cryoglobulins are abnormal serum proteins that precipitate at low temperatures (39.2° F[4° C]) and redissolve when warmed. Normally the serum level of these proteins should be negative.

The presence of cryoglobulins in the serum is associated with an immune system disorder. There are three types of cryoglobulins. **Type I monoclonal cryoglobulins** react to a single monoclonal immunoglobulin. They are most often seen in myeloma, Waldenström's macroglobulinemia, and chronic lymphocytic leukemia. Serum levels are generally higher than 5 mg/ml. **Type II mixed cryoglobulin** is a mixed monoclonal immunoglobulin that has antibody activity against a polyclonal immunoglobulin. Associated disorders include rheumatoid arthritis, Sjögren's syndrome, and mixed essential cryoglobulinemia. Serum levels are generally higher than 1 mg/ml. **Type III mixed polyclonal cryoglobulin** indicates immune responses to various antigens and the presence of circulating immune complexes. Common associated disorders include SLE, rheumatoid arthritis, Sjögren's syndrome, multiple infections (cytomegalovirus, mononucleosis, and endocarditis), poststreptococcal glomerulonephritis, chronic active hepatitis, and

leprosy. Serum levels often are lower than in type I or type II, at less than 1 mg/ml.

The cryoglobulin test involves collecting blood in a warm syringe until the blood clots. The blood sample is then separated by centrifugation and stored at 39.2° F (4° C) for 72 hours. It is observed for heat-reversible precipitation. If a precipitate forms, further evaluation by immunoelectrophoresis is recommended to identify cryoglobulin components.

INDICATIONS

To evaluate:
Raynaud-like vascular symptoms; autoimmune disorders; chronic and recurrent infections; pre–organ transplant
To detect: Cryoglobulinemia

PATIENT TEACHING

Explain that this test is used to detect antibodies in the blood that cause increased sensitivity to the cold. Instruct the patient to fast for 4 hours before the test is performed. Explain to the patient and family that this test involves a blood sample.

LYMPHOCYTE ASSAYS

Lymphocytes are T cells (cellular immunity), B cells (humoral immunity), and natural killer (NK) cells that together represent the primary cellular components of the immune system. Determination of the **absolute number** of lymphocytes from the WBC differential may be helpful. A lymphocyte count of less than 15% to 20% of the differential are considered abnormal and should be investigated further.

One of the tests used to evaluate overall in vivo immunocompetence and the immune system's ability to respond to a foreign antigen is the **delayed hypersensitivity skin test** (Figure 3-7). This test gauges immunodeficiency. The test involves injecting a small amount of antigen intradermally into the anterior surface of the forearm. Subcutaneous injections may cause dilution of the antigen and result in a false negative reading. To ensure an intradermal injection, 25- to 27-gauge needles on a tuberculin syringe should be used. The antigens are injected approximately 5 cm apart and are circled with a marking pen to facilitate later reading (Figure 3-7). A schematic drawing of the patient's forearm should be made, indicating the type and location of each antigen. Because signs of anaphylaxis (urticaria, hypotension, dyspnea, and disorientation) may occur within minutes of the antigen injection, it is important to have emergency equipment available before starting the test. At a minimum this equipment should include oxygen, intravenous (IV) epinephrine and Benadryl, oral and nasal airways, an Ambu bag, and IV fluids and supplies.

Delayed hypersensitivity reactions are read at 24, 48, and 72 hours. Areas of erythema and induration should be carefully measured at the widest point with a ruler. For consistency, the same health care provider should administer and read the skin reactions. Induration of 5 mm or more with erythema indicates a **positive response** and an intact cell-mediated immunity. A **negative response** is shown by lack of induration or erythema, indicating abnormal hypersensitivity. A state of hyporeactivity indicates the inability to react to **common skin antigens** and is known as **anergy.** Anergy is associated with immunodeficiency disorders such as cellular immunodeficiencies, severe combined immunodeficiency, AIDS, rheumatic diseases, and aging. Hyporeactivity should always be confirmed by retesting the patient with higher antigen concentrations.

More than 90% of normal individuals undergoing this type of test will respond to one of the antigens within 48 hours. A positive reaction to histoplasmin or purified protein derivative (PPD) indicates active infection or previous exposure to histoplasmosis or tuberculosis, respectively, and should not be used to evaluate anergy.

T-CELL AND B-CELL SURFACE MARKERS

Through extensive study of surface cell markers, three types of lymphocytes have been isolated: T cells, B cells, and natural killer (NK) cells. These cells can recognize antigens and can be isolated from one another for evaluation. To evaluate these cells more closely, lymphocytes are isolated either from other blood components through a cell separation process, or from tissue samples (tonsils, lymph nodes, bone marrow, or spleen). Their surface cell markers allow detection of the cellular subpopulations and assist in the diagnosis and monitoring of various immune disorders (Figure 3-8).

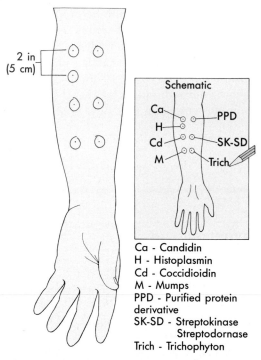

2 in (5 cm)

Schematic

Ca — PPD
H
Cd — SK-SD
M — Trich

Ca - Candidin
H - Histoplasmin
Cd - Coccidioidin
M - Mumps
PPD - Purified protein derivative
SK-SD - Streptokinase Streptodornase
Trich - Trichophyton

FIGURE 3-7
Delayed hypersensitivity skin testing to evaluate immunocompetence.

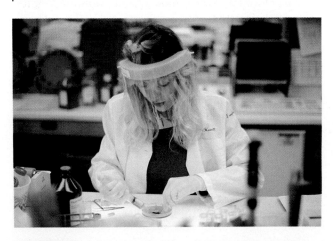

FIGURE 3-8
Medical technologist perfusing lymphocytes in preparation for differentiation of T and B cells.

Lymphocytes are identified by their **clusters of differentiation (CD)**, which are markers on their cell surfaces. Each of these CD markers reacts with a cluster of monoclonal antibodies, providing identification of the particular cell type. The results are expressed as a percentage of lymphocytes. It is necessary to obtain a WBC with a differential to determine absolute values.

T-CELL SUBSETS

All T cells express the CD3 marker. Major T-cell subsets are the helper T cells (CD4) and suppressor T cells (CD8). With the increasing incidence of AIDS, considerable interest has developed in the CD4/CD8 T-cell ratio. By using monoclonal antibodies, the normal ratio has been identified as 0.8:2.9 (Figure 3-9). Patients initially diagnosed with AIDS frequently demonstrate an elevation in the CD8 suppressor/cytotoxic T

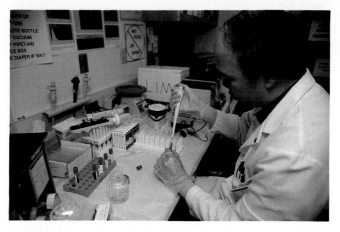

FIGURE 3-9
Medical technologist measuring T-cell subsets using monoclonal antibodies.

CLUSTER OF DIFFERENTIATION (CD) MARKERS

CD1
  Positive cells: Thymocytes, Langerhans' cells
  Used for developmental marker, cortical T (thymocytes)
CD2
  Positive cells: E-rosette receptor on T cells; NK cells
  First specific marker to appear; assists in differentiation of lymphoproliferative T-cell origin disorders from those of non-T-cell origin
CD3
  Positive cells: All T cells
  Used to detect cutaneous T-cell lymphoma; antibody to this marker has been used to inhibit T-cell activation (e.g., organ transplantation [OKT$_3$])
CD4
  Positive cells: T helper/inducer cells, monocytes
  Used to detect immunodeficiency disorders (decreased in AIDS); decreased in autoimmune (SLE) or immunoregulatory disorders; also used to differentiate lymphoproliferative disorders; participates in graft rejection in organ transplantation; decreased during infections; these cells control parasitic infections
CD5
  Positive cells: T cells; B-cell subsets
  B cells secrete autoantibodies and participate in the development of autoimmune disorders; assist in T-cell activation
CD6
  Positive cells: T cells
  Detected on malignant T cells

CD7
  Positive cells: Thymocytes, T cells, NK cells
  Detected in T-cell leukemias
CD8
  Positive cells: Suppressor/cytotoxic T-cell subset; NK cells
  Suppressor cells in autoimmune and immunoregulatory disorders may be deficient (MS, SLE); these cells assist in identification of lymphoproliferative disorders and participate in graft rejection in organ transplantation; this marker is used to monitor AIDS (transient increase in CD8 after initial exposure to the virus)
CD10
  Positive cells: PMN pre-B leukemia cells
  Previously called common acute lymphocytic leukemia antigen (CALLA), this marker used to identify tumor type and degree of malignancy
CD19
  Positive cells: All B cells
  Unknown; may be a differentiation marker
CD20
  Positive cells: B cells
  Used to identify B-cell tumors; may participate in B-cell activation
CD23
  Positive cells: Mature B cells
  Regulates B-cell growth

*Human leukocyte differentiation of antigens** nomenclature was initially established in 1983 to define cellular types and subtypes. **Cluster of differentiation (CD)** defines these cellular antigens on the basis of their cell surface markers. More than 80 individual molecules have been recognized. This table reviews the more important CD molecules. These markers may assist in the diagnosis and management of certain disorders.

Table 3-1

IMMUNOGLOBULINS

Class of immunoglobulin	Clinical significance	
	Increased level	Decreased level
IgG	IgG myeloma, bacterial infections, hepatitis A, glomerulonephritis, rheumatoid arthritis, SLE, AIDS	Agammaglobulinemia, IgA myeloma, IgA deficiency, chronic lymphocytic leukemia, type I dysgammaglobulinemia, lymphoid aplasia, combined immunodeficiency, common variable immunodeficiency, X-linked hypogammaglobulinemia
IgM	Hepatitis A and B, Waldenström's macroglobulinemia, trypanosomiasis, chronic infections, type I dysgammaglobulinemia, hepatitis, SLE, rheumatoid arthritis, Sjögren's syndrome, AIDS	Lymphoid aplasia, hypogammaglobulinemia, chronic lymphocytic leukemia, IgG myeloma, IgA myeloma, agammaglobulinemia
IgA	SLE, rheumatoid arthritis, IgA myeloma, glomerulonephritis, chronic liver disease	Ataxia, telangiectasia, hypogammaglobulinemia, acute and chronic lymphocytic leukemia, IgA deficiency, combined immunodeficiency, common variable immunodeficiency, X-linked hypogammaglobulinemia, agammaglobulinemia, IgG myeloma, chronic infections (especially upper respiratory type)
IgE	Atopic disorders: allergic rhinitis, allergic asthma, atopic dermatitis, Wiskott-Aldrich syndrome with eczema, parasitic infestation, hyperimmunoglobulin E	Associated with IgA deficiency, intrinsic (nonallergic) asthma
IgD	Eczema, skin disorders	Unknown

cells and a decrease in CD4 inducer/helper T cells, which results in a low CD4/CD8 ratio. As the disease progresses, there is a severe decrease in CD4 cells unless immunorestorative therapy (e.g., azidothymidine [AZT]) is effective, in which case CD4 cells would increase.

Other changes in T-cell subsets are reflected in viral infections as demonstrated by a marked increase in CD8 cells. With cytomegalovirus virus (CMV) and Epstein-Barr virus (EBV) infections, there is also a transient decrease in CD4 cells. T-cell subsets are also used to monitor both immunosuppressive therapy in organ transplantation and the effects of other drugs on the immune system.

T-cell subset ratios and absolute numbers or per-

Table 3-2

T-CELL SUBSETS AND B CELLS

T-cell subset	Percentage of lymphocytes	Absolute number of cells/μl
CD3 (total T cells)	70%-80%	565-2,585
CD4 (helper/inducer T cells)	29%-60%	359-1,725
CD8 (suppressor/cytotoxic T cells; few NK cells)	18%-42%	177-1,106
CD4/CD8 (helper/suppressor ratio)	0.8:2.9	
CD19 (total B cells)	10%-20%	75-545

EXAMPLES OF ALTERATIONS IN B-CELL AND T-CELL LEVELS

B cells	T cells
Increased level	*Increased level*
Chronic lymphocytic leukemia	Infectious mononucleosis
Multiple myeloma	Multiple myeloma
Waldenström's macroglobulinemia	Acute lymphocytic leukemia
DiGeorge syndrome	
Decreased level	*Decreased level*
Acute lymphocytic leukemia, immunodeficiency disorders	Congenital T-cell deficiency disorders (e.g., DiGeorge, Nezelof, and Wiskott-Aldrich syndromes)
	B-cell proliferative disorders (e.g., chronic lymphocytic leukemia, Waldenström's macroglobulinemia, AIDS)

centages of CD4 and CD8 can be used to monitor patients with immune disorders. However, because some NK cells express CD8, there is a risk of interfering with the CD4/CD8 ratio, rendering this test less useful in patients with congenital immunodeficiencies. Absolute numbers or percentages of CD4 are more helpful in monitoring a patient with AIDS.

Natural killer (NK) cells are also identified by using monoclonal antibodies. Function is determined by measuring their ability to kill specific target cells.

B-CELL SURFACE IMMUNOGLOBULIN

All B lymphocytes express on their cell surfaces immunoglobulin that can be readily detected by direct immunofluorescence using monoclonal antibodies.

FUNCTIONAL LYMPHOCYTE ASSAYS

Normal T- and B-cell counts do not ensure a competent immune system. For example, in SLE and rheumatoid arthritis, the normal numbers of T and B cells are present, but they are functionally incompetent.

PROLIFERATION ASSAYS

Proliferation assays evaluate lymphocytes' ability to proliferate and to recognize and react to antigens. There are two primary tests for assessing the functional status of lymphocytes: mitogen activation and antigen stimulation, and the mixed lymphocyte culture (MLC).

Mitogen activation and antigen stimulation are tests performed through the activation of B and T cells by mitogens or antigens. **Mitogens**, which are nonspecific plant lectins, are molecules that induce differentiation and division (mitosis). Different antigens and mitogens can be used to evaluate the proliferative response of both T and B lymphocytes. For example, phytohemagglutinin (PHA) and concanavalin A (con A) are mitogens that stimulate T lymphocytes, whereas pokeweed mitogen (PWM) stimulates primarily B lymphocytes and T cells only minimally. Antigens that are commonly used include purified protein derivative (PPD), mumps, tetanus toxoid, and streptokinase.

The procedure is basically the same for either an antigen or a mitogen assay. A blood sample from the patient is incubated with the mitogen or antigen for 3 to 5 days; most DNA synthesis takes place during this period. Also during this time a radioactive substance is added that becomes incorporated into the newly synthesized DNA. The uptake of the radioactive substance is measured in counts per minute (cmp). The cmp provides information on the rate of mitosis and can be compared to normal values.

Mixed lymphocyte culture (MLC) is the second proliferative assay and is used primarily in organ transplantation. This test measures the response of T lymphocytes to a foreign histocompatibility antigen on unrelated or "donor" lymphocytes or monocytes. The test is performed by irradiating the donor or stimulating cells to prevent DNA synthesis and proliferation. These irradiated cells are then cocultured with the recipient's lymphocytes. If the donor and recipient cells are not HLA-D region similar, the recipient's T cells will recognize the donor cells as foreign and proliferate. The more unlike the donor and recipient cells are, the greater the recipient T cell proliferation. This is a positive test result, demonstrating incompatibility between donor and recipient. Conversely, the more alike the donor and recipient cells are, the less T-cell proliferation will be evident, indicating a negative test result and therefore compatibility. This reaction is determined primarily at the HLA-D loci, which include HLA-DR, HLA-DQ, and HLA-DP antigens.

INDICATIONS FOR LYMPHOCYTE ASSAYS

To evaluate/monitor and diagnose: Immunodeficiency disorders; autoimmune disorders; infectious disease immunity; tumor immunity
Response to therapy
 Transplant immunology
To identify the source of malignant lymphocytes (lymphocytic leukemia, lymphoma)

NURSING CONSIDERATIONS

All T-cell subset specimens should remain at room temperature. *Do not* centrifuge.

PATIENT TEACHING

Explain to the patient and family the reason for the test and that a blood sample will be drawn.

HISTOCOMPATIBILITY TESTING

Histocompatibility testing identifies the **human leukocyte antigens (HLA),** which are present on all nucleated cells and most easily detected on lymphocytes. The HLA is the major histocompatibility complex in humans. Two methods are used for histocompatibility testing: tissue typing and cross-matching. Each of these methods encompasses a number of testing approaches that assess specific components of the HLA system. This discussion focuses on the major testing methods.

TISSUE TYPING

There are two primary methods of tissue typing: complement-dependent cytotoxic assay and mixed lymphocyte culture. In the complement-dependent test, the patient's lymphocytes are incubated with antisera to HLA for approximately 30 minutes. This allows time for the antibody to bind to the cell surface. Complement is added for 60 minutes. If the antibody has bound to the antiserum, complement components C1 through C9 will be activated and cause cell lysis. A dye is added to detect cell lysis. If the antibody has not bound to the surface of the cell, the cells will remain intact and appear clear and round under the microscope; this is considered a negative test result. If the antibody has bound to the surface of the cell and complement activation was sufficient to cause cell lysis, the dye will have accumulated in the cells, and they will appear red and swollen; this is considered a positive test result, meaning that 20% or more of the cells have been lysed (are dead). The particular serum that reacts with the cells identifies the HLA antigens on the cell surface.

CROSS-MATCHING

Cross-matching is done before organ transplantation (primarily kidney and heart) to prevent the risk of rejection after surgery. This test can detect the presence of antibodies in the recipient's serum that are directed against the HLA antigens of the potential donor. A number of testing methods are used to complete this assessment. Patients preparing for organ transplantation undergo four initial cross-matching tests: lymphocyte, T or B lymphocyte–enriched preparations, and preformed antibodies. To differentiate autoantibodies from antidonor antibodies, an auto-cross-match is performed.

The simplest, most common test is the standard cytotoxicity method. (Cytotoxicity is the process of cell lysis by antibody.) In this method the recipient serum is mixed with donor lymphocytes to assess the presence of preformed antibody directed against the donor antigens. If lysis occurs, preformed antibody is present. This is considered a positive reaction, and transplantation is deferred.

INDICATIONS

Organ transplantation; paternity testing; autoimmune disorders

PATIENT TEACHING

Explain to the patient and family why they are undergoing histocompatibility testing and that it requires a blood sample. Tissue typing is so called because blood is considered a tissue.

BONE MARROW ASPIRATION AND BIOPSY

Bone marrow aspiration and biopsy provide histologic and hematologic examination of the stem cells for all cellular components of the blood. Before the procedure, coagulation and platelet studies should be done to minimize the risk of bleeding. The biopsy generally is performed on an outpatient basis using a local anesthetic unless the patient is already hospitalized. The preferred site for both adults and children is the posterior iliac crest. The main exception to this is children under 1 year of age, in whom the preferred site is the tibia. Other bone marrow biopsy sites are the anterior iliac crest, spinous process, and sternum (the sternum is contraindicated in children because of the risk of cardiac and mediastinal perforation).

INDICATIONS

To diagnose: Metastatic carcinoma; granuloma; aplastic or megaloblastic anemia; differential diagnosis of thrombocytopenia; leukemia
To evaluate:
Immune and hematolymphatic systems; chronic anemia; chronic leukopenia; histologic nature of marrow
Other: Culture

CONTRAINDICATIONS: Bleeding

COMPLICATIONS

Bleeding at the site; infection at the site

NURSING CARE

In conjunction with the physician, obtain written consent. Children should have nothing by mouth for 4 to 8 hours before the procedure, depending on their age and the need for mask anesthesia or sedation. Administer sedation as ordered. Disinfect the patient's skin, and prepare a sterile field. After the procedure, apply pressure for 3 to 5 minutes and then an occlusive dressing. Monitor the site for bleeding, and check vital signs frequently. Keep the patient on bed rest for 1 hour, and administer analgesics as ordered or indicated.

PATIENT TEACHING

Explain the procedure and its purpose to the patient and family. Inform them that a local anesthetic will be used that will sting slightly when the medication is injected. Explain that the patient will feel pressure and some discomfort when the biopsy needle is inserted, and that it takes approximately 15 to 30 seconds to complete the procedure.

PERCUTANEOUS RENAL BIOPSY

Percutaneous renal biopsy is performed to obtain a specimen of core renal tissue for histologic examination by light and immunofluorescent microscopy. Before the procedure, the patient must have nothing by mouth for 6 to 8 hours and coagulation studies should be done to minimize the risk of bleeding. The patient is placed in a prone position with a small sandbag under the lower abdomen to provide support and ready access to the kidney. The area is injected with a local anesthetic. A small incision is made in the skin between the last rib and the iliac crest, with the assistance of ultrasonographic guidance. Renal tissue is removed by means of needle excision and immediately visualized under a hard lens to ensure that the specimen contains tissue from the renal cortex and medulla.

INDICATIONS

Suspected glomerular lesion (e.g., lupus nephritis)
To assess amyloid infiltration
To diagnose acute or chronic glomerulonephritis
To monitor controlled therapeutic new drug trials
To evaluate persistent hematuria or proteinuria

CONTRAINDICATIONS

Renal tumors; severe bleeding dyscrasias; severe hypertension; hydronephrosis; perinephric abscess; polycystic kidney disease

COMPLICATIONS

Bleeding; hypotension; hematoma; arteriovenous fistula; infection

NURSING CARE

In conjunction with the physician, obtain written consent. Determine whether the patient can hold his breath for short periods in order to cooperate during the procedure. Before the procedure assess coagulation studies, hematocrit, and platelets to minimize the risk of bleeding. Follow standard preoperative procedures. Start an IV line, and administer sedation as ordered. Disinfect the skin, and prepare a sterile field. Prepare necessary labels and tubes.

After the procedure, apply firm pressure (with gloves) to the incision site for at least 5 minutes. Apply a pressure dressing when the bleeding has stopped. Check vital signs every 15 minutes for 1 hour, every 30 minutes for 1 hour, and every hour for 8 hours unless there are indications of bleeding that require more frequent checks. The patient should remain on bed rest for 24 hours after the procedure, and a 6- and 12-hour hematocrit is recommended. Additional fluids should be administered to facilitate a mild diuresis, which will minimize colic pain and obstruction from clots in the renal pelvis and prevent dehydration. Urine output should be checked hourly for volume, blood, and pH. Administer non-aspirin-containing analgesics as ordered or indicated.

PATIENT TEACHING

Explain the biopsy and IV placement procedures and their purposes. Inform the patient and family that the procedure generally requires overnight admission. Tell them that a local anesthetic will be used that may sting slightly when injected. Prepare the patient for the possibility of pain when the biopsy needle is inserted and immediately after the procedure. Explain that it takes approximately 15 to 30 seconds to complete the procedure. Reassure the patient that analgesic medication will be available. Inform the patient and family that bed rest is generally required for 24 hours after the procedure. Inform them that mild hematuria is normal. Explain that blood will be drawn at least twice after the procedure, at 6 and 12 hours to monitor for risk of bleeding. Inform them that close monitoring by the nurse will continue for at least 12 hours after the procedure.

LYMPH NODE BIOPSY

Lymph node biopsy or **excision** generally is performed as a surgical procedure on an outpatient basis using a local anesthetic. The node is removed and evaluated for architectural structure and histologic characteristics. Usually the supraclavicular scalene region is recommended and the inguinal and axillary areas avoided because of the increased risk of local trauma and infection.

INDICATIONS

Staging of malignancies
Tumor diagnosis
To assess immunologic function in immunodeficiency disorders

CONTRAINDICATIONS: Bleeding dyscrasias

COMPLICATIONS: Bleeding and infection at the site

NURSING CARE

In conjunction with the physician, obtain written consent. Before the procedure, assess coagulation studies, hematocrit, hemoglobin, and platelets to minimize the risk of bleeding. The patient should have nothing by mouth for 6 to 8 hours before the procedure. Disinfect the skin, and establish a sterile field. After the procedure, monitor the patient for bleeding at the site and check vital signs until stable. Apply a sterile occlusion pressure dressing to the site.

PATIENT TEACHING

Explain the procedure and its purpose. Inform the patient that a local anesthetic will be used and that it may cause a slight sting when injected. Explain that he may feel some discomfort after the procedure when the anesthetic has worn off and that he will be sent home with appropriate analgesic medication. Inform the patient and family that a follow-up visit may be necessary to remove sutures.

SYNOVIAL BIOPSY

Synovial biopsy is the aspiration of synovial fluid, usually from the knee joint. It is performed on an outpatient basis in a surgical area using a local anesthetic. The biopsy specimen is obtained through a specialized needle and sent for histologic examination.

INDICATIONS

To assist in the differential diagnosis of various forms of arthritis
Bone malignancies

COMPLICATIONS

Joint effusion
Bleeding into the joint

NURSING CARE

In collaboration with the physician, obtain written consent. The patient should have nothing by mouth for 1 to 4 hours before the procedure. Assess coagulation studies, hematocrit, and platelets to minimize the risk of bleeding. Disinfect the skin, and establish a sterile field. After the biopsy, apply a sterile dressing with an elastic bandage. Monitor site for bleeding, edema, or pain. Apply ice and analgesics as ordered.

PATIENT TEACHING

Explain the procedure and its purpose to the patient and family. Explain that a local anesthetic will be injected, and may cause a slight stinging sensation. Teach the patient that she will feel a sense of pressure when the needle is inserted and mild discomfort after the anesthetic has worn off. Reassure her that analgesic medication will be ordered to assist in pain management. Caution the patient to minimize joint use for 24 hours after the biopsy to prevent bleeding or effusions.

OPHTHALMOLOGIC TESTS

Schirmer's test determines the amount of lacrimal tearing present. It is performed by placing small strips of filter paper (3.5 × 0.05 cm) in the conjunctival cul-de-sac behind the lower lids for 5 minutes. The results are determined by the amount of wetness to the strip of paper; 10 to 15 mm of wet paper is considered normal; less than this is considered abnormal (Figure 3-10).

A **rose bengal staining test** involves instilling a drop of 1% or 2% solution into the conjunctival sac. Patients with a deficiency in the aqueous portion of tears have punctate staining of the lower two thirds of the cornea and bright red staining of the bulbar conjunctiva.

INDICATIONS

Sjögren's syndrome (decreased tearing and staining)
SLE (when presented in conjunction with Sjögren's syndrome; decreased tearing and staining)
Sicca complex

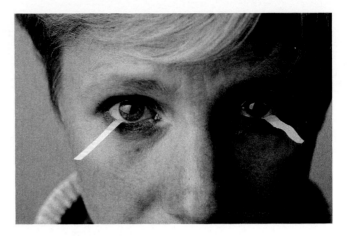

FIGURE 3-10
Schirmer's tear test.

PATIENT TEACHING

Explain the purpose and procedure of the test. Remove contact lenses before instillation of the rose bengal stain, which tends to discolor lenses.

Acquired Immunodeficiency Syndrome

Acquired immunodeficiency syndrome (AIDS) is characterized by dysfunction of cell-mediated immunity. The cell-mediated immune defect is manifested clinically as the development of recurrent, often severe opportunistic infections, such as *Pneumocystis carinii* pneumonia, or unusual malignancies, such as Kaposi's sarcoma.

EPIDEMIOLOGY

AIDS was first recognized in homosexual men in 1981. By 1983 the disease was appearing in many diverse groups, including intravenous drug users, Haitians, hemophiliacs, recipients of blood transfusions, infants of mothers at risk for AIDS, heterosexual sexual partners of people with AIDS, and Africans. However, it was not until the epidemiology of the disease was clearly defined that a hypothesis was formed to explain the pathogenesis of AIDS. It is now understood that AIDS is an infectious disease transmitted through intimate contact with body fluids, blood, or blood products. Specifically, it is acquired through sexual intercourse with an infected individual (anal or vaginal), by the injection or administration of infected blood or blood products (intravenous drug use or transfusions), or, with infants, from an infected mother.

In 1984 a breakthrough in AIDS research occurred almost simultaneously on two continents. In April Dr. Robert Gallo of the National Institutes of Health announced his discovery of the probable AIDS virus, which he called human T-cell leukemia virus, type III (HTLV-III). Four years earlier Gallo had discovered

HTLV, which is known to induce hematologic malignancies by infecting T cells and altering their genetic structure. In June 1984 Dr. Luc Montagnier and his colleagues at the Pasteur Institute in Paris announced that they had discovered the probable AIDS virus, a new human retrovirus called the lymphadenopathy-associated virus (LAV). HTLV-III and LAV later were determined to be the same virus; therefore in 1987 the virus was renamed the human immunodeficiency virus (HIV).

It is estimated that 5 million to 10 million people worldwide are infected with HIV. More than 250,000 cases of AIDS have already occurred, and in the next 5 years a million more cases are likely.

In the United States alone, approximately 1 million to 1.5 million individuals are infected with the virus. In the next few years, close to 400,000 cases of AIDS are predicted. According to the World Health Organization's Global Program on AIDS, patterns of AIDS distribution can be recognized in the world.[111] The United States is a member of the region that accounts for the greatest number of reported AIDS cases. Homosexual and bisexual men and intravenous drug users make up the highest percentage of infected individuals. The average age of men with AIDS is 25 to 45 years. The male-to-female ratio is about 10-15:1. Women account for only 11% of AIDS cases.

Children account for approximately 1.5% of AIDS cases, and the vast majority of these children are under 5 years of age. The primary mode of transmission in this group is perinatal exposure. Hemophiliacs account for most of the group between 5 and 13 years of age, mainly through transfusion-associated transmission.

Intravenous drug use is the major source of HIV transmission in women, heterosexual men, and, consequently, in infants through perinatal exposure.[79] There is also a disproportionately high percentage of AIDS cases among blacks and Hispanics, compared to their respective percentages in the general population, which may be due to intravenous drug use in these groups. The geographic distribution of the aforementioned groups, therefore, corresponds to the area with the greatest concentration of intravenous drug users, primarily the northeastern states.

CLINICAL MANIFESTATIONS

The signs and symptoms of AIDS vary greatly. Clinical manifestations depend on the degree of immunosuppression and the particular infection or neoplasm that develops secondarily. Nonspecific constitutional complaints may also occur and usually are exacerbated as the disease progresses.

Clinical manifestations of HIV infection have been referred to in the past as AIDS-related complex or condition (ARC). However, because there are no precise diagnostic criteria for this term, clinicians recently have described this phase of HIV infection as HIV disease. Among the illnesses common to HIV disease are persistent generalized lymphadenopathy, immune thrombocytopenic purpura, and hairy leukoplakia. Essentially, the term HIV disease is a way to describe immunosuppression in a person with high-risk behaviors who has not yet developed the sequelae of recurrent infections and/or neoplastic diseases. As many as 99% of these patients may develop AIDS eventually, and 50% will develop AIDS within 10 years of infection. Signs and symptoms of HIV disease include severe fatigue; malaise; weakness; persistent, unexplained weight loss; persistent lymphadenopathy; fevers; arthralgias; rigors; nocturnal diaphoresis; and persistent diarrhea. However, laboratory tests and other diagnostic measures to detect the virus are important, because such observations are nonspecific.

PATHOPHYSIOLOGY

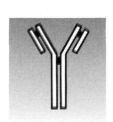

Viruses generally are successful pathogens because of their ability to invade host cells and use the metabolism and genetic material of the host cells to produce copies of themselves. HIV, a retrovirus, is no exception (Figure 4-1). A retrovirus is one that carries its genetic information on ribonucleic acid (RNA) chromosomes. However, deoxyribonucleic acid (DNA) is still needed for replication. HIV begins by binding to the T4 host cell,

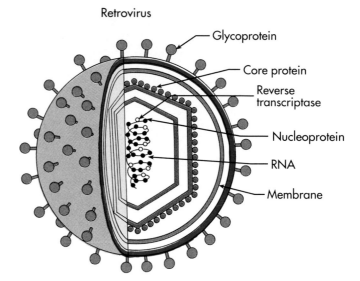

Retrovirus

- Glycoprotein
- Core protein
- Reverse transcriptase
- Nucleoprotein
- RNA
- Membrane

FIGURE 4-1
Retroviruses have been associated with AIDS. They are called retroviruses because they carry their genetic information on RNA rather than DNA chromosomes, producing a DNA copy during transcription with the enzyme reverse transcriptase.

then infecting the RNA core. An enzyme, reverse transcriptase, converts the viral genetic information into a single-strand DNA and then destroys the original RNA. The enzyme then makes a second DNA, using the first as a model. The double-stranded DNA travels to the cell nucleus, where another enzyme integrates it into the host cell's DNA.

Transcription of the provirus yields the viral genome and messenger RNA needed to direct production of new viral proteins. These assemble at the cell membrane, awaiting release by "budding." The virus can remain dormant indefinitely, but once the host T4 cell has been immunologically stimulated, the provirus will begin to reproduce. Replication may continue to the point of a cytopathic effect, meaning that the T4 cell membrane ruptures as a result of emerging "budding" virus (Figures 4-2 and 4-3). More circulating HIV particles infect more T4 cells. Eventually, the number of T4 cells is greatly reduced. The normal 2-to-1 ratio of T4 cells (helper T lymphocytes) to T8 cells (suppressor T lymphocytes) is now reversed; suppressor T mechanisms dominate.

Clinical findings are compatible with profound immunosuppression. Because T cell–mediated immunity is important in tumor surveillance and in defense against intracellular pathogens such as viruses, protozoa, mycobacteria, and fungi, deregulation in this component of the body's defensive network results in the development of AIDS characteristics.

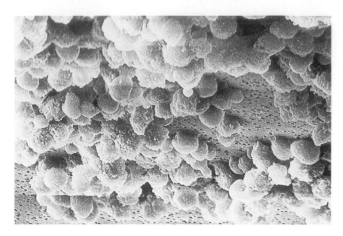

FIGURE 4-2
Scanning electron micrograph (SEM) of a population of AIDS-infected lymphocytes. (From the Centers for Disease Control, 1992.)

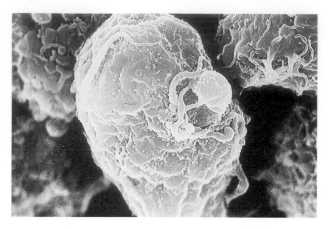

FIGURE 4-3
Scanning electron micrograph of HTLV-III—injected T4 lymphocytes, showing virus budding from the plasma membrane of the lymphocytes. (From the Centers for Disease Control, 1992.)

HUMAN IMMUNODEFICIENCY VIRUS (HIV) DISEASE

Persistent Generalized Lymphadenopathy

First recognized in homosexual men in the late 1970s, persistent generalized lymphadenopathy (PGL) is now described by the Centers for Disease Control (CDC) staging schema for HIV infection as palpable lymphadenopathy at two or more extrainguinal sites persisting for longer than 3 months without concurrent illness or conditions other than HIV exposure to explain the findings.[39] It remains unclear whether lymphadenopathy is a primary response to HIV infection or secondary to reactivation of an underlying viral infection, such as a herpes virus.[1] Although its true incidence is unknown, estimates suggest that persistent generalized lymphadenopathy is a very common manifestation of HIV infection.

PGL has a very high likelihood of progressing to AIDS, although the length of time it takes for AIDS to evolve ranges from a few years to longer than 5 years. Further investigation of the natural history of persistent generalized lymphadenopathy is needed to determine the rate of progression to AIDS.

Several factors appear to yield some predictive value, including clinical and laboratory data such as the presence of oral thrush or hairy leukoplakia, an elevated erythrocyte sedimentation rate, anemia, leukopenia, and other blood dyscrasias.[1] All of these seem to increase the likelihood of disease progression. Nevertheless, many individuals with persistent generalized lymphadenopathy can function normally for many years without harmful sequelae. Of note is the common observation among clinicians that lymph nodes tend to disappear just before AIDS develops. This supports the idea that lymphadenopathy represents an appropriate response to initial HIV infection, but that exhaustion of the immune system causes the nodes to disappear about the same time that AIDS takes complete control.[1]

Frequently the onset of lymphadenopathy occurs 1 to 2 months after a flulike illness. Most patients then describe symptoms such as fevers, night sweats, fatigue, headaches, cough, weight loss, and diarrhea. On examination the axillary, inguinal, and posterior cervical nodes are found to be involved in almost all patients. They are firm, nontender, larger than 1 cm in diameter, and sometimes visible under the skin.

On a computed tomography (CT) scan, splenomegaly, enlarged retroperitoneal lymph nodes, and rectal mucosal thickening (chronic proctitis) are repeatedly seen. Routine hematology and chemistry studies can help determine clinical condition and evaluate the progression toward AIDS.

Therapy for persistent generalized lymphadenopathy must augment the immune system since, as stated earlier, the condition represents an appropriate immune response to HIV infection; on the other hand, activated lymphocytes may encourage further HIV attack. Therefore one suggestion has been to treat the lymphadenopathy with immune modulation and antiviral therapy. Some trials have taken place with drugs such as alpha-interferon, isoprinosine, ribavirin, and suramin, but none of these pharmacologic agents has demonstrated therapeutic efficacy to date. The only agent that has shown any benefits is zidovudine (Retrovir, AZT). Early

CRITERIA FOR DIAGNOSING AIDS IN ORDER TO ESTABLISH UNIFORMITY IN REPORTING AIDS CASES

I. Without laboratory evidence of HIV infection

Candidiasis of the esophagus, trachea, bronchi, or lungs

Extrapulmonary cryptococcosis

Cryptosporidiosis, with diarrhea persisting longer than 1 month

Cytomegalovirus disease of an organ other than the liver, spleen, or lymph nodes in a patient over 1 month of age

Infection with herpes simplex virus, causing a mucocutaneous ulcer that persists longer than 1 month; *or* bronchitis, pneumonitis, or esophagitis of any duration affecting a patient over 1 month of age

Kaposi's sarcoma affecting a patient under 60 years of age

Lymphoma of the brain (primary) affecting a patient under 60 years of age

Lymphoid interstitial pneumonia and/or pulmonary lymphoid hyperplasia affecting a child under 13 years of age

Disseminated *Mycobacterium avium* or *Mycobacterium kansasii* disease (at a site other than or in addition to the lungs, skin, or cervical or hilar lymph nodes)

Pneumocystis carinii pneumonia

Progressive multifocal leukoencephalopathy

Toxoplasmosis of the brain, affecting a patient over 1 month of age

II. With laboratory evidence for HIV infection

Bacterial infections, multiple or recurrent, affecting a child under 13 years of age

Septicemia, pneumonia, meningitis, bone or joint infection, or abscess of an internal organ or body cavity caused by *Haemophilus* or *Streptococcus* organisms or by other pyogenic bacteria

Disseminated coccidioidomycosis (at a site other than or in addition to the lungs or cervical or hilar lymph nodes)

Isosporiasis, with diarrhea persisting longer than 1 month

Kaposi's sarcoma at any age

Lymphoma of the brain (primary) at any age

Non-Hodgkin's lymphoma of B-cell or unknown immunologic phenotypes; small, noncleaved (Burkitt's) lymphoma; and immunoblastic sarcoma histologic types

Mycobacterioses, including disseminated or miliary tuberculosis (at a site other than or in addition to the lungs, skin, or cervical or hilar lymph nodes)

Salmonella (nontyphoid) septicemia, recurrent HIV wasting syndrome ("slim" disease)

III. Diagnosed presumptively

Candidiasis of the esophagus

Cytomegalovirus retinitis with loss of vision

Kaposi's sarcoma

Lymphoid interstitial pneumonia and/or pulmonary lymphoid hyperplasia affecting a child under 13 years of age

Disseminated mycobacterioses

P. carinii pneumonia

Toxoplasmosis of the brain affecting a patient over 1 month of age

From Centers for Disease Control.[38]

intervention may help delay the progression from HIV disease to full-blown AIDS.

AIDS Encephalopathy

AIDS encephalopathy, more recently referred to as AIDS dementia complex (ADC), is a primary infection of the brain by the human immunodeficiency virus. The virus has been isolated from brain tissue, cerebrospinal fluid, and spinal cord and peripheral nerve tissue. It is estimated that as many as 90% of AIDS patients have some degree of dementia.

The early effects of HIV on the brain are described

as diffuse pallor and mild vacuolation of the white matter, often accompanied by a mild perivascular lymphocytic reaction. Inflammation is present, often associated with reactive astrocytosis of variable degree. In more advanced stages, myelin pallor and cell reactions generally increase in prominence. Vacuolar myelopathy is also common in patients with an advanced pathologic condition of the brain. The exact mechanisms by which these changes in the brain cause HIV-related dementia continue to be investigated.

An insidious onset (anywhere from weeks to months) of cognitive impairment characterizes the early stage of this progressive dementia. Symptoms range from subtle alterations in memory to frank confusion and disorientation. Behavioral disturbances include apathy, lethargy, or withdrawal. These symptoms frequently mimic depression. Early motor deficits may include ataxia, leg weakness, tremor, and loss of fine-motor coordination. In the most advanced stage of the disease, patients suffer from severe dementia, mutism, incontinence, and paraplegia.

The absolute method to determine the diagnosis is brain biopsy. However, because of the poor prognosis, this usually is not done. Computed tomography or magnetic resonance imaging (MRI) can show a distinctive pattern of cerebral atrophy and ventricular enlargement.

There is no known effective treatment for AIDS dementia complex. Mean survival time is 3 to 7 months. It is important, therefore, to rule out completely other treatable causes of central nervous system disease. Neurologic manifestations could also be due to an opportunistic infection caused by organisms such as cytomegalovirus. Regardless of the cause, supportive care is essential.

Immune Thrombocytopenic Purpura

Immune or idiopathic thrombocytopenic purpura (ITP) is an autoimmune process that prematurely destroys platelets. It was first noted as an AIDS-related condition among homosexual men in 1982. It is unclear whether the condition is a direct response to HIV or results from other, unknown causes. Similar to persistent generalized lymphadenopathy, over the course of time patients with ITP have an increased risk of developing AIDS. Thrombocytopenia along with lymphadenopathy heightens the risk. It has also been observed in ITP that the platelet count approaches normal about the time that AIDS takes over.

HIV-related immune thrombocytopenic purpura seems to involve the development of antibodies to one's own platelets. Two hypotheses attempt to explain the mechanism by which this occurs. One possible explanation is that, because of abnormal regulation of immunity in AIDS, the large numbers of B cells and immunoglobulins present may react with self-tissues or blood components. Another theory suggests that an unknown mechanism disguises the body's own platelets as foreign. The sites of platelet destruction are the spleen and the liver. Clinical features include easy bruising and petechiae in most patients, as well as occasional nasal, gingival, and rectal bleeding. Major bleeding as a complication has not been observed in these patients. Some patients with immune thrombocytopenic purpura may not have any physical signs or report any symptoms. Others may have simultaneous conditions such as persistent generalized lymphadenopathy, hairy leukoplakia, or thrush. Laboratory tests show platelet counts that average 20,000 cells/mm^3, although the range varies from 3,000 cells/mm^3 to 75,000 cells/mm.^{3}

Treatment does not seem to be a necessity. Despite markedly low platelet counts, patients respond about the same with or without therapy. The standard treatment is splenectomy or steroid therapy, or both. Steroids do achieve favorable platelet counts in HIV-infected patients. Oral prednisone slows the peripheral destruction of platelets. However, once the drug has been tapered off, the platelet count drops again. Splenectomy may also achieve some success. No further immunosuppression has occurred with either treatment. Currently, as long as no serious bleeding has occurred, close monitoring is recommended instead of treatment.

Oral Hairy Leukoplakia

In 1981 in San Francisco, a unique, oral white lesion appeared among a group of homosexual men. Since then oral hairy leukoplakia (OHL), as it has been called, has been identified in other individuals engaging in high-risk behaviors. The disorder is highly predictive of progression to AIDS. One study of 155 patients with oral hairy leukoplakia who did not have AIDS showed that after 31 months of follow-up, 83% had developed AIDS, most with *Pneumocystis carinii* pneumonia (PCP) as their first manifestation. The Centers for Disease Control lists oral hairy leukoplakia in the HIV classification schema as a specific secondary infectious disease.

Although initially misdiagnosed as candidiasis, oral hairy leukoplakia later implicated the Epstein-Barr virus from biopsy and suggested the possibility of a second virus, the human papillomavirus. **For picture of hairy leukoplakia of the tongue, see Color Plate 4, page x.** Whatever the cause, the condition is a virally induced epithelial hyperplasia. Oral hairy leukoplakia resembles thrush; in fact, the lesions often are colonized with *Candida* organisms. However, oral hairy leukoplakia does not rub off and has several other distinguishing characteristics. It is a painless, white, raised lesion that often appears on the lateral margins of the tongue, often with projections off it that make it look "hairy." It can be smooth or corrugated, thin or thick. It can appear on one or both lateral margins of the tongue, on the dorsal and ventral surfaces, and on the buccal mucosa and the floor of the mouth. The lesion may be present in one or more small areas or in a single large area.

Diagnosis is based on clinical appearance and histopathologic tests. A thorough examination is essential, using both hands to carefully inspect a well-lit oral cavity and to palpate any lumps or indurations. Until a biopsy is performed, failure to respond to antifungal therapy may be considered an optional way to confirm the diagnosis. Noninvasive diagnostic methods are being investigated.

There is no known agent available to eradicate oral hairy leukoplakia. It usually is not symptomatic, but if candidiasis is present, antifungal therapy may lessen the related discomfort. Acyclovir (Zovirax) is under investigation as a possible therapy for oral hairy leukoplakia. Oral and topical antiviral drug regimens are in the developmental stage.

OPPORTUNISTIC INFECTIONS

Pneumocystis carinii Pneumonia

Pneumocystis carinii pneumonia (PCP) is the most common opportunistic infection recognized in patients with AIDS (Figure 4-4). More than half of AIDS patients develop PCP initially, and one third to one half develop recurrent PCP within 12 months. More than 75% ultimately have PCP at some point during the course of the disease.

P. carinii is a one-celled protozoan that is ubiquitous in the environment. Usually a benign flora in healthy individuals, it becomes an aggressive pathogen in immunocompromised hosts. Infestation can result in death from respiratory failure. Until the advent of AIDS, *P. carinii* pneumonia was considered a rare complication affecting cancer patients receiving chemotherapy, transplant recipients, other patients receiving immunosuppressive therapy, malnourished patients, premature infants, and patients with congenital defects of cellular immunity.

Probably spread person to person via the respiratory route, this opportunistic organism assaults pulmonary tissue, resulting in diffuse, bilateral, interstitial infiltrates and alveolar infiltration by exudates of many clumped organisms or cysts.

P. carinii pneumonia usually is slow to manifest itself, requiring anywhere from 2 weeks to 8 months. Early symptoms often include increasing dyspnea on exertion, nonproductive cough, and weight loss. Fever

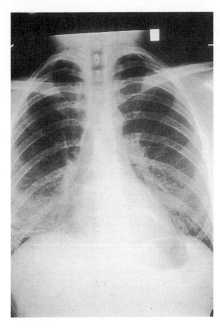

FIGURE 4-4
Pulmonary pneumocystosis. Chest x-ray showing interstitial infiltrates as the result of *Pneumocystis carinii* pneumonia. (From the Centers for Disease Control.) (Courtesy Jonathan W.M. Gold, M.D., New York, N.Y.)

sometimes is present, with or without chills. Chest x-rays are unremarkable, initially revealing only nonspecific interstitial infiltrates, if anything. Lung fields generally are clear upon auscultation and percussion. Abnormal findings of pulmonary function studies, specifically decreased diffusing capacity for carbon monoxide, and increased air flow rates may be the only signs confirming early suspicions of infection. Arterial blood gas measurements may be low or normal. Gallium lung scans may be helpful if used with a grading system for assessing scan activity. Definitive diagnosis is obtained from bronchoscopy with transbronchial lung biopsy or bronchoalveolar lavage (or both) or, in rare cases, from open lung biopsy. Before bronchoscopy, sputum induction may yield a sample that, if accurately evaluated, identifies the presence of protozoa. However, sputum results are not always conclusive.

The latter course of *P. carinii* pneumonia can be rapid and associated with clinical findings indicating respiratory failure. AIDS patients with untreated *P. carinii* pneumonia develop life-threatening pulmonary insufficiency as a result of extensive pulmonary consolidation. The chest x-ray shows gross bilateral consolidation, or "whiteout."

Two drugs are available to treat *P. carinii* pneumonia. The first-line defense is trimethoprim-sulfamethoxazole (Bactrim, Septra) given intravenously and later orally. Pentamidine isethionate (Pentam 300) is the second drug of choice. It is administered intramuscularly or intravenously for a minimum of 10 days.

New antibiotic treatments for *P. carinii* pneumonia continue to be evaluated. These include a dapsone-trimethoprim regimen and difluoromethylornithine (DFMO), an inhibitor of polyamine synthesis. In addition, using steroids in certain cases of *P. carinii* pneumonia may help prevent or suppress the inflammatory response of the host.

Pharmacologic intervention usually decreases the mortality associated with *P. carinii* pneumonia. Seventy percent of patients respond well to treatment. However, AIDS patients tend to clear the organism very slowly despite therapy, and relapses are common. Also, because AIDS patients' chances of survival from subsequent episodes of infection are greatly diminished, prolonged treatment often is required. Furthermore, since subsequent episodes increase the morbidity of *P. carinii* pneumonia, much work is being done on prophylactic therapy. Currently the CDC recommends either trimethoprim-sulfamethoxazole or aerosolized pentamidine for PCP prophylaxis.

Toxoplasmosis

The infection toxoplasmosis is caused by a protozoal parasite of the Coccidia order, *Toxoplasma gondii*. *T. gondii* is an opportunistic pathogen found in the past to infect patients with hematologic malignancies, collagen-vascular diseases, and organ transplantations. Common to humans and animals, especially cats, it has a worldwide distribution. Most American adults were exposed to *T. gondii* as children. In AIDS, toxoplasmosis is the major cause of central nervous system disease, next to HIV infection itself. The incidence in the United States is 2% to 13%, depending on the risk group and geographic location.

Common clinical signs include fever, lethargy, seizures, and weakness. However, a vast array of neurologic signs and symptoms may be present, ranging from headaches to hemiparesis, which may appear gradually or develop all at once.

Diagnosis may be made by a computed tomography (CT) scan of the brain. The abnormalities seen may be single or multiple, deep, ring-enhancing intracerebral lesions, although, on occasion, CT scans will be nonspecific. In these situations magnetic resonance imaging (MRI) might be more helpful. Regardless, MRI or CT findings should be supported by specific clinical symptoms.

Brain biopsy is one definitive method of diagnosis that usually is not undertaken unless absolutely necessary. Instead, an empiric trial of therapy is given to see if lesions or symptoms diminish in patients with strong clinical and radiologic evidence for cerebral toxoplasmosis.

The treatment of choice is a combination of sulfadiazine and pyrimethamine (Fansidar) administered orally, usually for the patient's lifetime, to prevent relapse. Clindamycin (Cleocin) is used instead of sulfadiazine for patients allergic to sulfa drugs or intolerant of the sulfadiazine-pyrimethamine combination. Clindamycin can be used alone or with pyrimethamine.

Therapy should bring about marked improvement in approximately 2 weeks. Meaningful survival for as long as 1 year after diagnosis has been reported. Early rehabilitative efforts such as speech and physical therapy programs are beneficial for patients with focal neurologic manifestations. Follow-up neurologic examinations and CT or MRI scans are important to evaluate therapy and to identify new opportunistic infections or other central nervous system disorders.

Cryptosporidiosis

Cryptosporidium muris is an intestinal protozoan of the Coccidia order. Lacking host specificity, it has been found in mammals, birds, reptiles, household pets, and, more recently, humans. The first reported human case was in 1976. The disease, called cryptosporidiosis, causes a severe but self-limited diarrheal syndrome that lasts 10 to 20 days. It is a communicable disease that can pass from animal to man (e.g., through the water supply or while working with animals) or from person to person (e.g., infected individual to caregiver, between children at day care centers, or through sexual contact). The route of infection is fecal-oral contamination. In AIDS patients, cryptosporidiosis probably develops as a reactivation of an earlier undiagnosed infection. Documented enteritis caused by *C. muris* that lasts longer than 1 month is diagnostic for AIDS. It occurs most frequently in children and homosexual men.

The pathogenesis of cryptosporidiosis currently is unclear. It is known that *C. muris* cryptosporidia infect the microvillus border of the small intestine. Furthermore, the organism has been identified along other mucosal surfaces throughout the gastrointestinal tract and even the bronchi. It is characterized by villous atrophy and fusion, loss of epithelial cells, and minimal inflammation. Permanent damage from prolonged infection may result in continued diarrhea and malabsorption despite the absence of protozoa.

The AIDS diarrheal syndrome caused by *C. muris* consists of profuse, watery diarrhea along with anorexia, nausea, vomiting, fatigue, malaise, low-grade fever, and occasionally abdominal pain and cramps. Massive fluid loss from diarrhea (up to 20 liters per day) leads to dehydration, electrolyte disturbances, malabsorption, extreme weight loss, and possibly death.

Concurrent infections with other enteric pathogens such as *Shigella* and *Salmonella* organisms are possible. Less often, bronchitis (aerosol transmission) and cholecystitis are caused by *C. muris* infection.

The diagnosis of cryptosporidiosis is based on the finding of *C. muris* cysts in the stool. This test is done using modified acid-fast staining techniques on stool specimens. Biopsies of the gastrointestinal tract or bronchioles may be necessary on occasion and may reveal the organism attached to the microvilli.

Treatment should be aimed at symptom control, since cryptosporidiosis has evaded most attempts at eradication. Combination antiperistaltic, antispasmodic, and bulk agents, along with fluid and electrolyte replacement, are essential. Nonsteroidal antiinflammatory drugs may alleviate symptoms. Nutritional consultation will be needed to explore options for a patient who is severely compromised.

Isosporiasis

Isosporiasis is another intestinal infection caused by a similar protozoan, *Isospora belli*. This organism also invades the microvillus of the small intestine, producing severe protracted diarrhea. It can occur alone or concurrently with cryptosporidiosis. Infection with *Isospora* organisms that persists longer than 1 month is diagnostic for AIDS. The clinical picture resembles the diarrheal syndrome described for cryptosporidiosis.

The life cycle of *I. belli*, the histologic changes in the small bowel, and diagnostic tests with stool stains and biopsies are analogous to those for cryptosporidiosis. However, the morphology distinguishes between *I. belli* and *C. muris*. *I. belli* cysts are oval, not round, much larger, and contain two sporoblasts instead of four sporozoites.

Isosporiasis responds with some degree of success to trimethoprim-sulfamethoxazole (Bactrim, Septra). Therefore although isosporiasis is not as common as cryptosporidiosis, it is important to recognize the possibility of *I. belli* infection. Continual therapy for the patient's lifetime is required, because the recurrence rate of isosporiasis is high. Symptomatic treatment is necessary, just as in cryptosporidiosis.

Candidiasis

Candida albicans is the organism most often implicated in oral fungal disease. It is a yeast that is ubiquitous in the environment. Usually benign, *C. albicans* often inhabits the gastrointestinal, genitourinary, or respiratory tracts of humans. In fact, it can live as a commensal organism in some of these areas, primarily the oropharynx. Colonization is not unusual and not a problem unless overgrowth leads to tissue invasion and damage. Factors that may predispose an individual to candidiasis include antibiotic therapy or other treatments that diminish normal host flora, radiation or other treatments that disrupt skin and mucosal barriers, diabetes mellitus, Addison's disease or other illnesses that alter hormonal and nutritional systems, and immature, compromised, or suppressed immune systems such as in infants, AIDS/HIV infection, and steroid therapy or chemotherapy.

In AIDS/HIV disease, candidiasis of the oropharynx and candidiasis of the esophagus represent two common findings. Only candidal esophagitis is diagnostic for AIDS. Less often, *C. albicans* infects the integumentary, pulmonary, and lower gastrointestinal systems, as well as the genitalia, but rarely disseminates. Oral candidiasis among persons engaging in high-risk behaviors may be a predictor of the development of AIDS.

The development of candidiasis begins when *C. albicans* attaches to the mucous membranes, followed by colonization. This progresses in AIDS/HIV patients to tissue invasion. Inflammation follows, bringing aggregates of neutrophils to the site. The combined result (tissue invasion and inflammation) is tissue damage from cellular destruction and death.

For picture of oral candidiasis, see Color Plate 6, page xi.

At least three oral presentations are possible. The most common in AIDS/HIV patients is pseudomembranous candidiasis, or thrush. It has the characteristic appearance of white, creamy or curdy plaques scattered throughout the oropharynx. The plaques scrape off easily, revealing a bright red, bleeding surface. In contrast, atrophic candidiasis looks red and smooth and usually is seen on the palate and dorsum of the tongue. At worst, it may involve erosion and fissures of the oral mucosa. Angular cheilitis (involvement of the lips) may occur simultaneously or alone.

Symptoms of oral candidal injections include soreness, burning, and changes in taste; symptoms of esophageal infection include dysphagia, nausea, vomiting, and retrosternal pain. In rare cases, severe candidiasis can cause gastrointestinal bleeding.

Candidal infections can also involve fingernails or toenails and the skin or mucous membranes, especially the skin folds such as the axillae, groin, and perianal areas. Symptoms include an erythematous rash; lumpy, fissured nails; and yellow-brown granulomatous lesions.

A diagnosis of oral candidiasis can be made from examination of a Gram stain or potassium hydroxide suspension of smears, showing the presence of yeast. Routine culture can determine the species and colony count. A high count suggests active infection. Biopsies of suspected lesions can also be tested with Gram's stain and may show the presence of yeast. Appropriate procedures for obtaining the biopsy may be necessary, such as upper endoscopy for esophagitis. If dissemination is a concern, fungal blood cultures may be helpful, although these sometimes give a false-negative result. Dissemination is confirmed when *C. albicans* is isolated from two different organs or systems.

Several antifungal medications are effective in treating candidal infections, including nystatin (Nilstat, Mycostatin), ketoconazole (Nizoral), clotrimazole (Mycelex, Lotrimin), and amphotericin B (Fungizone).

Cryptococcosis

The common soil fungus *Cryptococcus neoformans* is ubiquitous in the environment. It is particularly associated with pigeons. It enters the host by means of inhalation into the respiratory tract. Asymptomatic pulmonary infections are common. However, the organism most often is discovered as the cause of fungal infection in the central nervous system. The bloodstream facilitates its spread to this area. Humans most susceptible to cryptococcosis are patients with baseline ill health or a dysfunctional cell-mediated immune system. These patients include organ transplant recipients, diabetics, persons on long-term corticosteroid therapy, persons with lymphoma, and persons with AIDS.

In AIDS patients, symptoms similar to meningitis dominate the clinical picture. Intense, intermittent headaches; moderate, irregular fevers; and general malaise come on slowly without notice. Over time the headaches worsen, especially with activities that increase intracranial pressure, and they do not respond to routine analgesics. Less commonly other symptoms develop, such as intolerance to light and sound, stiff neck, loss of appetite, and altered mental status. Occasionally patients have no symptoms or neurologic changes. In AIDS patients the mortality rate for initial infections is 17%.

Less frequently, cryptococcosis manifests as a pulmonary infection in patients with AIDS. The initial symptoms are much the same as those already described, lacking specificity. Also, disseminated disease should be expected in AIDS patients. It can occur almost anywhere in the body (e.g., the skin, heart, kidneys, liver, and bone marrow).

Diagnosis of cryptococcal meningitis requires demonstration of a positive cryptococcal antigen titer or fungal culture in cerebrospinal fluid (CSF), or both. The CSF sample is obtained through lumbar puncture and may also reveal increased protein and low or normal glucose. Computed tomography (CT) scans and magnetic resonance imaging (MRI) may be helpful in ruling out other causes with similar clinical findings. Serum cryptococcal antigen tests may prove positive; the more

specific the serologic test, the better the chance of isolating the organism.

For pulmonary cryptococcosis, a chest x-ray and bronchoscopy with bronchial lavage and transbronchial biopsy determine the diagnosis.

Amphotericin B (Fungizone) is the treatment of choice. However, the drug's severe toxicities have become well known since it was first used almost 40 years ago. Drug toxicity is related to the rate of infusion, the cumulative dose of the drug, and the patient's baseline renal function. The oral agent flucytosine (5FC, Ancobon) is also a drug of choice, although using it alone may allow resistant organisms to flourish. Recently, ketoconazole (Nizoral), although known not to enter cerebrospinal fluid, has been found to be as effective as amphotericin B in improving survival and preventing relapses in patients who can tolerate this drug.

Lifelong maintenance therapy generally is required for cryptococcosis, because relapses are very common, especially during the first year after diagnosis, and with each relapse, the mortality rate climbs.

Histoplasmosis

Histoplasma capsulatum is another common soil fungus. This dimorphic organism frequents the environment, especially in areas with large concentrations of birds. In the United States, it is endemic in the Ohio River Valley region. Here 80% of the general population demonstrate positive skin tests for histoplasmosis, indicating past asymptomatic infection. This disease can cause a focal, self-limited, pulmonary infection or a disseminated syndrome. The former is most often observed in immunocompetent hosts, the latter in patients with AIDS. Overall most AIDS patients experience reactivation of an old focus of infection, which then disseminates.

Histoplasmosis is transmitted through inhalation of spores released by *H. capsulatum*. These spores easily reach the smaller bronchioles and alveoli, where infection is established. From the lungs, dissemination occurs rapidly via the bloodstream.

Patients initially may have fevers, chills, malaise, fatigue, and wasting syndrome; a respiratory component may be present. Nearing total dissemination, a picture similar to septic shock appears, involving high fevers, tachycardia, hypotension, hepatosplenomegaly, coagulopathy, and pulmonary, hepatic, and renal failure.

Isolating the organism from blood or tissue or both constitutes the diagnosis. Serologic tests without a positive blood or tissue culture do not mean much, because they do not distinguish between past and current disease. In some cases invasive procedures such as bronchoscopy or open lung biopsy may be needed to confirm a diagnosis.

The treatment of choice is amphotericin B (Fungizone), and maintenance therapy is required to prevent relapse. Ketoconazole (Nizoral) in doses of 400 to 600 mg per day may be sufficient to achieve continued suppression of disease.

Mycobacterial Disease

Mycobacterium avium-intracellulare (MAI) is ubiquitous in the environment. *M. avium* and *M. intracellulare* are rod-shaped, aerobic, gram-positive, acid-fast bacteria that are rarely seen apart; hence the term "*Mycobacterium avium* complex" (MAC) has been coined to describe this bacterial couplet. It is commonly found in soil and water and in a variety of birds and mammals, particularly barnyard animals. However, in the barnyard, chickens and pigs are the only targets of actual disease. Humans can be infected via either the respiratory tract or the gastrointestinal tract from ingestion of contaminated water. Before the emergence of AIDS, disease occurred only in rare cases in persons with chronic lung disease or who were immunosuppressed as a result of chemotherapy, corticosteroid therapy, or malignancy. However, with AIDS, MAI infection is most likely a reactivation of a formerly acquired infection. It is a frequent pathogen in AIDS patients and usually is not susceptible to known treatment. Disseminated MAI infection is one of the indicator diseases for AIDS. The diagnosis of MAI disease often marks the beginning of a slow, insidious physical decline.

Once inside the host, *M. avium* complex disseminates through the bloodstream. It can infect many different sites, including the lungs, blood, lymph nodes, bone marrow, liver, and gastrointestinal tract. Tissue changes often do not include the usual granuloma formation of tuberculosis (nodular aggregation of inflamed tissue) because of the lack of cell-mediated immunity in HIV infection.

Fever, weight loss, fatigue, and malaise, although not specific for MAI infection, describe the usual clinical picture. Gastrointestinal infection gives rise to symptoms such as abdominal cramping and pain, diarrhea, and anorexia.

Laboratory data include chronic anemia and declining complete blood counts. Pancytopenia frequently occurs as a result of bone marrow invasion. Liver function tests and erythrocyte sedimentation rates are elevated. Catabolic breakdown occurs as wasting ensues.

A definitive diagnosis is made by positive culture of *M. avium* complex from at least one extrapulmonary site. Colonization in the lungs, which can occur even in immunocompetent persons, does not constitute disseminated disease. Blood is a common source to culture, since venipuncture yields easy access. Otherwise, biopsy of the suspected site is the method used to obtain the specimen for culture. It may take up to 6 weeks to identify the organism on culture media, because it has a slow reproductive cycle.

While culture reports are awaited, if the tissue smear tests positive for acid-fast bacillus (AFB) and the organism resembles *M. avium* complex under the microscope, treatment can begin. However, a positive AFB test or culture from a lung source should be presumed *Mycobacterium tuberculosis* until determined otherwise. In this case tuberculosis precautions and treatment should be initiated. When the actual diagnosis is made, therapy can be modified accordingly.

Multiple drug resistance makes MAI infection difficult to treat. Combinations of various drugs demonstrate some degree of effectiveness against the disease. Isoniazid (INH) and ethambutol (Myambutol) continue to be the mainstays of pharmacologic intervention. In addition, clofazimine (Lamprene), an antileprosy drug; rifabutine (Ansamycin), a more potent rifampin derivative; streptomycin; and cycloserine (Seromycin) have been used to treat MAI infection.

Cultures may remain positive for as long as 1 to 2 months into therapy. Because relapse is a strong possibility, some degree of maintenance therapy should be followed. Also, managing the symptoms of the AIDS patient with MAI infection should be a primary focus of the treatment plan.

Tuberculosis

Mycobacterium tuberculosis is an acid-fast, aerobic, nonsporulating, rod-shaped bacterium responsible for the disease tuberculosis. Tuberculosis has been a worldwide plague of mankind for centuries, especially in areas of malnutrition and poor sanitary conditions. In this century the prevalence of tuberculosis in many Western countries has been substantially reduced. Unfortunately, however, in regions of the world such as the Far East and the tropics (Haiti), it still reigns. Furthermore, unknown thousands of individuals with the disease have escaped detection or have not been adequately treated after diagnosis. With the advent of AIDS, the downward trend in tuberculosis cases in the United States has stopped, primarily because of new cases among HIV-infected intravenous drug users and Haitians. The presence of *M. tuberculosis* in at least one extrapulmonary site in an individual with laboratory evidence of HIV infection is diagnostic for AIDS.

The primary mode of transmission is through inhalation of droplet nuclei from coughs or sneezes of infected individuals. Ingestion and direct inoculation are possible but less common ways the bacteria can be transmitted. Pulmonary tuberculosis occurs in about 50% of patients. Extrapulmonary sites may involve the bone marrow, kidneys, brain, lymph nodes, gastrointestinal tract, or practically any other body site.

Predisposing or secondary causes of tuberculosis relate to environmental factors such as overcrowding and poor ventilation, as well as the ability of the host's cell-mediated immune system to activate a response. This explains why HIV-infected individuals, who have altered cell-mediated immunity, are more at risk of developing tuberculosis.

The pathologic condition of the infection and disease occurs in three stages—initial, or primary, infection, latency, and postprimary disease. In the initial infection, the bacilli invade the tissue at the portal of entry and multiply, creating a small inflammatory lesion. Almost immediately the lymphatic system and the bloodstream carry bacilli to the lymph nodes and throughout the body, where they produce more inflammatory lesions. Some phagocytosis of tubercle bacilli occurs at these sites, producing suppuration and necrosis in the central portion of the lesion. Within 3 to 12 weeks an immune response stimulates fibroblasts to form a dense, connective tissue enclosure and a noncaseating granuloma. The focal lesions continue to harbor viable tubercle bacilli, with the potential for reactivation under conditions of decreased host resistance, such as in HIV infection. Individuals with successful encapsulation of all the lesions as a direct result of immune response are in a period of latency. The length of time they will remain disease free depends on their ability to maintain specific and nonspecific resistance. For 5% to 15% of infected persons, however, host responses are inadequate to contain the infection. Necrosis and cavitation continue in the lesions, forming caseation. The lesions may rupture, spreading necrotic residue and bacilli throughout the tissue and the body. Disseminated bacilli establish new focal lesions that progress through the stages of inflammation, noncaseating granulomas, and caseating necrosis.

The AIDS patient with pulmonary tuberculosis has a productive, purulent cough, fever, fatigue, and other nonspecific constitutional complaints. However, disease symptoms vary, depending on the body tissue affected. Disseminated or extrapulmonary infection has a greater incidence in AIDS patients.

Sputum smears for acid-fast bacillus and culture should be obtained more than once. However, biopsy of nodular lesions is more likely to provide histopathologic evidence of acid-fast organisms than sputum smears. Specimens from clinically indicated areas can also be cultured.

Because AIDS patients may be unable to activate a skin response even if infected with *M. tuberculosis*, purified protein derivative (PPD) skin testing is useful only with control antigens, which help reveal anergy.

Chest x-rays may show cavitation, tubercle formation, or a miliary pattern typical of pulmonary tuberculosis. Granulomas may not be present, since this depends on a cell-mediated immune response, which is deficient in HIV infection. Diffuse pulmonary infiltrates associated with hilar or mediastinal adenopathy can be a helpful radiologic clue.

Clinically, tuberculosis in AIDS patients responds readily to therapy, and patients have few adverse reactions. The standard treatment is three-drug therapy with isoniazid (INH), ethambutol (Myambutol), and rifampin (Rifadin) over 9 to 12 months. Long-term maintenance, perhaps for the patient's lifetime, should be considered, since reactivation is always possible. These patients are not considered infectious 24 hours after therapy has begun. Symptom management is also an important aspect of treatment.

LYMPHOCYTIC INTERSTITIAL PNEUMONIA

Lymphocytic interstitial pneumonia (LIP) is diagnostic for AIDS in children. It is defined as diffuse infiltration of alveolar walls by mature lymphocytes, plasma cells, and reticuloendothelial cells. The disease is associated with various immune deficiencies and autoimmune diseases, especially Sjögren's syndrome. Lymphocytic interstitial pneumonia affects at least half of children with AIDS but few adults. The cause is unknown; it may be an expression of HIV, or it may represent the pulmonary component of another illness. The histology of lymphocytic interstitial pneumonia in AIDS differs from that in patients without AIDS. With AIDS, instead of mature lymphocytes and plasma cells encircling the bronchioles and vessels, atypical lymphocytes actually invade the bronchioles, thereby creating the pulmonary infiltrate.

LIP is a chronic, progressive, interstitial lung disease. Symptoms consist of dyspnea and nonproductive cough, with or without fever. The respiratory rate is increased, and breath sounds are normal or decreased. Occasionally basilar rales may be present. Other signs include generalized lymphadenopathy, enlargement of the salivary glands, and hypergammaglobulinemia. The chest x-ray reveals a diffuse miliary pattern similar to that of tuberculosis. Pulmonary physiology resembles *P. carinii* pneumonia: restrictive lung volumes with decreased diffusing capacity associated with hypoxia and respiratory alkalosis.

The diagnosis is confirmed by open lung biopsy, which reveals lymphocytic alveolar infiltration.

No particular therapy has proven effective in treating LIP. However, pediatric AIDS patients with the disease have a better prognosis than those with opportunistic infections. Some spontaneously clear the pneumonia without relapsing for over 2 years. Steroid therapy has been suggested in progressive LIP, but responses have been inconsistent.

VIRAL DISEASES

Many of the viral disease seen in AIDS patients belong to the family Herpesviridae. They include cytomegalovirus (CMV), herpes simplex virus (HSV), varicella-zoster virus (VZV), and Epstein-Barr virus (EBV). These are all endemic in the world and frequently cause morbidity in the immunocompetent host. Each of these DNA viruses produces a primary cytolytic infection in host cells and then establishes a nonproductive latent phase for the life of the host; the virus can be reactivated from this latent phase with stimulation. Normally the cellular immune system keeps this under control, but in immunocompromised individuals, these viruses can cause significant morbidity and mortality.

Cytomegalovirus Infection

Cytomegalovirus (CMV) infects about half of the adults in the United States; in other countries, especially those less developed, the number is definitely higher. The virus is transmitted perinatally, through blood transfusions, organ transplantation, and sexually. Saliva is probably a mode of transmission also, as evidenced by the unusually high prevalence of CMV among children who interact in close environments such as school, day care, and like settings. Venereal transmission is noted to be more common among homosexual men than among heterosexuals.

CMV has been suggested as a possible cofactor for AIDS, besides being an infection in itself. One study found that a higher level of CMV antibodies determined who developed AIDS from a group of sexually active homosexual men known to be seropositive for HIV.[47] Also, increasing evidence, including a serologic association between CMV and Kaposi's sarcoma (KS), implies that CMV may have a role in the pathogenesis of Kaposi's sarcoma. Furthermore, CMV infection alone, with or without symptoms, shows an inverted ratio of helper T to suppressor T cells, indicating increased susceptibility to other infections.

CMV appears to target lymphocytes or mononuclear cells. Total body dissemination follows by way of the bloodstream. Inflammatory changes can occur in many organs and systems but are most commonly seen in the lungs, liver, and central nervous system. Infection results in characteristic intranuclear and intracytoplasmic inclusion bodies and cell enlargement, or cytomegaly.

Primary infections usually are asymptomatic. If symptoms are present, they appear as general fatigue and malaise or more specifically as respiratory illness, hepatitis, or mononucleosis. In AIDS, reactivation of latent CMV infection as a result of suppressed cellular immunity produces serious, often disseminated disease. In fact, if no underlying immune pathologic condition is present, this illness is diagnostic for AIDS; 90% of AIDS patients develop CMV infection during their illness. As many as 25% may experience life- or sight-threatening infections. Some of the possible infections in AIDS patients are retinitis, pneumonitis, esophagitis, colitis, and encephalitis.

Retinitis caused by CMV infection is the major cause of visual loss in AIDS patients. Symptoms include painless, blurred vision, floaters, and decreased visual field, usually worse in one eye. Examination of the retina shows large white granular areas often associated with hemorrhage and edema and following a vascular distribution. The diagnosis should be distinguished from cotton wool spots and confirmed by an ophthalmologist. Untreated, retinitis leads to blindness in both eyes. Although treatment will halt the disease, it may not stop the deterioration in vision, because scarring and thinning of the afflicted area increase susceptibility to retinal detachment.

The diagnosis is made by tissue biopsy with histologic evidence of virus-mediated damage or by detecting CMV antigen or nucleic acid in tissue. Cultures alone are not conclusive because of the high degree of viral shedding that occurs.

The only drug of choice for treatment is dihydroxypropoxymethylguanine (DHPG), more commonly known as ganciclovir (Cytovene). Ganciclovir, an acyclovir derivative, has demonstrated ability to inhibit replication of CMV as well as other herpes viruses.

Herpes Simplex Infection

The two types of herpes simplex virus, type 1 (HSV-1) and type 2 (HSV-2), have infected 50% to 90% of the general population, depending on geographic location. Highly developed nations tend to have a lower incidence. Exposure to HSV-1 (orolabial infection) primarily occurs during childhood. HSV-2 (genital infection) is transmitted by sexual contact. Although each virus usually is associated with its respective anatomic site, either can infect any body site. Homosexual men have a greater seroprevalence than do heterosexuals, meaning that this group is at increased risk for acute infection. Furthermore, if an individual is immunosuppressed, especially through a defect in cellular immunity such as AIDS, more frequent and more severe herpetic outbreaks can be expected. These outbreaks frequently are complicated by bacterial and fungal superinfections. Ulcerative HSV infection that lasts longer than 1 month is diagnostic for AIDS.

Transmission occurs through direct inoculation of infected droplets from ulcerative lesions with a susceptible mucosal surface or a break in the skin. Asymptomatic individuals excreting the virus may transmit herpes, but this is not an efficient method. The incubation period varies from 2 to 12 days. Replication occurs in cells of the epidermis and dermis. Infection then establishes itself in sensory or autonomic nerve cells near the entry site. Viral particles travel via the axons to the nerve-cell bodies in the ganglia, where replication continues. Migration along peripheral sensory nerves, as well as local viral spread, expands the infection to other areas. Latency is established in the neural tissues following the primary infection, thus providing a route for recurrence. Stimulation such as trauma, stress, ultraviolet light, and immunosuppression often reactivates HSV. This results in transport of the virus to the body surface, where replication begins again. Prodromal symptoms such as paresthesia, itching, or tingling frequently are felt in the area of impending eruption.

For picture of primary perineal herpes, see Color Plate 5, page x. In the patient with AIDS, orolabial or genital herpes as a primary infection consists of vesicles that rapidly coalesce and rupture to form large ulcers. Chronic lesions can form, since the healing process takes longer than normal. Recurrences of increased severity are common as immunity continues to decline. Progressive ulcerations, severe local pain, and prolonged viral shedding are common in AIDS. Diagnosis of either orolabial or genital herpes should be confirmed by viral culture despite the appearance of the lesions. Infection with one HSV type activates specific antibodies that are partly cross-reactive with the other. This does not offer complete protection against the alternate virus but does decrease the number and severity of infections.

Chronic perianal HSV ulcers were one of the first manifestations of AIDS observed in 1981. Pain and itching are the predominant symptoms. On examination, shallow perianal ulcers can be seen that may coalesce to form connecting lesions along the gluteal crease up to and including the sacrum. Care should be taken not to misdiagnose these lesions as decubiti. Any suspicious ulceration should undergo culture. HSV proctitis is also common in AIDS. Typical symptoms include rectal pain, constipation, and spasms of the anal sphincter. Sigmoidoscopy will show diffuse, shallow, ulcerative lesions and a fragile mucosa. Again, the diagnosis should be made by biopsy and viral culture.

HSV encephalitis appears in AIDS as a subacute illness with subtle neurologic abnormalities. However, acute infection can occur and eventually may result in death. Diagnosis is difficult, because tests and cultures may be negative or nonspecific. Brain biopsy often is the only way to confirm the diagnosis but is rarely used because the hazards are too great. Empiric therapy is an option when a diagnosis has not been confirmed.

Acyclovir (Zovirax), an antiviral agent, is considered the treatment of choice for HSV infection. It acts by inhibiting viral DNA polymerase. Intravenous acyclovir is indicated for patients with severe or extensive mucocutaneous HSV infection and for patients with dissemination, visceral organ infection, or neurologic complications. Topical acyclovir is less beneficial but can be used for patients who do not require intravenous therapy or who cannot tolerate the oral route.

HSV lesions should be kept clean and dry. Mild soap and water are sufficient to prevent secondary infection. Analgesics help control the discomfort.

Varicella-Zoster Infection

Varicella-zoster virus (VZV) reaches a seroprevalence in the general population of nearly 100% by 60 years of age. Approximately 2.8 million primary cases occur each year. Most outbreaks occur before age 9, although age distributions are different in regions outside the United States. Reactivation of the virus is called herpes zoster, or shingles. It is most common among the elderly.

The mode of transmission for chickenpox is inhalation of infectious droplets via the respiratory tract. Zoster, although not as contagious, can be transmitted through contact with open lesions. Local replication occurs at the port of entry. Viremia follows, with dissemination to the skin and viscera. The incubation period lasts an average of 2 weeks. Hosts are considered infectious from 1 to 2 days before the vesicles form until 4 to 5 days after crusting has occurred. It may be at this time that the virus establishes latent infection, while the normal ratio of helper T to suppressor T cells is reversed. The virus hibernates in one or more ganglia until cellular immunity dwindles as a result of stress, trauma, infection, immunosuppression, or other events; it then travels via the nerve to the skin. Reactivation usually involves a single dermatome of a sensory nerve. Vesicles typically appear on dermatomes of the trunk, although other areas are possible.

As in the general population, most AIDS patients have already had chickenpox and therefore are not susceptible to primary infection. However, they are susceptible to herpes zoster. The initial clinical signs and symptoms are similar to those in an immunocompetent individual; that is, radicular pain develops first, followed by an erythematous rash over one to three dermatomes. The maculopapular rash progresses to fluid-filled vesicles, which merge to form bullae. Eventually crusting occurs, followed by reepithelization. Inflammation of the nerve roots causes significant pain and discomfort that may last indefinitely (postherpetic neuralgia). A clinical diagnosis is easily made, because the presentation is so characteristic. In addition, the virus can be cultured from the lesions.

Complications and visceral dissemination are common in AIDS patients with varicella-zoster infection. Herpes zoster ophthalmicus (infection of the cornea) occurs when reactivation involves the ophthalmic branch of the trigeminal nerve. This may result in corneal scarring and permanent visual loss. Central nervous system dissemination to the spinal cord or meninges may lead to meningitis, myelitis, or local palsies, any of which may be fatal. Encephalitis may also result from central nervous system dissemination. Onset varies from 1 to 2 weeks up to 3 months after zoster development. Diagnosis is difficult, because the symptoms are similar to herpes virus encephalitis. Brain biopsy may be necessary, or an empiric trial of acyclovir can be initiated.

Primary or recurrent varicella-zoster infections can be treated effectively with intravenous acyclovir (Zovirax), which shortens the duration of viral shedding, halts formation of new lesions, enhances healing, and alleviates acute pain.

As with herpes simplex, the lesions should be kept clean and dry to prevent superinfection. Extensive lesions can be soaked with aluminum acetate (Burow's) solution three to four times daily. Treatment with analgesics may relieve some of the discomfort.

Progressive Multifocal Leukoencephalopathy

Progressive multifocal leukoencephalopathy (PML) is a central demyelinating disease caused by the papovavirus JC. Those at risk for developing the disorder are patients with lymphoproliferative or myeloproliferative diseases, patients with chronic granulomatous disorders associated with suppression of the cell-mediated immune response (e.g., systemic lupus erythematosus, tuberculosis, sarcoidosis, AIDS), and transplant recipients, because of the suppression of cellular immunity. First described in AIDS patients in 1982, the incidence of PML has been increasing ever since.

The papovavirus JC, usually nonpathogenic to intact immune systems, enters the central nervous system (CNS) cells of AIDS patients, replicates, and causes cytodegenerative changes. It is slow growing but relentless in its pursuit of oligodendrocytes, which are stripped of myelin from their membrane sheaths.

PML causes a slow, progressive deterioration of mental acuity that results in dementia. It may or may not be associated with other neurologic deficits, which slowly progress until death occurs. Symptoms range from mild confusion and forgetfulness to blindness, aphasia, ataxia, hemiparesis, and even coma. Patients also have speech and memory difficulties, hyperreflexia, and gait and coordination disturbances.

Diagnostic tests include computed tomography (CT) scans or magnetic resonance imaging (MRI), an electroencephalogram (EEG), and brain biopsy. The characteristic CT scan shows low-density lesions without contrast enhancement, mass effect, or associated edema. Electroencephalograms exhibit foci of slow wave activity in different locations of the brain. Brain biopsy yields a definitive diagnosis, but many patients do not consider it an option because of the poor prognosis and lack of treatment for PML. To date, all therapeutic regimens for PML have been unsuccessful.

MALIGNANCIES

Kaposi's Sarcoma

Named after a turn-of-the-century dermatologist, Kaposi's sarcoma (KS) is a malignant tumor of the endothelium, the layer of epithelial cells that lines the cavity of the heart, blood vessels, lymphoid tissue, and serous cavities. In its most benign form, KS usually is limited to the skin, particularly of the lower extremities. Lesions are characteristically soft, vascular, bluish-purple, painless areas of discoloration. They may be macular or papular or may appear as plaques, keloids, or ecchymotic areas. In this classic form the course of the disease usually is indolent, with a high rate of survival at 10 years. Until recently this form affected only select groups. In the United States these groups included Jewish and Mediterranean men between 40 and 70 years of age and severely immunocompromised individuals such as organ transplant recipients and cancer patients receiving immunosuppressive drug therapy. The disease was rare; fewer than 40 cases were reported to the Centers for Disease Control between 1976 and 1980.

Late in 1980, physicians in New York City began to notice an alarming increase in the number of patients with Kaposi's sarcoma; approximately 30 cases were reported over a period of months.

For pictures of Kaposi's sarcoma, see Color Plates 1 to 3, page x.

Two findings were disturbing to investigators. First, KS was appearing in apparently healthy people, not individuals with known histories of or predispositions for immunosuppression. Moreover, these patients were sexually active homosexual men between 25 and 50 years of age. For unknown reasons, KS continues to occur more often among homosexual men than in members of other AIDS risk groups.

The second disturbing fact was that the form of Kaposi's sarcoma described by clinicians was not the classic, chronic form limited to the skin. Rather, the syndrome mimicked the invasive form previously detected only in a population inhabiting central Africa. It initially was characterized by diffuse cutaneous spread of lesions to the upper extremities and trunk. In addition, multi-

---

STAGING SYSTEM OF KAPOSI'S SARCOMA

Stage	Description
I	Cutaneous, locally indolent
II	Cutaneous, locally aggressive with or without regional lymph nodes
III	Generalized mucocutaneous or lymph node involvement
IV	Visceral

Subtypes

A—No systemic signs or symptoms

B—Systemic signs: 10% weight loss or temperature over 37.8° C (100° F) orally, unrelated to identifiable source of infection and lasting longer than 2 weeks

From Laubenstein.[99]

STAGING WORKUP FOR KAPOSI'S SARCOMA

Skin:	Photographs and biopsies of representative lesions
Nodes:	Biopsy of accessible nodes, CT scan of abdomen and pelvis
GI:	Endoscopy, colonoscopy, contrast studies
Lung:	Bronchoscopy (if chest x-ray is abnormal)
Bone:	Bone scan when alkaline phosphatase level is elevated

From Laubenstein.[99]

---

centric lesions were found in the endothelium of the gastrointestinal tract and other organs such as the lungs, liver, viscera, bones, and lymph nodes. Although Kaposi's sarcoma in AIDS patients tends to resemble the aggressive African form, the degree of systemic and cutaneous involvement varies. It is possible that the invasiveness of KS reflects the degree of immunodeficiency.

Certain cofactors for the development of KS have been suggested. Studies have revealed cytomegalovirus (CMV) DNA in the nucleus of KS cells, implicating a viral role in the disease. Evidence continues to accumulate supporting the possibility of CMV as a cofactor. However, other viral or genetic factors may contribute to the pathogenesis of the disease; the exact cause remains unknown.

Kaposi's sarcoma is a malignant tumor of the endothelium or lymphatic vessel wall. Proliferation of small, incompletely formed blood vessels lined by unusually large cells results in dilated vascular spaces that permit extravasation of red blood cells into them. The amount of extravasation determines the lesion's color or shade.

Lesions may appear on almost any skin surface, including the palms, soles, and genitalia. They commonly are multicentric, meaning that several primary tumors may arise at the same time. They are oval or elongated and range in color from pink to violet to red-brown. The trunk, arms, head, and neck, including the oral cavity, frequently are affected. The lesions do not blanch with direct pressure, and they cause pain only if the tumor impinges on organs or nerves or if tissue invasion has caused structural damage.

Typically, as the disease advances to the end stage, the skin lesions coalesce, and spreading involvement of the lymph system causes localized edema, which can progress to anasarca. Invasion of lung tissue leads to respiratory distress.

Kaposi's sarcoma in previously healthy individuals under 60 years of age is diagnostic for AIDS, as is a diagnosis of KS in previously healthy individuals over 60 years of age who are known to be HIV positive. In 30% to 35% of AIDS patients, Kaposi's sarcoma is the first manifestation of AIDS. The diagnosis is based on biopsy of suspicious tissue or skin lesion; thus the various locations will require appropriate methods to obtain the specimen for biopsy (e.g., oral mucosal lesions will require oral surgery, pulmonary tissue will require a bronchoscopy, rectal lesions will require an endoscopy).

The current staging system serves as a means to compare the research results on AIDS patients with those from patients with Kaposi's sarcoma across the country as the latter are evaluated before therapy is begun (see box). This system has two drawbacks: (1) patients with AIDS-related Kaposi's sarcoma usually are in an advanced stage of KS at the time of diagnosis (stage III or stage IV), and (2) the staging system does not include the degree of underlying immune deficiency. The presence of subtype B symptoms when assessing prognosis and treatment has been found to predict the clinical course and should be considered during staging.

Generally, AIDS patients with Kaposi's sarcoma have a milder immunodeficiency. However, severe immunosuppression and invasive KS carry a poor prognosis, although survival rates are longer than for patients with recurrent opportunistic infections. The average length of survival is 18 months, but the range varies from less than 12 months to 5 years.

Based on clinical assessment of the patient and the patient's preferences, therapy ranges from no treatment at all to palliative radiation or a full course of chemotherapy or both. Surgical excision is rare, given the dissemination of the disease. In early Kaposi's sarcoma no treatment is necessary for asymptomatic disease. Cosmetic radiation may be applied to aesthetically displeasing facial lesions, such as on the tip of the nose. In more advanced stages, palliative radiation therapy may be useful for large, erosive oral lesions, painful lesions of the feet, or swollen lower extremities. The dose of radiation varies from 1,800 to 3,000 rad. Adverse reactions affect the site being irradiated.

Chemotherapy is the conventional therapy for KS. Whether to use single agents or several regimens should be decided by whatever is most likely to control the tumor without exacerbating the underlying immune dysfunction. Many chemotherapeutic agents for cancer have been used to treat AIDS-related KS. The list includes vinblastine (Velban), vincristine (Oncovin), bleomycin (Blenoxane), doxorubicin (Adriamycin), etoposide (VePesid, VP-16), and methotrexate (Folex, Mexate).

Experimental therapy consists of immune modulators and antiviral drugs. Immune modulators are still undergoing trials and testing, except for alpha-interferon, which has shown activity comparable to that of vinblastine. The various immune modulators include alpha- and gamma-interferon, isoprinosine, cimetidine, thymic hormones, and interleukin-2.

Antiviral drugs, namely zidovudine (Retrovir, AZT), are also being considered as possible therapy for Kaposi's sarcoma. Zidovudine is being tested as a treatment for early KS.

Lymphomas

Lymphomas are malignant disorders of the lymphoid tissue, which consists of either lymphocytes or reticular cells. These disorders include lymphosarcoma, reticulum cell sarcoma, Burkitt's lymphoma, and Hodgkin's disease. They are identified by histologic differences and have come to be classified as either non-Hodgkin's or Hodgkin's lymphoma. Persons at increased risk for non-Hodgkin's lymphoma (NHL) are individuals with congenital immunodeficiency, those who are immunosuppressed because of transplants, and persons with autoimmune disorders such as systemic lupus erythematosus. In 1984 a relationship was established between non-Hodgkin's lymphoma in homosexual men and AIDS/HIV disease. In contrast to non-AIDS NHL, AIDS-related NHL is clinically aggressive, with frequent involvement of extranodal sites, bone marrow, and the central nervous system. The overall prognosis is poor.

Lymphocytes normally respond to antigens brought into the lymph node via the lymphatic channels. The malignancy of lymphoma involves proliferation of these lymphocytes inside the node, which alters the structure and function of the node. Immune dysregulation, viral activation, and exogenous stimulation may conspire to enhance this lymphomagenesis in AIDS. Both cellular and humoral systems activate a response to antigens and also modulate the immune response over time. Any disruption of normal immunoregulatory circuits could lead to uncontrolled lymphoproliferation.

Viral activation may occur because of certain viruses that have been suspected of causing indefinite lymphoproliferation of their respective target lymphocytes. These viruses include the Epstein-Barr virus (EBV), which is closely associated with African Burkitt's lymphoma, and possibly the human T-cell leukemia virus, type 1 (HTLV-1) retrovirus, associated with certain rare T-cell malignancies, such as adult T-cell leukemia and Sézary syndrome.

Exogenous stimulation occurs when continuous antigen invasion provokes the immune system into constant defense, such as when individuals receive blood transfusions, abuse intravenous drugs, or have chronic infections or neoplasia.

Painless, rubbery, enlarged lymph nodes usually are the first clinical sign. The neck, axillae, and inguinal areas are the most common sites of initial involvement. As the disease advances, malignant cells travel via the lymph system to other nodes, eventually invading organ systems. These typically include the spleen, liver, gastrointestinal tract, skin, lungs, central nervous system, and, classically, the bone marrow. Patients with non-Hodgkin's lymphoma show a wide variety of symptoms. These depend on the site or sites of involvement and whether the involvement is nodal or extranodal. Pain may be a primary symptom as the enlarged lymph nodes begin to press on surrounding organs and structures.

A lymph node biopsy is done to confirm diagnosis. Once identified, the disease is classified as low, intermediate, or high grade, based on histologic criteria set forth by the Working Formulation of Non-Hodgkin's Lymphomas for Clinical Usage (The Non-Hodgkin's Lymphoma Pathologic Classification Project, 1982). In addition, staging is done to determine the extent of the disease and to establish parameters for following the patient's response to therapy. To accomplish staging, a number of tests must be performed, including bilateral bone marrow biopsy and aspiration, lumbar puncture, chest x-ray, computed tomography (CT) scan, and blood tests. Despite its specific design for Hodgkin's disease (and therefore some limitations with non-Hodgkin's lymphoma), the Ann Arbor staging system for Hodgkin's disease is accepted in staging patients with NHL (see box).

ANN ARBOR STAGING SYSTEM (1971)

Stage I   Involvement of a single lymph node region or of a single extralymphatic organ or site

Stage II   Involvement of two or more lymph node regions on the same side of the diaphragm, **or** localized involvement of an extralymphatic organ or site and of one or more lymph node regions on the same side of the diaphragm

Stage III Involvement of lymph node regions on both sides of the diaphragm, possibly with localized involvement of an extralymphatic organ or site, or involvement of the spleen, or both

Stage IV   Diffuse or disseminated involvement of one or more extralymphatic organs or tissues with or without associated lymph node enlargement

From American Joint Committee on Cancer, 1983.

AIDS-related lymphoma most often appears as high grade, stage III or stage IV. This is a rapid-growing malignancy that responds well, at least initially, to chemotherapy. Agents frequently used include cyclophosphamide (Cytoxan), vincristine (Oncovin), methotrexate (Folex, Mexate), etoposide (VePesid, VP-16), cytarabine (Cytosar-U, ARA-C), bleomycin (Blenoxane), and steroids. These drugs are much more effective in multiple-treatment regimens and therefore are rarely used alone.

Radiation is used primarily to control localized disease, to treat patients unable to tolerate chemotherapy, and to offer palliative treatment.

Despite intervention, the prognosis is poor due to inadequate bone marrow reserve, leukopenia, a high relapse rate, and complicating, sometimes fatal, opportunistic infections.

Primary Central Nervous System Lymphoma

Primary malignant lymphomas are rare, space-occupying tumors of the central nervous system (CNS). They are most commonly seen in immunosuppressed individuals, especially transplant recipients and AIDS patients. The pathogenesis is not entirely clear. One theory is that normal immune regulation is inactive in the central nervous system. Thus with chronic antigenic stimulation, transformed cell proliferation leads to lymphoma.

Patients usually manifest confusion, lethargy, and memory loss. They may also experience headaches, seizures, cranial nerve palsy, hemiparesis, or dysphasia.

Computed tomography (CT) scans or magnetic resonance imaging (MRI) will reveal several enhancing intracranial lesions. A definitive diagnosis requires brain biopsy. However, in many cases this is deferred because of the extremely poor prognosis of CNS lymphoma (survival is 2 to 6 months).

Without confirmation of a diagnosis, often an empiric trial of pyrimethamine and sulfadiazine is initiated, since the clinical symptoms resemble CNS toxoplasmosis. If this treatment fails, primary CNS lymphoma is considered. Although no therapy has proven effective against this malignancy, recent data show a small degree of improvement with radiation treatment.

DIAGNOSTIC STUDIES AND FINDINGS

Diagnostic Test	Findings
Laboratory blood tests	
Enzyme-linked immunosorbent assay (ELISA)	Positive for antibodies against HIV; usually repeated to confirm result
Western blot analysis	Positive for antibodies against HIV; usually performed to confirm ELISA
P24 antigen test	Positive for circulating HIV antigen
HIV culture	Positive for reverse transcriptase activity in T lymphocytes (60-day incubation)
Complete blood count (CBC) and differential	
White blood cell count (WBC)	Decreased (leukopenia)
Lymphocyte count	Decreased (lymphocytopenia)
Neutrophil count	Decreased (neutropenia)
Platelets	Decreased (thrombocytopenia)
Red blood cell (RBC) count	Decreased (anemia)
Hematocrit (Hct)	Decreased (anemia)
Hemoglobin (Hb)	Decreased (anemia)

DIAGNOSTIC STUDIES AND FINDINGS—cont'd

Diagnostic Test	Findings
Erythrocyte sedimentation rate (ESR)	Elevated
Serum protein level	Increased, especially globulin
Albumin/globulin ratio	Decreased
Liver function tests (LFT)	Elevated
Hepatitis screen	Demonstrates carrier state or active disease (positive for hepatitis B surface antigen)
T-cell studies	Numbers and function reduced; helper T/suppressor T <1:2
B-cell studies	Numbers and function normal or increased
Natural killer (NK) cell activity	Usually depressed
Skin tests	Decreased or no response (anergy)
Serologic antigen test	Detection of cryptococcosis
Viral titers	Documented exposure or elevated titers to HSV, hepatitis, EBV, CMV
Other laboratory tests	
Stool test for ova and parasites	Used to detect a variety of parasites, including *Giardia lamblia, Cryptosporidium muris*
Modified acid-fast stain	*C. muris* identified in stool is
Acid-fast bacillus (AFB) stain	confirmation of mycobacterial diseases
Potassium hydroxide (KOH) preparation of yeast	Confirmation of *Candida* organisms
Cultures	Identification of polymicrobial infections
Biopsies	Evaluation of neoplasia, disseminated diseases, viral invasion
Electron microscopy	Detection of oral viruses associated with hairy leukoplakia
Other tests and procedures	
Ophthalmic examination	Confirmation of CMV retinitis, HZV conjunctivitis, lesions
Electroencephalogram (EEG)	Evidence of slow wave activity due to progressive multifocal leukoencephalopathy (PML)
Sputum induction	Used to detect bacterial and protozoal pneumonias
Pulmonary function tests (PFT)	Used for early detection of interstitial pneumonia, *P. carinii* pneumonia
Chest x-ray	Used for initial evaluation of respiratory complaints and to detect pneumonia, pneumonitis, pulmonary infiltrates, etc.
Gallium scan	Used for early detection of interstitial pneumonias and organ enlargement
Computed tomography (CT) scan and magnetic resonance imaging (MRI) study	Used to evaluate changes in mentation and fever of unknown origin and to detect organ or node enlargement, PML, meningitis, and toxoplasmosis
Arterial blood gases (ABGs)	Low or normal with pneumonia
Endoscopy	Used to identify systemic or disseminated disease
Lumbar puncture (LP)	Used to evaluate changes in mentation and fever of unknown origin; useful for PML, meningitis, and encephalopathy
Bronchoscopy (bronchial lavage or transbronchial biopsy)	Used to confirm causative agents of pneumonias or to identify disseminated diseases; useful for PCP, pulmonary Kaposi's sarcoma, and CMV pneumonitis

MEDICAL MANAGEMENT

The goals in the medical management of AIDS are to quickly detect and treat opportunistic infections and neoplastic disease, to manage signs and symptoms, and to prevent complications from treatment. The ultimate objective for treatment of AIDS is to reconstitute the immune system. However, all attempts to correct the underlying immune defect, including bone marrow transplantation, have been unsuccessful. The closest medical science has come to rejuvenating the immune system has been with the drug zidovudine (Retrovir, AZT).

MEDICAL MANAGEMENT—cont'd

GENERAL MANAGEMENT

Code status: Discuss code status at the earliest appropriate time.

Risk factors: Reduce risk factors for infection, such as malnutrition and exposure to infectious sources or invasive procedures (e.g., contaminated equipment, frequent venipuncture, Foley catheterization); obtain appropriate immunizations.

Hygiene: Maintain personal hygiene, including optimum skin integrity with intact oral mucosa.

Fluid and electrolytes: Maintain adequate hydration, particularly during acute febrile episodes and with administration of nephrotoxic medications or with individuals who have chronic diarrhea. Replace electrolytes for imbalances caused by dehydration, especially from chronic diarrhea. Transfuse for treatment of symptomatic anemia.

Nutrition: Maintain optimum nutritional status by providing a high-calorie, high-protein diet, by using supplemental feedings if needed, and by using parenteral alimentation if necessary.

Safety: Maintain safety (especially fall precautions), and frequently reorient the patient with CNS disturbances.

Pulmonary: Provide chest physiotherapy, postural drainage, positioning, and oxygen therapy in conjunction with antimicrobial therapy if needed for pulmonary infections.

Activity: Maintain a regular program of rest and exercise; encourage physical therapy if patient is immobilized and speech therapy if he is aphasic. Provide uninterrupted periods of sleep whenever possible.

Pain management: Administer analgesics as needed to minimize discomfort and pain; assist with alternative therapies and selection of distracting measures.

Support services: Coordinate assistance of appropriate support services, such as social worker, clergy, psychologist or psychiatrist, clinical nurse specialist, and support groups, and involve significant others (partner and family) in care. As discharge nears, refer patient to professional support services as well as to local support groups for home care and follow-up.

SURGERY

Placement of a venous access device, such as a Hickman catheter, to facilitate frequent blood drawing, hyperalimentation, transfusions, and administration of chemotherapy.

Surgical intervention for treatment of malignancies in certain cases.

Splenectomy for immune thrombocytopenic purpura in some instances.

RADIATION

Palliative or cosmetic radiation treatment in malignancies; also to control localized disease and to treat patients unable to tolerate chemotherapy.

DRUG THERAPY

Directed at treatment of opportunistic diseases associated with AIDS; antiviral and immune modulation therapies are undergoing experimentation. The following is a list of disorders often seen in AIDS with the corresponding drugs used to treat each disorder.

Pneumocystis carinii pneumonia: Trimethoprim-sulfamethoxazole (Bactrim, Septra); pentamidine isethionate (Pentam 300); dapsone-trimethoprim.

Toxoplasmosis: Pyrimethamine (Daraprim); sulfadiazine (synergistic with pyrimethamine; together known as Fansidar); clindamycin (Cleocin) for patients intolerant of sulfadiazine.

MEDICAL MANAGEMENT—cont'd

Cryptosporidiosis: Spiramycin (Rovomycin).

Candidiasis: Nystatin suspension (e.g., Mycostatin) for oral thrush; clotrimazole lozenges (e.g., Mycelex troche, Lotrimin) for oral thrush; ketoconazole (Nizoral) (e.g., for esophageal candidiasis); amphotericin B (IV for candidiasis septicemia).

Cryptococcosis: Amphotericin B (Fungizone); flucytosine (Ancobon, 5FC); ketoconazole (Nizoral).

Amphotericin B specifications: central line preferred, usually mixed with hydrocortisone and heparin; often initiated first with a test dose; requires premedication with dyphenhydramine, acetaminophen, and meperidine to prevent severe adverse reactions; used to treat disseminated candidiasis, aspergillosis, and histoplasmosis.

Mycobacterial diseases: Rifabutine (Ansamycin); clofazimine (Lamprene).

Tuberculosis: Isoniazid (INH); ethambutol (Myambutol); rifampin (Rifadin); pyrazinamide (PZA); cycloserine (Seromycin); streptomycin.

Viral diseases: Gancyclovir (Cytoven, DHPG) for CMV; acyclovir (Zovirax) for HSV or VZV.

Antiviral medications under investigation: Dideoxycytine (ddC); trisodium phosphonoformate (Foscarnet); AL721 (Active Lipid); dextran sulfate; CD4 (synthetic); castanospermine; peptide T; ribavirin (Vilona, Virazole); ampligen; iscador; carrisyn (Acemanna, ACE-M); compound Q (GLQ-223).

HIV infection: Zidovudine (Retrovir, AZT); ddI (Videx).

Kaposi's sarcoma/lymphoma: Vinblastine (Velban); vincristine (Oncovin); bleomycin (Blenoxane); doxorubicin (Adriamycin); etoposide (VePesid, VP-16); methotrexate (Folex, Mexate); interferon alfa-2A (Roferon-A); cytarabine (Cytosar-U, ARA-C); cyclophosphamide (Cytoxan).

Immune modulators under investigation: Recombinant alpha-interferon; recombinant beta-interferon; gamma-interferon; interleukin-2 (IL-2); imreg; imuthiol (DTC); isoprinosine.

UNIVERSAL PRECAUTIONS

Medical history and examination cannot reliably identify all patients infected with HIV or other bloodborne pathogens, such as hepatitis B virus. Therefore *all* patients should be assumed to be infectious. Nurses and other health care workers should consistently follow universal precautions when they are exposed to blood, certain other body fluids (amniotic, pericardial, peritoneal, pleural, synovial, and cerebrospinal fluids and semen and vaginal secretions), or any body fluid visibly contaminated with blood.

1. Routinely use appropriate barrier precautions to protect skin and mucous membranes from exposure to blood or other body fluids to which universal precautions apply (i.e., gloves for potential contact with blood or body fluids; masks or protective eyewear and/or gowns when splash or splatter is anticipated).
2. Wash hands and other skin surfaces immediately and thoroughly if contaminated with blood or body fluids to which universal precautions apply (i.e., always wash hands after removing gloves; wash hands before and after any patient or specimen contact).
3. Take precautions to prevent injuries from needles, scalpels, and other sharp instruments. Needles should *not* be recapped, purposely bent, or broken by hand, removed from disposable syringes, or otherwise manipulated by hand. Sharp items should be placed in puncture-resistant containers for disposal; these containers should be located as close as practical to the use area.
4. Resuscitation equipment should be available in areas where the need for resuscitation is predictable.
5. Health care workers with exudative lesions or weeping dermatitis should refrain from all direct patient care and handling of patient care equipment until the condition resolves.

From Centers for Disease Control.[36]

1   ASSESS

ASSESSMENT	OBSERVATIONS
General complaints	Daily fever spikes (39°-40° C [102.2°-104° F]) with or without chills; recurrent night sweats; malaise, weakness, anorexia, weight loss, fatigue, headache
Head, ears, eyes, nose, and throat (HEENT)	Visual acuity changes or loss of vision; white or red raised lesions in oral cavity; difficulty swallowing, throat pain; palpable lymph nodes
Neurologic	Behavior changes; memory loss, inability to concentrate, confusion, apathy, withdrawal, lethargy; impaired communication, aphasia; peripheral neuropathy; neuromuscular incoordination; pain
Musculoskeletal	Gait disturbances, ataxia; weakness; edematous extremities
Cardiovascular	Tachycardia secondary to fever; hypotension or orthostatic blood pressure changes secondary to dehydration; irregular heart rate secondary to electrolyte imbalance
Pulmonary	Dyspnea; cough (productive or nonproductive); distant or decreased breath sounds
Gastrointestinal	Difficulty eating secondary to oral discomfort; anorexia; nausea, vomiting; diarrhea, incontinence; weight loss; abdominal cramping or pain
Genitourinary	Blisters or sores on genitalia; decreased urine output secondary to dehydration; incontinence
Integumentary	Rash (especially facial); red-violet, raised lesions; petechiae; palpable lymph nodes; persistent nocturnal diaphoresis; elevated skin temperature secondary to fever; poor turgor secondary to dehydration; anal or perianal blisters

2   DIAGNOSE

NURSING DIAGNOSIS	SUBJECTIVE FINDINGS	OBJECTIVE FINDINGS
Potential for infection related to immune deficiency, bone marrow suppression, effects of chemotherapy or radiation, malnutrition, frequent venipunctures, immobility, or environmental pathogens	Reports fevers, recurrent night sweats; complains of malaise, weakness, lack of appetite, weight loss, fatigue, headache	Reversed helper T/suppressor T ratio; decreased T cells; <1,000 cells/mm; elevated temperature; malnutrition; decreased mobility; stress

NURSING DIAGNOSIS	SUBJECTIVE FINDINGS	OBJECTIVE FINDINGS
Potential for transmitting infection related to high-risk behaviors and lack of knowledge regarding modes of transmission	Reports sexual activity without the use of safe sex practices; shares needles when using drugs; has a sexual partner who shares needles; received multiple blood transfusions prior to 1985; experiences feverish episodes and night sweats frequently; complains of skin lesions and small lumps around the neck and cervix; complains of extreme fatigue; complains of mouth and throat discomfort	History of probable exposure to HIV; blood test for HIV is positive; body secretions, excretions, or exudates contain viable pathogens; fever; lymphadenopathy; skin lesions; dark circles under the eyes; pale skin; oral thrush
Potential for injury related to CNS disease, mental status changes, neuromuscular impairment, debilitation, dehydration, or medication reactions	States unrealistic expectations of self; complains of sluggishness, extreme weakness, poor vision, poor coordination, and tremors; others report confusion, inability to care for self	History of falls; neurologic impairment; sedative effects of medication; visual disturbances; seizures; apraxia; ataxia
Impaired gas exchange related to pulmonary infection or malignancy, increased secretions, hypoxemia, cough, decreased lung volume, or radiation to lung	Complains of worsening shortness of breath, productive or nonproductive cough, fever with or without chills, fatigue	Dyspnea; rapid, shallow respirations, distant or decreased breath sounds; elevated temperature; chest x-ray: infiltrates or miliary pattern; PFT: decreased diffusing capacity for carbon monoxide; gallium scan: diffuse uptake; ABGs: P_{O_2} 60-100 mm Hg; sputum sample or lung biopsy reveals viral, protozoal, or bacterial infection or malignancy
Pain related to infections, lymphadenopathy, impingement of KS lesions, frequent venipunctures	Complains of discomfort under arms or in groin because of enlarged nodes; complains of fevers, headaches, muscle aches, stiff neck; reports tender, painful lesions of mouth, lips, genitalia, and perirectal region; complains of discomfort in areas where KS tumors are pressing on body organs or nerves; complains of stomach cramping or pain	Palpable, enlarged lymph nodes (especially axillary and groin); vesicles, open lesions, or crusted lesions of the oral, genital, and perirectal areas; internal KS invasion; signs of meningitis or other CNS involvement; abdominal infection
Altered thought processes related to CNS infection or involvement, hypoxemia, fever, stress, medication reactions	Complains of headache, stiff neck, malaise; reports sluggishness, forgetfulness; others report confusion, disorientation, memory loss, and change in personality	Cognitive dysfunction, mental status changes, neurologic impairment; signs of meningitis or other CNS disease; elevated temperature; low P_{O_2}; CT/MRI: brain lesions
Diarrhea related to GI infection or malignancy, chemotherapy or radiation, or medication reactions	Complains of many watery stools of large quantity each day, stomach pain and cramping, weakness, lack of appetite; reports inability to reach bathroom quickly enough because of urgency of diarrhea or decreased sensation	Signs of dehydration: poor skin turgor, pallor, hypotension, orthostatic blood pressure changes, tachycardia; electrolyte imbalance; tenderness on abdominal palpation; hyperactive bowel sounds; stool quantity loss up to 20 L/day; perianal excoriation; incontinence; stool examination or intestinal biopsy reveals viral, protozoal, or bacterial infection or malignancy

→ > >

NURSING DIAGNOSIS	SUBJECTIVE FINDINGS	OBJECTIVE FINDINGS
Altered nutrition: less than body requirements related to GI infection or malignancy, nausea, vomiting, anorexia, dysphagia, stomatitis, effects of chemotherapy, radiation, or medication reactions	Complains of inability to eat because of mouth or throat discomfort, stomach cramping, or pain; reports lack of appetite, nausea, vomiting, diarrhea, and weight loss	Wasting syndrome; cachexia; abdominal tenderness on palpation; abdominal bloating; abnormal bowel sounds; profuse diarrhea (up to 20 liquid stools per day); biopsy or culture reveals microbial infection or malignancy
Hyperthermia related to infectious processes (especially HIV, mycobacterial, or protozoal infections), medication reactions	Reports persistent fevers that may not respond to aspirin or acetaminophen; complains of recurrent night sweats, fatigue, malaise	Elevated temperature: 38°-41° C (100.4°-108.8° F); flushed skin color; tachycardia; diaphoresis, leukocytosis; elevated ESR; positive cultures
Fluid volume deficit related to nausea, vomiting, malabsorption, quantity of diarrheal stools, insensible losses, or systemic infections	Complains of thirst, dry mouth, dry skin, nausea, vomiting, diarrhea; reports weight loss, lack of appetite, fevers; complains of dizziness and lightheadedness, especially when standing	Signs of dehydration: poor skin turgor, pallor, hypotension, orthostatic changes, tachycardia; oliguria or anuria; liquid stools up to 20 L/day; recurrent diaphoresis; increased Hct, BUN, creatinine, specific gravity; electrolyte imbalance
Potential for impaired skin integrity related to malnutrition, immobility, edema, incontinence, frequent diarrheal stools, KS lesions, cutaneous candidiasis, herpes blisters, other skin infections, side effects of chemotherapy or radiation	Reports unexplained bruises in various body locations, skin rash, open sores or blisters or redness on most any area; complains of rectal discomfort, swollen arms and/or legs; reports difficulty getting up and around (especially to the bathroom), weight loss, lack of appetite, nausea, vomiting, and diarrhea	Red-violet, raised KS lesions of skin or mucous membranes that do not blanch with pressure; erythematous skin rash; stomatitis; signs of dehydration or malnourishment; herpetic vesicles on oral mucosa or genitalia; perianal excoriation; reddened pressure points; edematous extremities if tumors block circulation
Altered oral mucous membrane related to oral infection or malignancy, side effects of chemotherapy or radiation	Complains of dry mouth, soreness or burning in mouth or throat; reports changes in taste; points to white spots or reddened areas in mouth, especially on tongue	White patches anywhere in the oral cavity—may or may not easily scrape off to reveal a bleeding surface; may appear creamy and curdled or raised with hairlike projections, or smooth with fissures; diagnostic tests may reveal viral, fungal, or malignant causes

NURSING DIAGNOSIS	SUBJECTIVE FINDINGS	OBJECTIVE FINDINGS
Potential for injury related to bleeding due to decreased circulating hemostatic mechanisms (thrombocytopenia), bone marrow depression, and medication reactions	Complains of easy bruising, prolonged bleeding from minor cuts, frequent nose-bleeds, bleeding gums, rectal bleeding; reports dizziness upon standing	Hemorrhagic spots on the skin such as petechiae, purpura; bleeding from mucous membranes (epistaxis, gingival, rectal); low platelet counts: <20,000-80,000 cells/mm^3; palpable spleen; orthostatic changes
Activity intolerance related to weakness, fatigue, arthralgias, myalgias, CNS involvement, side effects of therapy, dyspnea, fever, malnutrition, or fluid and electrolyte imbalances	Complains of weakness, fatigue, shortness of breath, malaise, tremors in extremities; reports difficulty walking and impaired co-ordination and balance	Psychomotor incoordination: ataxia, dysmetria, dysdiadochokinesia, apraxia; paralysis of limbs, dyspnea, muscle atrophy, inability to perform minor activities without considerable assistance
Fatigue related to disease process, weakness, adverse reactions to medication, neuromuscular changes, insomnia, anxiety, or stress	Reports exhaustion from minimal activity; complains of shortness of breath, weakness, insomnia, and irritability	Dyspnea on even mild exertion; inability to perform an activity for more than a few minutes without resting; sunken eyes; extreme anxiety
Anxiety related to diagnosis, fear of death or dying, fear of hospitalization, perception of unknown threat, knowledge deficit, multiple changes and losses—family role change, sense of self, job, loss of control, social stigmatization and isolation	Expresses fear, anger, denial, hostility; appears restless, agitated, nervous, and irritable; complains of insomnia and forgetfulness; reports loss of financial security and a sense of loneliness	Impaired concentration; inability to process information; unrealistic expectations; inability to communicate effectively; repetition of questions; sleeps only for short intervals despite sedatives and quiet environment
Body image disturbance related to diagnosis of KS or presence of other lesions, wasting syndrome, motor dysfunction, side effects of chemotherapy, depression, social stigmatization and isolation	Expresses concern about appearance; describes loss of friends, loved ones, family; expresses anger and hostility; reports feeling useless and burdensome	Withdrawal; reluctance or refusal to participate in care; depression; loss of self-esteem; passive, nonassertive behavior

→ › › ›

NURSING DIAGNOSIS	SUBJECTIVE FINDINGS	OBJECTIVE FINDINGS
Impaired home maintenance related to knowledge deficit concerning local resources, activity intolerance, self-care deficit, inadequate finances and/or support systems	Reports living alone and having few available resources and limited financial means; demonstrates inability to care for self	Extreme weakness and fatigue; activity intolerance, which makes activities of daily living (ADL) very difficult; minimal income; lack of connection with local resources and potential support systems
Alteration in sexual patterns related to fear of disease transmission; alteration in self-concept; severed relationships; activity intolerance	Reports changes in sexual activity and social behaviors; states recent loss of significant other; complains of inability to care for self, fatigue, and increasing weakness	When seen in clinic, comes alone; when hospitalized, has few or no visitors; never the same individuals visit; appearance is unkempt; activity tolerance is poor; is dyspneic with minimal exertion
Ineffective family coping related to anxiety, fear of infection or stigma, long-term dysfunctional relationships, and demands of providing care	Reports that family/significant others are reluctant and anxious about providing home care; patient expresses concern about how they are coping with the disease	Family/significant others do not visit; no one available to take responsibility for home care; phone calls from family and significant others demonstrate their lack of understanding about the disease

3   PLAN

Patient goals

1. The patient will be free of opportunistic infections and their complications.
2. HIV will not be transmitted to patient contacts or health care providers.
3. The patient will remain free from accidental injury or falls.
4. The patient will maintain adequate gas exchange to support body function.
5. The patient will have no signs of pain or discomfort; the patient will demonstrate methods of coping with pain.
6. The effects of altered thought processes on the patient's life will be minimized.
7. The patient will obtain maximum control of diarrhea and remain comfortable; complications of diarrhea will be minimized.
8. The patient will maintain adequate nutrition to maintain body functions.
9. The patient will maintain a normal temperature; patients with fever will remain comfortable and safe.
10. Fluid and electrolyte balance will be maintained.
11. The patient will obtain adequate fluids to maintain body functions.
12. The patient will maintain intact skin integrity.
13. The patient will maintain intact oral mucous membranes.
14. The patient will demonstrate no signs of excessive bleeding.
15. The patient will engage in activity as tolerated.
16. The patient will obtain adequate rest.
17. The patient will cope effectively with anxiety using individual strategies.
18. The patient will demonstrate increased acceptance of body image and improved self-concept.
19. Patient and partner will be provided with support and counseling to enable resumption of safe sexual practices.
20. Family/significant others will maintain mutual support and adapt to changing demands placed on them.
21. The patient will acknowledge local resources and support systems to facilitate management at home.
22. The patient will increase knowledge regarding transmission and prevention of AIDS/HIV as well as the disease process, life-style implications, and therapy.

4 IMPLEMENT

NURSING DIAGNOSIS	NURSING INTERVENTIONS	RATIONALE
Potential for transmitting infection related to immune deficiency, bone marrow suppression, effects of chemotherapy or radiation, malnutrition, frequent venipunctures, immobility, or environmental pathogens	Assess and monitor skin integrity, oral mucosa, rectum, injection sites, and pressure areas for evidence of redness and breakdown.	Promotes early detection and intervention to prevent skin breakdown that would increase the risk of infection.
	Monitor vital signs q 4 h or as indicated.	Elevated temperature, heart rate, and respiratory rate may indicate an infection; immunosuppression may alter responses; and sepsis may develop without fever.
	Monitor WBC and differential.	Elevated WBC may indicate an infection; decreased neutrophil count indicates increased risk for infection.
	Initiate neutropenia precautions when level is $<500 \text{ mm}^3$.	To protect patient from environmental microorganisms.
	Use strict aseptic technique for all invasive procedures; wash hands before providing care.	To prevent infection.
	Practice universal precautions (see box, page 77).	To prevent transmission of microorganisms while performing care.
	Restrict contact with individuals having infectious diseases.	To decrease risk of infection.
	Administer antimicrobials as prescribed and monitor response.	Prophylactic therapy decreases risk of infection; to maintain blood levels; to determine drug effectiveness.
	Provide a clean environment.	To reduce exposure to environmental organisms.
	Protect patient from injury and promote bodily hygiene.	To minimize susceptibility to infection.
	Promote optimum fluid and nutritional intake.	Adequate diet supports immune functioning and minimizes the risk of infection from debilitation.
	Encourage ambulation; if patient is unable, reposition every 1 to 2 hours as indicated.	Immobility promotes respiratory compromise, increasing the risk of infection.
Potential for transmitting infection related to high-risk behaviors and lack of knowledge regarding modes of transmission	Instruct patient/significant others in methods of preventing transmission of HIV and other pathogens.	To minimize the risk of disease transmission and provide patient and significant others with accurate information.
	Refer patient/significant other to available resources for counseling, support, and information.	Resources are needed to assist patient/significant other with needed services such as applying for disability insurance and special housing and obtaining emotional and respite care.

→ 〉 〉

NURSING DIAGNOSIS	NURSING INTERVENTIONS	RATIONALE
	Use universal blood and body fluid precautions at all times when caring for the patient.	To minimize the risk of transmitting the disease.
Potential for injury related to CNS disease, mental status changes, neuromuscular impairment, debilitation, dehydration, or medication reactions	Assess risk factors: seizures, motor dysfunction, confusion, weakness, diarrhea, sedation.	Early identification of risk factors enables precautions to be initiated.
	Initiate fall precautions and evaluate need for assistive devices (walker, cane).	To prevent falls and injury.
	If patient is at risk, initiate seizure precautions.	Seizures may increase the risk of injury.
	Structure the environment to promote patient safety (e.g., use safety bars, good lighting, eliminate clutter); provide instruction on home safety; counsel patient about driving, riding a bike; refer to public transportation; closely supervise disoriented patient and while smoking; keep objects (e.g., commode) within reach; encourage patient to ask for help with activities.	To prevent accidents and injury.
	Monitor orthostatic blood pressure before ambulating patient.	To check for hypotension; to prevent dizziness and reduce falling.
	Monitor fluid status (daily weight, intake and output).	To assess and monitor for dehydration.
	Evaluate and monitor for effects of sedation; assist with movement if patient is drowsy or unsteady.	Drowsiness or unsteadiness contributes to impaired mobility and increases the risk of injury.
	Refer patient to physical therapist and/or exercise physiologist for evaluation, development of an exercise plan, and instruction on environmental safety aids.	Physical therapist and exercise physiologist provide expertise to the health care team and assist in the development of an individualized plan of care.
Impaired gas exchange related to pulmonary infection or malignancy, increased secretions, hypoxemia, cough, decreased lung volume, or radiation to lung	Assess and monitor breathing patterns and breath sounds.	To detect respiratory complications.
	Assess and monitor changes in behavior (e.g., irritability, agitation), level of consciousness, and skin color.	Changes in behavior, decreased level of consciousness, and pale or cyanotic skin color may indicate hypoxia.
	Encourage patient to report cough and progressive dyspnea.	To promote early detection and treatment of respiratory complications (these symptoms indicate worsening condition).
	Provide chest physiotherapy, postural drainage, suction if necessary.	To aid in opening airways and mobilizing secretions.

NURSING DIAGNOSIS	NURSING INTERVENTIONS	RATIONALE
	Monitor arterial blood gas levels (ABGs).	To determine acid-base balance and need for oxygen.
	In collaboration with the physician administer humidified oxygen and monitor effectiveness.	To minimize risk of hypoxia; ideally Pa_{O_2} >90 mm Hg and oxygen saturation >95%.
	Monitor complete blood count (CBC).	To determine amount of hemoglobin to carry oxygen; elevation in WBC may indicate the presence of infection.
	Position in Fowler's to facilitate breathing; teach and encourage use of incentive spirometer; teach pursed-lip or diaphragmatic breathing.	To improve lung expansion.
	Keep suction and artificial airway at bedside.	To prevent aspiration; debilitation and weakness may inhibit effective airway clearance.
	Administer antibiotics, antitussive/expectorants as ordered and monitor response.	To facilitate resolution of pulmonary infection; to promote removal of secretions.
	Provide preprocedural care and teaching (e.g., bronchoscopy, sputum induction, pulmonary function tests, ABGs, lung biopsy).	To decrease anxiety and provide informed consent.
	Teach patient and family relaxation techniques.	To minimize risk of hyperventilation as a result of anxiety due to difficulty in breathing; to incorporate family into care.
	Teach energy-conserving behavior (e.g., slip-on shoes; sit while ironing).	To decrease oxygen demands and respiratory effort.
	Encourage smoking cessation.	Smoking increases the risk of pulmonary infections.
Pain related to infections, lymphadenopathy, impingement of KS lesions, frequent venipunctures	Assess and monitor pain: location, onset, duration, precipitating and alleviating factors, character, and frequency; ask patient to describe intensity on a scale of 1 to 10.	To guide selection of appropriate therapy; to identify changes in pain and need for reevaluation of treatment.
	Administer antiinflammatory and/or analgesic agents as ordered and indicated; monitor response.	To provide pain relief and comfort; to decrease metabolic demands and respiratory effort.
	Implement use of alternative therapies (e.g., massage, backrubs, visualization, self-hypnosis, meditation, diversional activities).	To alter pain perception.
	Provide thermal therapy to affected muscles and joints as needed.	Causes vasodilation and relaxation of muscles; may decrease pain and provide comfort.

→ › ›

NURSING DIAGNOSIS	NURSING INTERVENTIONS	RATIONALE
	In collaboration with physician consider central venous access placement for frequent blood work.	To eliminate pain of daily (or more frequent) blood work.
Altered thought processes related to CNS infection or involvement, hypoxemia, fever, stress, medication reactions	Assess and monitor mental and neurologic status.	To establish baseline; early recognition of altered thought processes facilitates promotion of patient safety.
	Monitor WBC with differential and temperature.	Elevations in WBC and temperature may indicate infection.
	Administer antibiotics as ordered.	To treat the infection.
	Monitor ABGs, oxygen saturation, level of consciousness, and behavior; administer oxygen as indicated.	To assist in identifying hypoxia; to promote prompt intervention and treatment.
	Provide a structured environment with familiar surroundings.	To minimize disorienting stimuli and confusion.
	Encourage patient to have familiar objects close; encourage frequent visits by familiar people; reorient often and to new occurrences in environment; provide clues for orientation (clock, calendar, radio).	Tangible reminders aid memory and support reality orientation.
	Give simple directions or explanation, one at a time using short words and sentences.	To simplify complex messages and minimize confusion; to promote understanding and orientation.
	When speaking, face the patient, listen with interest, call by name.	Maintains reality, expresses an interest, arouses attention; use of name promotes sense of identity and personal recognition.
	Involve significant others and family in care; ask for personal items to be brought in from home; encourage reminiscing.	To stimulate recollections; to increase feelings of security; familiar people promote orientation and memories.
	Encourage patient to write down things to be remembered on a note pad; keep a date book of planned activities and appointments.	To compensate for memory loss.
	Teach relaxation exercises.	To minimize and manage stress.
Altered nutrition: less than body requirements related to GI infection or malignancy, nausea, vomiting, anorexia, dysphagia, stomatitis, effects of chemotherapy, radiation, or medication reactions	Assess and monitor dietary habits and needs.	To assist in individualizing diet plan.
	Weigh patient daily while hospitalized and weekly in clinic.	Nutritional improvement may increase patient's weight.
	Auscultate bowel sounds three times daily.	To determine whether gastrointestinal peristalsis is present.

NURSING DIAGNOSIS	NURSING INTERVENTIONS	RATIONALE
	Monitor albumin.	To determine adequacy of visceral protein to support the immune system.
	Measure midarm circumference and triceps skinfolds.	To determine protein and fat stores, indicating presence of malnutrition.
	Encourage oral care before and after meals.	To remove unpleasant taste that may reduce appetite; to prevent oral infection and offer comfort.
	Monitor chewing and swallowing ability.	Decreased intake may be related to mouth and throat pain.
	Administer antiemetics before meals as ordered and monitor response.	To reduce nausea that may interfere with eating.
	Provide high-protein foods (e.g., fish, chicken, meat, tofu).	To support the immune system, tissue integrity, and repair.
	Administer vitamins as ordered.	To supplement the diet.
	Provide small, frequent, high-calorie meals.	Large meals act to distend gastric pouch, stimulating peristalsis.
	Consult nutritionist and plan diet with patient and significant others; incorporate favorite foods.	Expertise of the nutritionist will provide an individualized and adequate diet; incorporating significant others will help ensure that the plan continues at home.
	Implement dietary supplements as indicated.	To ensure an adequate diet.
	Routinely evaluate and determine the need for enteral feedings.	To promote optimal nutritional status.
	For patient who has difficulty swallowing, encourage small bites and to swallow only after food is completely chewed; if patient is unable, consider tube feedings.	To prevent aspiration; to promote adequate nutritional intake.
Diarrhea related to GI infection or malignancy, chemotherapy or radiation, or medication reactions	Assess and monitor elimination pattern; quality, quantity, frequency of stool; presence of blood, fat, or undigested food.	To establish baseline functioning; to assist in differential diagnosis; to facilitate selection of appropriate therapy.
	Assess and monitor bowel sounds.	Hypermotility and increased bowel sounds are common with diarrhea.
	Monitor intake/output, daily weight, vital signs, and evidence of hypovolemia (dizzy, orthostatic hypotension, decreased urine output, nausea, elevated hematocrit).	Hypovolemia as a result of diarrhea may cause inadequate tissue perfusion, renal dysfunction, or circulatory collapse.

→ › ›

NURSING DIAGNOSIS	NURSING INTERVENTIONS	RATIONALE
	Assess and monitor perianal skin condition; provide skin care after every stool; apply skin barrier or fecal bag as indicated.	Perianal irritation, excoriation, and pruritus may occur with diarrhea; proper skin protection will prevent breakdown.
	Monitor stool culture and (if performed) intestinal biopsy results.	To reveal presence of microorganism or malignancy; to facilitate identification of appropriate treatment.
	Administer antimotility agents and psyllium (Metamucil) as prescribed and monitor response.	To decrease intestinal motility; psyllium acts to absorb fluid and forms a soft water-retaining gelatinous residue in the lower bowel, has a demulcent effect on inflamed mucosa.
Hyperthermia related to infectious processes (especially HIV, mycobacterial, or protozoal infections), medication reactions	Assess and monitor vital signs q 2 to 4 h while patient is awake and as indicated.	Increased temperature, respiratory rate, and heart rate generally indicate an infection.
	Assess and monitor for dehydration (e.g., diaphoresis, poor skin turgor, dry mucous membranes, orthostatic hypotension, decreased urine output).	Significant fluid loss often accompanies a fever; perspiration reflects body's attempt to reduce temperature; as fever rises, water loss via skin increases.
	Change linen after diaphoretic episodes.	To promote comfort.
	Administer antipyretics and/or antimicrobials as ordered; monitor effectiveness.	To reduce temperature, promote comfort, and facilitate resolution of infection.
	In collaboration with physician evaluate need to discontinue other medication.	Fever may be an adverse drug reaction.
	In collaboration with physician consider alternating acetaminophen with aspirin or ibuprofen every 4 hours if platelet function is adequate, only in adults.	To capitalize on the benefits of different medications; to avoid toxicity from too frequent administration of one specific drug; aspirin has been implicated in Reye's syndrome in children with viral infections.
	Adjust environmental temperature for patient comfort; provide air conditioning, fan; remove excess clothing.	Body heat is lost through evaporation of sweat.
	Provide alcohol and tepid water sponge bath for temperature >39° C; initiate cooling blanket as ordered and monitor response; discontinue cooling blanket if shivering ensues.	May assist in controlling temperature; shivering causes body temperature to rise even higher.
	Encourage fluid intake as tolerated; in collaboration with physician evaluate need for IV fluid replacement.	To prevent dehydration.

NURSING DIAGNOSIS	NURSING INTERVENTIONS	RATIONALE
Fluid volume deficit related to nausea, vomiting, malabsorption, quantity of diarrheal stools, insensible losses, or systemic infections	Assess and monitor for signs of dehydration (e.g., orthostatic hypotension, weight loss, oliguria, tachycardia, dry mucous membranes, poor skin turgor).	To establish baseline and detect impending dehydration; to promote early recognition and treatment; dehydration may result in hypoperfusion of tissues and subsequent renal failure and circulatory collapse if not corrected.
	Assess types of fluids preferred and set up daily schedule for fluid intake; minimum intake for an adult is 1,500 ml/day.	To compensate for increased output; encourages patient participation in care; yields higher compliance; minimum fluid intake will meet basic body requirement; more is required if insensible loss is increased or diarrhea is present.
	Administer IV fluids and electrolytes as prescribed and monitor response.	To maintain adequate hydration and electrolyte balance.
	Assess and monitor behavioral changes, level of consciousness; initiate safety precautions as necessary.	Confusion may be present as a result of hypovolemia; protect from injury.
	Provide skin and mouth care daily and as necessary.	Dehydration promotes skin breakdown; daily skin and mouth care will minimize breakdown of susceptible tissues.
Potential for impaired skin integrity related to malnutrition, immobility, edema, incontinence, frequent diarrheal stools, KS lesions, cutaneous candidiasis, herpes blisters, other skin infections, side effects of chemotherapy or radiation	Assess and monitor skin integrity and status of any lesions daily.	To establish baseline and identify changes in skin or lesions early to allow for prompt intervention and treatment.
	Monitor patient's response to specific therapy in treating skin lesions (e.g., KS, *Candida*, herpes); observe changes in color, size, odor, and drainage.	To evaluate effectiveness of therapy.
	Encourage patient to perform meticulous daily hygiene; if patient is unable, perform activities until he is able; keep skin clean and dry; clean rectal area with warm soapy water after every bowel movement; apply moisturizing lotions; use sheepskin pads and elbow and heel protectors; change linens as needed.	To prevent irritation and infection; to prevent pressure sores from developing and provide comfort.
	Encourage use of mild hypoallergenic, nondrying soaps for skin cleansing, and massage with oils and lotions.	Cleans skin and keeps it soft and pliable; promotes venous return, increases vascular tone, and minimizes edema.
	Reposition or ambulate patient q 1 to 2 h.	To alter area of pressure, minimizing tissue injury; to improve circulation, muscle tone, and joint motion and promote activity.
	Encourage and maintain adequate nutrition and hydration.	To promote a positive nitrogen balance and an optimal nutritional state; to prevent skin breakdown and promote healing.

→ > >

NURSING DIAGNOSIS	NURSING INTERVENTIONS	RATIONALE
	Implement care of pressure sores as indicated.	To prevent further tissue damage; necrosis and/or infection can occur quickly in the AIDS/HIV patient.
	Use appropriate beds and appliances (e.g., air or flotation mattresses).	To provide protection and improve circulation by changing the amount of pressure on skin and/or eliminating pressure.
Altered oral mucous membrane related to oral infection or malignancy, side effects of chemotherapy or radiation	Assess and monitor condition of oral mucosa and patient's account of limitation imposed on oral hygiene and eating.	HIV infection allows oral lesions to occur and may be the first sign of infection and immunosuppression.
	Encourage careful, gentle oral hygiene with a soft brush, toothettes, or salt/baking soda; encourage patient to use mouth wash before and after meals and at bedtime.	Oral cavity is an excellent medium for growth of organisms; routine gentle hygiene prevents spread of lesions; promotes comfort, and minimizes bleeding.
	Provide topical lip balm as needed.	To prevent chapping and cracking of lips; to provide comfort.
	Administer antiinfective agents and/or topical anesthetic agents as prescribed and monitor response.	To promote comfort and healing.
	Consult with nutritionalist and evaluate need for diet-consistency modification and supplements.	Soft, mild diet reduces gum irritation; supplements may be required to meet daily caloric needs.
	Counsel patient to avoid very hot or cold foods or fluids and those that are acidic or spicy.	To prevent irritation.
	For patient undergoing chemotherapy or oral radiation, encourage prophylactic oral hygiene.	To prevent stomatitis, which is a common side effect of these therapies.
	Refer patient to a dentist for routine oral care.	Routine dental visits will minimize periodontal disease.
Potential for injury related to bleeding due to decreased circulating hemostatic mechanisms (thrombocytopenia), bone marrow depression, and medication reactions	Assess and monitor vital signs and orthostatic blood pressure every 2 h or as indicated; monitor for signs of internal bleeding (e.g., tachycardia, hypotension, pallor, anxiety, restlessness).	Changes in vital signs (e.g., increased heart rate, decreased blood pressure, particularly while standing) may indicate hypovolemia, and a rapidly changing condition.
	Assess and monitor body surface for ecchymoses, petechiae, and hematomas.	Increase in number and size of such areas demonstrates continual bleeding.
	Monitor urine, stool, and emesis for blood.	To determine the onset or resolution of a GI bleed; gross evaluation of amount of bleeding.

NURSING DIAGNOSIS	NURSING INTERVENTIONS	RATIONALE
	Monitor platelets, hematocrit, and hemoglobin.	Decreased platelet count increases the risk of bleeding; decreased hematocrit and hemoglobin may indicate extent of bleeding.
	Implement safety precautions for patients with low platelet counts (<20,000 cells/mm^3) (varies between centers; generally no injections, fall precautions, no razors, no rectal temperatures, avoid aspirin, use stool softeners).	To minimize risk of bleeding.
	Instruct patient, family, and significant others about safety precautions.	To encourage participation of supportive individuals and to promote safety continued at home.
	Monitor hematologic effects of medications.	Zidovudine and other medications can suppress bone marrow activity.
Activity intolerance related to weakness, fatigue, arthralgias, myalgias, CNS involvement, side effects of therapy, dyspnea, fever, malnutrition, or fluid and electrolyte imbalances	Assess and monitor degree of activity intolerance; observe for manifestations of intolerance (e.g., tachypnea, tachycardia, increased fatigue and weakness).	To evaluate patient's abilities and guide therapeutic intervention.
	Assist with activities of daily living as necessary.	To preserve strength, minimize hypoxemia, help maintain motivation and a sense of self, and meet patient's needs without causing undue fatigue.
	Consult with physical therapist, exercise physiologist, and/or occupational therapist.	Expertise of other health care team members will facilitate the development of an individualized plan of activity that is well tolerated.
	Encourage regular exercise and a balance between activities and rest.	To minimize loss of muscle tone; to promote circulation and maximum functioning; to prevent exhaustion.
	Structure environment to conserve energy (e.g., keep frequently used items within reach; commode at bedside); provide information on energy-saving techniques to be used at home (e.g., grab bar for toilet and bath; sit to perform activities; slip-on shoes; microwave cooking).	To decrease energy demands and preserve optimum functioning; to facilitate adjustment to level of function and to promote independence.
	Monitor tolerance for visits and phone calls; in collaboration with the patient, set limits.	To conserve energy; to provide patient with control over environmental factors; to maintain active participation in care.
	In collaboration with physician provide appropriate treatment for underlying causes of activity intolerance, such as pain, infections, sleeplessness, or malnutrition, and monitor effectiveness of therapy.	Any factor that contributes to activity intolerance should be evaluated and alleviated or minimized to promote optimum functioning; monitoring for effectiveness will determine if underlying cause is contributing to altered activity.

NURSING DIAGNOSIS	NURSING INTERVENTIONS	RATIONALE
Fatigue related to disease process, weakness, adverse reactions to medication, neuromuscular changes, insomnia, anxiety, or stress	Assess and monitor level of fatigue by noting time spent in activity before feelings of exhaustion.	To guide therapeutic interventions; to facilitate optimal plan for daily routine; to identify factors that may help decrease "spent energy."
	Assist patient in identifying factors related to fatigue (e.g., anxiety, financial worries, relationship concerns, depression) and most effective tactics to deal with the causes.	Identification of contributing causes of fatigue will guide interventions to alleviate these causes; will promote sense of control and emphasize efficient use of energy.
	Assist patient in developing a balance between rest and activity.	To minimize fatigue; to promote independence; to allow time to restore energy.
	Allow for periods of uninterrupted sleep.	Uninterrupted periods of sleep should be long enough to allow all stages of sleep to occur, normally a minimum of 3 to 4 h; sleep minimizes fatigue.
	In collaboration with physician evaluate need for mild sedation at night to promote sleep; monitor effectiveness.	To promote rest and sleep; mild sedation may enhance length and quality of sleep.
Anxiety related to diagnosis, fear of death or dying, fear of hospitalization, perception of unknown threat, knowledge deficit, multiple changes and losses—family role changes, sense of self, job, loss of control, social stigmatization and isolation	Assess and monitor level of anxiety in terms of behavior and statement (mild, moderate, severe, panic).	To provide appropriate assistance, level of anxiety must be determined.
	Provide an atmosphere of individual acceptance; engage in honest, consistent communication with patient.	To establish trust and confidence; to promote relaxation.
	Avoid false reassurance, but encourage hope.	Maintaining hope promotes general well-being and helps the patient feel less helpless.
	Provide opportunities for patient to express feelings; use indirect, open-ended communication.	To help patient to identify and verbalize perceived threats; indirect and open-ended communication facilitates discussion.
	Encourage patient to identify factors that increase anxiety and to generate alleviating solutions.	To support coping, problem solving, and decision making in resolving anxiety-provoking factors.
	Employ simple words and repetition when communicating with patient.	Anxiety hinders one's ability to decipher complex messages.
	Provide accurate information about AIDS/HIV, procedures, and related treatment.	To ease fear and anxiety about the unknown and enable patient to make decisions based on knowledge.
	Teach anxiety-controlling techniques (e.g., relaxation, deep breathing, guided imagery, talking).	To gain control over anxiety and enhance coping.

NURSING DIAGNOSIS	NURSING INTERVENTIONS	RATIONALE
	Encourage patient to participate in care as much as possible.	To promote independence and control over activities, minimizing anxiety.
	Keep room door open at night and a light on; visit frequently and touch as appropriate.	To decrease feelings of isolation and loneliness.
	Involve hospital and community resources and encourage use.	Multiple services may assist patient, family, and significant others in dealing with anxiety and developing methods of coping.
	Refer to community organizations for support.	Support is essential through all stages of the illness; will assist in minimizing anxiety, promote coping, and foster independence.
	In collaboration with physician and patient, determine the need for psychopharmacologic intervention.	Psychoactive medications may assist in relieving anxiety.
Body image disturbance related to diagnosis of KS or presence of other lesions, wasting syndrome, motor dysfunction, side effects of chemotherapy, depression, social stigma and isolation	Assess and monitor self-concept in terms of statements and behavior.	To guide therapeutic intervention and referrals.
	Create an atmosphere of acceptance, encourage expression of feelings, and refrain from negative criticism.	To establish trust and confidence in order to assist patient to improve self-image.
	Acknowledge body changes; assist patient to focus on identifying strengths and accomplishments.	To promote restoration of self-image by validating reality while encouraging and reinforcing positive individual qualities.
	Involve family and significant others in nonjudgmental listening, acceptance, and support.	To reestablish relationships and reinforce commitment and support.
	Encourage participation in activities suited to ability and level of tolerance.	Being successful at something enhances self-esteem.
	Have personal items and clothes brought in from home.	Identification of items from home stimulates recollections and increases one's sense of self.
	Problem solve with patient to arrive at methods of improving body image (e.g., wig, makeup, clothing, participation in a group activity, increasing independence).	To facilitate decision making and promote a positive body image.
	Direct patient to appropriate resources (e.g., support group, clergy, social worker, psychologist, psychiatrist, AIDS/HIV clinic counselor).	Use of resources and support groups may facilitate development of a positive body image.

NURSING DIAGNOSIS	NURSING INTERVENTIONS	RATIONALE
Impaired home maintenance related to knowledge deficit concerning local resources, activity intolerance, self-care deficit, inadequate finances and/or support systems	In collaboration with patient and significant others, identify home care needs (e.g., assistance with ADLs, cooking, transportation, medication, administration).	To guide therapeutic intervention.
	Refer to social worker for assistance with finances.	Expertise of health care team will promote independence and facilitate home maintenance.
	Provide patient with a list of community resources and the function of each.	To provide patient with resources to assist in home maintenance.
	Inform patient about available AIDS/HIV support groups and encourage participation.	These groups provide opportunity for sharing experiences, offer mutual support and practical advice, and enhance ability to cope with disease as friendships develop.
	Assess need for home equipment (e.g., oxygen, commode, walker); arrange delivery; arrange transportation home from hospital (e.g., ambulance, medivan).	To ensure smooth transition from hospital to home environment and facilitate adequate provision of home care.
	Contact professional nursing services if needed for home care.	Nursing care delivered at home assists patients in maintaining optimum function.
	Encourage patient, family, and significant other to participate in discharge planning process.	To increase awareness of resources and how they are utilized; to decrease anxiety about discharge; to promote independence and control.
Alteration in sexual patterns related to fear of disease transmission; alteration in self-concept; severed relationships; activity intolerance	Assess and monitor patient and partner concerns about sexual activity; provide information regarding disease transmission and the use of safe sex practices.	To minimize the risk of disease transmission; to reduce the chance of acquiring other sexually transmitted diseases that would further weaken the immune system.
	Instruct patient and partner in activities that promote intimacy (e.g., touching, hugging, massage).	Physical touch may promote intimacy and reduce feelings of shame and abandonment.
	Discuss alternative sexual techniques that do not involve exchange of body fluids, such as mutual masturbation and fantasy.	Alternative techniques may help provide sexual satisfaction without risk of disease transmission.
	Provide information regarding support groups or counselors.	To obtain assistance with adjusting to effects of HIV/AIDS on sexuality and self-concept.
Ineffective family coping related to anxiety, fear of infection or stigma, long-term dysfunctional relationships, and demands of providing care	Establish rapport with family and significant others; assess strengths and weaknesses in coping with patient's illness and providing care.	To guide therapeutic interventions and promote functioning of family and significant others.
	Allow family and significant others to verbalize their feelings through active listening and indirect and open-ended communication.	Verbalizing one's feelings may assist in gaining insight into one's perception of family function; understanding may promote acceptance and minimize dysfunction.

NURSING DIAGNOSIS	NURSING INTERVENTIONS	RATIONALE
	Refer family and significant others to local HIV/AIDS family support groups.	Families and significant others may benefit from interacting with people in a similar situation; support groups may provide helpful information, support, and understanding.
	Teach family and significant others about the disease and its transmission.	To relieve anxiety regarding transmission through casual contact.
	Instruct family and significant others in patient care activities in anticipation of discharge; provide them information about community resources and respite care.	To enable family and significant others to care for the patient at home and be familiar with community resources for respite care to minimize stress.

5 EVALUATE

PATIENT OUTCOME	DATA INDICATING THAT OUTCOME IS REACHED
New infectious processes have been prevented or minimized.	There is no evidence of inflammation. WBC is within normal limits.
HIV infection is not transmitted.	Patient contracts to maintain practices that will prevent the transmission of the disease; all health care workers observe blood and body fluid precautions; patient contacts and health care workers are not exposed to HIV (no positive test).
Injury has been prevented or minimized.	There are no falls or other causes of injury. Patient asks for assistance with movement when necessary.
Optimal respiratory status is maintained.	There are no symptoms associated with respiratory distress.
Pain is managed or minimized.	Patient reports that pain has been reduced to a tolerable level or resolved; patient can now perform activities, since pain is under control.
Thought processes are within functional limits.	Patient verbalizes increased awareness by responding appropriately to questions assessing orientation and mentation.
Frequency and consistency of stools are within normal limits.	Frequency of stools is reduced, and soft formed consistency returns.
Optimal nutritional status is maintained.	Albumin and total protein are within normal limits; weight is improving for patient's height and build.

PATIENT OUTCOME	DATA INDICATING THAT OUTCOME IS REACHED
Regulation of body temperature is maintained.	Temperature is within normal limits; patient has no fever, chills, diaphoresis, or flushing.
Fluid volume is adequate to maintain normal body functioning.	There are no signs of dehydration; electrolytes have returned to normal, and intake and output are balanced.
Skin integrity remains intact.	Dermatologic signs and symptoms have improved or are controlled; circulation to affected part is uncompromised.
Intact oral mucosa is maintained.	Mouth and throat pain is diminished or absent; there are no signs of mucosal breakdown.
Bleeding episodes have been prevented or minimized.	There are no ecchymoses, petechiae, or signs of internal bleeding.
Activity tolerance has increased.	Patient participates in daily activities and uses energy conservation measures.
Level of fatigue has decreased.	Patient reports energy level sufficient to maintain usual routine.
Anxiety level has diminished.	Patient verbalizes understanding of own anxiety and demonstrates methods to manage it.
Patient will demonstrate a positive body image.	Patient participates in own hygiene and grooming; he verbalizes realistic expectations and acknowledges personal strengths.
Patient is able to obtain sufficient and adequate care at home.	Patient demonstrates knowledge of local support systems and resources and completes plans for adequate living arrangements.
Patient and significant other engage in safe and satisfying sexual activity.	Patient and significant other state methods for safe sex practices and verbalize feelings of sexual satisfaction; both state available resources that may be accessed as needed.
Family and significant others maintain mutual support and adapt to the changing demands placed on them.	Patient, family, and significant others interact in constructive ways to promote caring and support; family is supportive without denying patient power over decision making; family and significant others demonstrate the ability to provide home care and list resources from which they can obtain help if needed.
Knowledge is acquired through individual learning experiences.	Patient verbalizes accurate information about diagnosis and treatment.

PATIENT TEACHING

1. Provide information about AIDS/HIV, disease transmission, and therapy. Teach the importance of obtaining up-to-date factual information.
2. Explain the importance of meticulous hygiene.
3. Explain the importance of regular oral care before breakfast, after meals, and at bedtime.
4. Encourage patient to avoid accidental injury to skin or mucous membranes and to inspect all wounds for signs of infection.
5. Teach safety precautions when the patient is at risk for bleeding.
6. Encourage limiting contact with individuals who have infections.
7. Stress the fact that smoking further limits resistance to respiratory infections.
8. Teach methods of self-assessment for recurrent infections.
9. Encourage the patient to keep a diary of symptoms and treatment.
10. Stress the importance of regular follow-up by a physician or nurse practitioner familiar with AIDS/HIV disease.
11. Teach a balanced program of rest and exercise as tolerated.
12. Teach pursed-lip, diaphragmatic breathing exercises to decrease respiratory effort required.
13. Teach energy conservation measures to decrease effort needed in daily activities.
14. Review the principles of a balanced diet. Encourage the use of dietary supplements, such as Ensure, for weight gain. Encourage daily intake of a multivitamin.
15. Encourage avoidance of recreational drugs and excessive alcohol.
16. Review the signs and symptoms of anxiety. Encourage use of positive and effective anxiety-control techniques.
17. Teach relaxation techniques to ease anxiety.
18. Review safe sex guidelines: decrease number of partners—preferably to one, avoid contact with anonymous partners, explore alternative sexual activities that limit direct contact with mucous membranes and prevent transmission of secretions, avoid direct oral-genital contact, always use condoms, inform previous and prospective partners of HIV-positive status; if the patient is a woman, advise her to seek counseling to discuss issues surrounding pregnancy.
19. Remind patient to refrain from donating blood, plasma, sperm, or body organs.
20. Stress the importance of notifying any health care provider (e.g., physician, dentist, nurse) of HIV infection.
21. Stress importance of medical alert identification.
22. Explain home care to patient, family, and significant others. Instruct them in the care of a venous access device, hyperalimentation, or tube feeding, as indicated.
23. Teach the purpose, dose, administration, and desired and untoward effects of every medication.
24. Review available resources and encourage use.

HOME CARE

Home health care and hospice care are often preferred alternatives to hospitalization. Assessments of the desires of the patient and family/significant others and of the home environment are essential. Patient and home caregiver teaching includes:

- Maintenance of central lines for IV therapies
- Self-administration of aerosolized pentamidine therapy
- Instruction in how to maintain ALDs at the highest level (i.e., hygiene for the bedridden patient)
- Assistance with obtaining community resources for help. These include but are not limited to: income assistance, food stamps, home-delivered meals, transportation, support groups for patient and caregiver, legal assistance, housekeeping assistance, chore services, respite help for the caregiver, and help with shopping.
- Assistance with modification of the environment and obtaining equipment that will facilitate care in the home, conserve energy, and promote independence. Useful equipment includes tub seat, hand-held shower, bathtub and shower safety strips and rails; adaptive utensils for eating, dressing, and bathing; walker or wheelchair; hospital bed; and bedside commode. Refer to an occupational therapist if accessible for additional guidance.

Persons with AIDS can care for pets if some precautions are followed. It is important to keep the animal well so that it cannot transmit zoonotic infections to the person with AIDS. Pets should be restricted to indoors or to walks on a leash, fed commercial pet foods, examined periodically by a veterinarian, and kept free of fleas. Cat litter should be discarded by a person who is not at risk. A person with AIDS who must handle litter should wear gloves and mask during the process.

From Grimes D: *Infectious diseases*, St Louis, 1991, Mosby–Year Book.

CHAPTER 5

Immunodeficiency Diseases

Immunodeficiency diseases are disorders characterized by an inadequate number or impaired function of one or more components of the immune system. Immunodeficiency disorders are classified as B-cell immunodeficiencies (humoral mediated), T-cell immunodeficiencies (cell mediated), combined B- and T-cell immunodeficiency, phagocytic dysfunction disorders, and disorders of complement deficiencies.

B-cell immunodeficiency generally reflects a decreased level of one or more of the immunoglobulin classes and is referred to as hypogammaglobulinemia. These patients generally are at risk for developing infections from pyogenic microorganisms such as *Streptococcus* and *Staphylococcus*. However, they also are at risk for infections such as *Pneumocystis carinii* or live virus vaccine–induced infections.

ANERGY
Anergy is the inability of an individual with a T-cell immunodeficiency to produce an adequate delayed hypersensitivity skin reaction.

T-cell immunodeficiency involves an inadequate amount or a dysfunction of T cells. These patients have minimal immunity against fungal and viral infections. They are at risk for severe and fatal reactions to normal childhood diseases such as varicella and to vaccinations with live viruses. Individuals with cell-mediated immunodeficiencies are especially at risk for opportunistic infections from such organisms as *Candida albicans* and *P. carinii* and for the development of graft-versus-host disease (GVHD) after transplantation or lymphocyte transfusion.

T cells facilitate B-cell growth and maturation into antibody-secreting plasma cells; thus T-cell deficiency disorders often are associated with abnormal B-cell function, which stems from the decreased level of primarily helper T cells.

Combined B- and T-cell immunodeficiency diseases are the most severe, having a profound effect on both B- and T-cell immunity. Because most of these disorders result from the under-development or absence of essential immune mechanisms, an individual with primarily a combined T- and B-cell immunodeficiency is at risk for developing nearly every type of infection.

Abnormalities in T-cell immunity often are accompanied by altered B-cell immunity.

Phagocytic dysfunction is caused by either extrinsic or intrinsic factors. Extrinsic factors include (1) a deficiency of opsonins caused by a decrease in antibodies and complement components; (2) suppression of circulating neutrophils and altered neutrophil chemotaxis caused by a deficiency or alteration in the complement components; (3) a decrease in the amount of lymphokines (which trigger phagocytic cells); and (4) interference with phagocytic numbers and activity as a result of immunosuppressive medications. Intrinsic phagocytic disorders are caused by a defect in the metabolic pathways of phagocytic cells responsible for killing bacteria.

Characteristically patients with phagocytic disorders are at risk for developing mild to severe bacterial infections, which may be fatal. They are generally not at risk for viral or protozoal infections.

Disorders arising from abnormalities in the complement system produce a variety of effects, ranging from recurrent infections to autoimmune disorders. The absence of an inhibitor or deficiency of a specific complement component can result in an array of disorders with varying severity.

INFECTIONS ASSOCIATED WITH IMMUNODEFICIENCIES

Immunodeficiency disorder	Associated susceptibility (examples of microorganisms)
B cell (humoral mediated)	Pyrogenic organisms (e.g., *Streptococcus, Staphylococcus, Pseudomonas, Haemophilus influenzae,* and pneumococci); infections often are recurrent (chronic or acute) and severe
T cell (cell mediated)	Mainly fungal and viral organisms; these patients are very susceptible to opportunistic infections (e.g., *C. albicans* and *P. carinii*) and are more susceptible to developing GVHD after transfusion of lymphocytes or transplantation
Combined T- and B-cell mediated	Fungal, viral, protozoal, bacterial organisms

EXAMPLES OF OPPORTUNISTIC INFECTIONS

Classification	Specific type of microorganism/disease
Bacterial	Tuberculosis, *Mycobacterium avium-intracellulare,* salmonellosis
Fungal	Aspergillosis, candidiasis, coccidioidomycosis, cryptococcosis, histoplasmosis
Protozoal	Cyrtophorida, giardiasis, *P. carinii* pneumonia, toxoplasmosis
Viral	Cytomegalovirus (CMV), progressive multifocal leukoencephalopathy, herpes simplex virus (HSV), Epstein-Barr virus (EBV)

DiGeorge Syndrome (Thymic Hypoplasia)

DiGeorge syndrome, or **thymic hypoplasia,** comprises a set of congenital abnormalities that include hypoplasia or absence of the thymus and parathyroid glands, abnormalities of the ear and facial structures, and congenital heart disease. DiGeorge syndrome results from interference with normal embryonic development of the pharyngeal pouches and leads to various degrees of thymic dysplasia and cellular immunodeficiency.

EPIDEMIOLOGY

DiGeorge syndrome is a rare disease, and the exact incidence and prevalence are unknown. A chromosomal abnormality occasionally has been found, but most infants with DiGeorge syndrome have normal chromosomes and their congenital abnormality is felt to be sporadic. Males and females are affected equally by DiGeorge syndrome.

PATHOPHYSIOLOGY

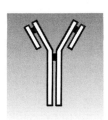

The pathophysiology of DiGeorge syndrome involves not only the immune system but also several organs that develop at the same time as the thymus during fetal life. The type of immunodeficiency and T-cell abnormalities that result from this syndrome depends partly on whether the thymus is absent or hypoplastic.

During the sixth through tenth weeks of intrauterine life, the thymus, parathyroid, thyroid, heart, and certain facial features develop from cells in the first through sixth branchial pouch area of the maturing embryo. However, in DiGeorge syndrome interference with normal development during this time leads to abnormalities in these structures.

The primary purpose of the thymus is to provide the necessary environment for T-cell maturation. Normally the thymus migrates to the anterior mediastinum by week 12 of gestation. In DiGeorge syndrome the thymus is either aplastic or hypoplastic, and in 75% of patients no thymus tissue can be located. As a result of abnormal thymus development, an isolated, cellular immunodeficiency state occurs. The absolute lymphocyte count generally is normal, but the B-cell count is elevated and the T-cell count decreased. Occasionally T-cell immunity improves spontaneously for unknown reasons; these patients are considered to have partial DiGeorge syndrome.

Factors that may promote this abnormal development of the thymus include exposure to teratogens, cytogenetic abnormalities, and mendelian disorders.

DiGeorge syndrome is categorized as a T-cell (cell-mediated) immunodeficiency disorder.

Cardiovascular defects are characteristic of this syndrome, with type B interrupted aortic arch and truncus arteriosus accounting for more than 50% of cardiac lesions. Various other types of outflow cardiac malformations have also been reported in children with DiGeorge syndrome, including a right-sided aortic arch, double aortic arch, tetralogy of Fallot, and atrial or ventricular septal defects. Cardiac malformations are the most common cause of death in these children. Cardiac abnormalities may be manifested by a murmur, congestive heart failure, or dysrhythmias.

Prominent facial anomalies described in DiGeorge syndrome include micrognathia (unusually small jaw), hypertelorism (wide-set eyes), blunted nose, low-set ears with notched pinna, short philtrum of the lip (fish shaped), and antimongoloid slant to the eyes. Moderate to severe mental retardation also is often seen; however, this is not well studied.

Other nonimmunologic abnormalities of DiGeorge syndrome are the result of tissues or organs derived either from the branchial pouches or that have developed or migrated between the sixth and twelfth weeks of embryogenesis. Abnormalities that may be present include esophageal atresia, tracheoesophageal fistula, bifid uvula, and hypothyroidism.

If these patients survive infancy, they generally are more susceptible to infections, especially chronic rhinitis, recurrent pneumonia, candidal infections, and diarrhea.

CLINICAL MANIFESTATIONS

The clinical features of DiGeorge syndrome result from the abnormal development of the thymus, parathyroid, heart, and certain facial structures. The immunologic features of DiGeorge syndrome include congenital hypoplasia or absence of the thymus, lymphopenia (reflecting a decrease in the number of T cells), and a de-

---

PRIMARY FEATURES OF DIGEORGE SYNDROME

Cellular immunodeficiency
Hypoparathyroidism with hypocalcemia
Abnormal facial features
Malformation of cardiac outflow tract

---

crease or absence of T-cell function. Because B cells are somewhat dependent on T-cell function, the levels and functioning of antibodies vary.

Since the thymus is responsible for T-cell maturation, these patients are particularly susceptible to opportunistic pathogens (e.g., fungi, viruses, and *P. carinii*), similar to infants with severe combined immunodeficiency disease.

The parathyroid is the primary organ responsible for regulating serum calcium. In DiGeorge syndrome the parathyroid demonstrates a congenital hypoplasia. As a result of hypoparathyroidism, patients often present with or develop hypocalcemia, hyperphosphatemia, and low parathormone levels. These changes in the infant's electrolytes during the first few hours to two weeks after birth tend to cause neonatal tetany and to place the child at additional risk for seizures. Thus the initial presentation of DiGeorge syndrome in early infancy does not necessarily relate to the immunodeficiency state, but rather to the hypoparathyroidism.

COMPLICATIONS

Failure to thrive
Anorexia, diarrhea, weight loss
Recurrent infections
Opportunistic infections (variety of sites)
Severe hypocalcemia
Seizures
Developmental delay
Graft-versus-host disease (with nonirradiated transfusions)
Malignancies
Autoimmune disease
Cardiac failure
Death

DIAGNOSIS

The hypoparathyroidism and cardiac defects associated with DiGeorge syndrome account for early diagnosis. DiGeorge syndrome is suspected in an infant with persistent hypocalcemia or hypocalcemia that does not respond to usual therapy in association with cardiac defects, especially aortic arch abnormalities. The suspicion increases with findings of abnormal facies (hypertelorism, micrognathia, low-set and externally rotated ears). Abnormal findings on T-cell studies confirm the diagnosis. However, if the immunologic studies are normal and other findings are suggestive of DiGeorge syndrome, the infant's T-cell numbers and function, as well as calcium, should be monitored at least until 1 year of age to confirm or disprove the diagnosis.

NURSING CARE

See pages 125 to 138.

DIAGNOSTIC STUDIES AND FINDINGS

Diagnostic Test	Findings
Total lymphocyte count	Normal or decreased
Immunofluorescence	
B lymphocytes	Increased or normal
T lymphocytes	Decreased
T-cell function using specific mitogens, phyto-hemagglutinin (PHA)-specific antigens, or allogenic lymphocytes	Decreased or absent T-cell function
B-cell function	Usually normal or decreased response to vaccinations
Immunoglobulin levels	Normal or decreased
Skin tests	Usually negative
Calcium	Decreased
Phosphorus	Increased
Parathormone	Decreased or absent
Chest x-ray	Absent thymic shadow, not conclusive evidence; may be cardiomegaly with cardiac disease
Echocardiogram/ECG	Findings vary, depending on cardiac abnormality

MEDICAL MANAGEMENT

Initial medical management of the infant with DiGeorge syndrome is directed toward controlling and correcting metabolic and cardiac abnormalities.

GENERAL MANAGEMENT

Institute seizure control and protection: Seizures may develop as a result of hypoparathyroidism and hypocalcemia.

Monitor electrolytes: Specifically check calcium and phosphorus.

Monitor immunologic studies: Institute serial monitoring, specifically T- and B-cell numbers and function.

Immunizations: Ensure that no live attenuated viral vaccines (e.g., MMR) and no live oral polio vaccines are given to patient or family members (oral polio virus shed in the stool).

Nutrition: Provide age-appropriate diet with adequate calories to promote growth.

Monitor growth and development: Encourage special educational programs as appropriate.

ECG monitoring: Observe for potential cardiac complications.

Oxygen therapy: Use as indicated by severity of cardiac abnormality or pulmonary infection.

Monitor blood products: Ensure that all blood products are CMV negative and have been irradiated (1500 rad) to minimize the risk of CMV and graft-versus-host disease.

MEDICAL MANAGEMENT—cont'd

DRUG THERAPY

Calcium gluconate IV to treat and prevent seizures.

Calcium PO to maintain normal calcium levels.

Vitamin D supplements to facilitate calcium absorption.

Parathyroid hormone.

Anticonvulsants; type and dosage are dictated by seizures and infant response dosages are regulated by blood levels and infant response.

Antibiotics directed at the specific microorganism; may institute prophylaxis (e.g., trimethoprim-sulfamethoxazole or pentamidine) to prevent *P. carinii* pneumonia.

Cardiac drugs are dictated by the patient's clinical status.

Varicella immunoglobulin for chickenpox exposure; with an outbreak of chickenpox treat with acyclovir IV.

SURGERY

Fetal thymus transplants have been performed in the past.

Thymosin in conjunction with thymus epithelial transplantation.

Cardiac surgery to repair congenital abnormalities.

Chronic Mucocutaneous Candidiasis

Chronic mucocutaneous candidiasis is associated with a defect in T-cell immunity, which results in increased susceptibility to chronic candidal infections with or without endocrinopathy.

PATHOPHYSIOLOGY

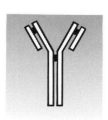

The syndrome of chronic mucocutaneous candidiasis (CMC) is a family of related disorders characterized by an immunoregulatory deficiency. Chronic mucocutaneous candidiasis is associated primarily with a selective T-cell immunity disorder that results in an increased susceptibility to candidal infections. B-cell immunity generally is not affected, allowing normal antibody response to candidal infections. CMC affects males and females equally and has a familial tendency, suggesting an autosomal recessive inheritance. The disorder may appear as early as 1 year of age or may be postponed until the second decade.

CMC is associated with the development of idiopathic endocrinopathies, which are thought to be the result of an autoimmune process. Approximately one fifth of patients with CMC develop an associated endocrinopathy such as diabetes mellitus or deficient parathyroid, thyroid, or adrenal functioning.

CLINICAL MANIFESTATIONS

CMC is a progressive disorder that may appear initially with either a chronic mucocutaneous candidiasis or with the development of an idiopathic endocrinopathy.

If a chronic candidal infection occurs first, it may take years before any clinical indications of endocrinopathy appear.

Candidal infections usually involve the mucous membranes, scalp, skin, and nails. Vaginal candidiasis is often reported in older patients. The most common candidal infections of the mucous membranes are thrush, esophagitis, balanitis, and vulvovaginitis. Itching may be extremely intense, with burning particularly around the vulva and anus. Intertrigo (superficial dermatitis on exposed skin surfaces) and paronychia (nail) are the most common disorders affecting the skin; these conditions often are associated with a dermatophyte infection. Associated clinical features of CMC include alopecia, blepharitis, cheilosis, corneal ulcers, depigmentation, keratoconjunctivitis, and pulmonary fibrosis.

The lesions of CMC are superficially denuded, beefy red areas in the body folds (e.g., in the groin, under the breasts, in the angles of the mouth, in the umbilicus, and behind the knees). These denuded erosions may be surrounded by satellite vesicopustules, with whitish, curdlike concretions on the surface of the lesions. These are seen particularly in the oral and vaginal mucous membranes. Erosions of the paronychial and interdigital areas may also occur.

Severe forms of the disease produce a horn formation with thick, plaquelike, hyperkeratotic scales (*candidal* granuloma) that often are distributed in a "stocking-glove" fashion on the skin or nails or both.

These patients generally are not susceptible to *systemic* candidal infections or to other infectious agents. CMC is rarely life threatening, but fulminant systemic infections have been observed in patients with severe T-cell dysfunction.

Endocrinopathies often are associated with CMC and generally involve the parathyroid, thyroid, adrenal,

> **Addison's disease** is a rare disorder thought to stem from an autoimmune process. It is caused by the destruction of the adrenal cortices, leading to adrenal insufficiency as characterized by a chronic deficiency of cortisol, aldosterone, and adrenal androgens. Clinical findings may include fatigue, weakness, myalgias, muscle stiffness, weight loss, anorexia, diarrhea, nervousness, irritability, emotional changes, hypotension, and pigment changes of the skin (increased freckles, vitiligo).

and/or pancreatic glands. Common symptoms seen in conjunction with endocrinopathy are related primarily to hypocalcemia and tetany secondary to hypoparathyroidism and Addison's disease (see box). A variety of other, less common endocrinopathies are also observed, including diabetes mellitus, hypothyroidism, pernicious anemia, adrenocorticotropic hormone (ACTH) deficiency, and ovarian failure.

COMPLICATIONS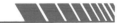

Addison's disease (major cause of death)
Nephrotoxicity secondary to long-term drug therapy
Psychologic difficulties with severe skin infections
Systemic *candidal* infection (rare)
Hypoparathyroidism
Hypocalcemia with seizures

NURSING CARE

See pages 125 to 138.

DIAGNOSTIC STUDIES AND FINDINGS

Diagnostic Test	Findings
Microscopic examination of skin scales or curd	*Candida* organisms
Total lymphocyte count	Normal, but decreased activity
Delayed hypersensitivity skin test to *Candida* antigen	No response
Activation of migration inhibitory factor (MIF) in response to *Candida* antigens	Decreased or absent
Suppressor T cells	Decreased
Neutrophil function	Normal
Serum immunoglobulins	Normal or increased; possible selective absence of IgA
Precipitating or agglutinating antibodies to *Candida* organisms	Present

DIAGNOSTIC STUDIES AND FINDINGS—cont'd

Diagnostic Test	Findings
Serum calcium	Decreased with hypoparathyroidism
Serum phosphorus	Elevated with hypoparathyroidism
Parathormone	Low or absent with hypoparathyroidism
Blood sugar	May be increased with diabetes mellitus and decreased with Addison's disease
Plasma cortisol, plasma adrenocorticotropic hormone (ACTH), neutrophils, eosinophils, serum blood urea nitrogen (BUN), and potassium	With Addison's disease: low plasma cortisol, high ACTH, neutropenia, and eosinophilia; elevated BUN and potassium

MEDICAL MANAGEMENT

GENERAL MANAGEMENT

No treatment currently is available to prevent idiopathic endocrinopathy. The patient with CMC should have close follow-up and monitoring for the development of idiopathic endocrinopathy.

Institute HIV testing: Chronic mucocutaneous candidiasis may be the first sign of HIV infection.

Encourage obesity control: Obtain dietician's help in identifying patient's ideal weight and a program of weight management, to minimize excess body folds and areas of possible infection.

Assist in managing hyperhidrosis (excessive perspiration): Keep body parts exposed to air and as dry as possible; using deodorant for sensitive skin or baking soda may be helpful; have patient avoid heat, moisture, and occlusive clothing, since they increase the risk of CMC developing, and recommend natural fabrics such as cotton.

Avoid all live or attenuated viruses: Household members should not receive oral polio vaccine (which is shed in the stool).

Provide psychiatric support: Patient may need additional assistance in coping with CMC.

Treat associated diabetes mellitus: Provide a modified diet, oral antihyperglycemic agents, and insulin if necessary.

DRUG THERAPY

Oral antifungal therapy

Clotrimazole (e.g., Mycelex), adults: 1.5 million U PO 3-5 times a day; children: 100,000 U PO qid.

Clotrimazole troches may be effective in controlling oral thrush (oral candidiasis); ketoconazole, 200 mg qd for 10 days.

Ketoconazole (Nizoral), 200 mg qd PO to treat thrush or esophagitis; will eradicate lesions (fungicidal); monitor liver function studies during administration.

Local treatment for nails and skin

Ciclopirox cream 1%; nystatin cream, 100,000 U/g; or miconazole, ketoconazole, or clotrimazole cream or lotion, 3-4 times a day; systemic therapy may be necessary.

MEDICAL MANAGEMENT—cont'd

1% gentian violet or carbol-fuchsin paint (Castellani's paint), 1-2 times a week, alternating.

Vulval and anal mucous membranes

Vaginal candidiasis: miconazole cream (Monistat 7), one applicator hs for 7 days; or clotrimazole (Gyne-Lotrimin, Mycelex-G), one suppository vaginally per day for 7 days; or terconazole vaginal cream (Terazol 7) or suppositories (Terazol 3), once a day for 7 days; or nystatin, one vaginal suppository (100,000 U) bid for 7 days.

1% gentian violet or carbol-fuchsin paint may be used 1-2 times a week.

Systemic intervention

Amphotericin B, IV for systemic infections; monitor renal function.

Flucytosine (e.g., Ancobon) may be added to amphotericin B for a potential synergistic antifungal activity in severe cases; 50-150 mg/kg/day PO in 4 divided doses; monitor renal function.

Other drug therapies

Acyclovir to prevent concurrent viral infections; antibacterial agents for prophylaxis; analgesics for pain relief; antipruritics for relief of itching; calcium and vitamin D supplements for hypoparathyroidism; anticonvulsants for seizures related to hypoparathyroidism.

SURGERY

Fetal thymus transplant has been used in the past in refractory cases (depends on federal regulation of fetal tissues).

X-Linked Agammaglobulinemia

X-linked agammaglobulinemia (X-LA) is primarily a B-cell (humoral mediated) immunodeficiency found in boys; it is characterized by the absence of B cells in the peripheral blood, an IgG level under 200 mg/dl, low to absent IgM, IgA, IgE, and IgD, and the absence of functional serum immunoglobulins and normal cell-mediated immunity.

EPIDEMIOLOGY

X-LA was first described 30 years ago in a boy brought for treatment of infections at 6 months of age. He was found to have no B cells, absent immunoglobulins IgM, IgA, IgE, and IgD, and low levels of IgG. The prevalence of the disease in the United States is virtually unknown, but estimates from the United Kingdom suggest that 1 in every 100,000 will be born with the disease.[4]

X-LA is an X-linked disease. Women who carry this genetic disease have a normal immunologic status, and it is not yet possible to detect which women carry the abnormal gene. The abnormal gene has not yet been identified; it is located on the short arm of the X chromosome. Prenatal diagnosis may be limited to sex difference, noted by amniocentesis, and affected males can be detected in utero by the absence of B cells in their blood. It is important to refer these families for prenatal diagnosis and counseling.[186]

PATHOPHYSIOLOGY

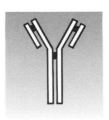

The development of plasma cells is well understood. Two sources of B-cell precursors have been proposed: gastrointestinal tract–associated lymphoid tissue (GALT) and the stem cells in fetal liver and bone marrow. Before becoming plasma cells capable of producing antigen-specific immunoglobulin, developing B cells pass through several stages of differentiation, which can be recognized by the presence of certain cell surface markers, such as surface Ig and the receptor for the Fc portion of the Ig molecules. It is thought that in the normal process of B-cell ontogeny, pre-B cells and immature B cells come into contact with factors that influence their development and maturation.

The immune dysfunction in X-LA is the failure of pre-B cells to differentiate into mature B cells, resulting in the absence of B lymphocytes and plasma cells. This defect is thought to be the result of (1) an intrinsic defect in the B-cell lineage itself, which has not had the necessary trigger to terminally differentiate, or (2) the result of stem cells or pre-B cells that have not had the necessary trigger in the bone marrow to terminally differentiate.[186]

CLINICAL MANIFESTATIONS

The onset of symptoms in X-LA usually occurs at about 5 months of age, but many children are not diagnosed until 2 or 3 years of age. During the last trimester of pregnancy, maternal IgG is transferred through the placenta, providing the newborn with protection for the first few months of life. As the levels of maternally transferred immunoglobulins drop, and with exposure to pathogens, an infant with X-LA becomes susceptible to infection. The availability and use of treatment, as well as the infant's response to treatment, may alter the age of onset of symptoms.

X-LA is suspected when a male infant or child has frequent bacterial infections or recurrent sinopulmonary infections that respond poorly to treatment. These infections usually cause otitis media, pneumonia, sinusitis, and meningitis. The organisms commonly responsible are *Staphylococcus* sp., *Streptococcus pneumoniae*, *Escherichia coli*, and *Haemophilus influenzae*. However, children with X-LA are also susceptible to viral infections. They are at increased risk for protozoal and enteroviral infections despite having normal T-cell numbers and functioning.

These patients occasionally have a malabsorption disorder often related to *Giardia lamblia* infestation. They also are known to develop dental decay, chronic conjunctivitis, and eczematoid skin infections.

Physical findings in patients with X-LA may include undeveloped or no tonsils or lymph nodes and the physical appearance of being undernourished. Quantitative testing reveals total serum immunoglobulins under 250 mg/dl, with low or no levels of all classes (IgG, IgM, IgA, IgE, and IgD). In X-LA the B-cell level usually is less than 1%.

Serum immunoglobulins vary with age and must be measured against age-appropriate norms. IgA and IgM do not usually appear until after birth, and IgG in children under 18 months of age may represent passively transferred maternal immunoglobulin. Additionally, low levels of immunoglobulins may represent a prolonged hypogammaglobulinemia of infancy. If this is the case, a normal number of B cells will be present and serum immunoglobulins will gradually increase to normal by 2 years of age.

Children with X-LA, even with normal T-cell numbers and functioning, are at greater risk for viral infections, live virus vaccine–induced polio, and echovirus. Death is most frequently caused by pulmonary disease or sepsis with severe viral infections. However, an infant with uncomplicated X-LA who is treated with intravenous immunoglobulin, appropriate prophylactic antibiotics, and episodic therapy for infections will survive to adulthood.

It is thought that early, aggressive treatment with intravenous immunoglobulin and antibiotic therapy improves the prognosis in patients with X-LA, such that most affected children can lead normal lives. Individuals in their second decade are surviving with this diagnosis.

COMPLICATIONS
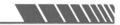

Dental caries
Chronic otitis media with possible loss of hearing
Chronic sinusitis
Pneumonia and other pulmonary diseases, leading to chronic lung disease
Failure to thrive from gastrointestinal infections
Encephalitis or meningitis
Live virus vaccine–induced infections
Malignancy
Dermatomyositis-like disease
Other infections

NURSING CARE

See pages 125 to 138.

DIAGNOSTIC STUDIES AND FINDINGS

Diagnostic Test	Findings
Laboratory	
Complete blood count with differential	WBC low or normal; lymphocyte count low or normal
Immunoglobulins (Ig)	Total Ig <250 mg/dl; IgG <200 mg/dl; IgG subclasses low to absent; IgA, IgM, IgE low to absent
Quantitative T- and B-cell studies	T cells, normal number and functioning; B cells, 0-<1%

DIAGNOSTIC STUDIES AND FINDINGS—cont'd

Diagnostic Test	Findings
Qualitative B-cell function studies	No antibody formation after stimulation with specific antigen
Immunization titers (immunizations are done with tetanus toxoid, to quantitate antibody responses, and pneumococcal polysaccharide [after 18 mo] to test antibody response to polysaccharide antigens)	Minimal response
Cultures	May be positive for the following:
Sinopulmonary	*Staphylococcus* sp., *Streptococcus pneumoniae, Haemophilus influenzae, Branhamella catarrhalis*
Gastrointestinal	*Giardia lamblia*
Meningitis/encephalitis	Echovirus
Radiologic studies	
Computed tomography (CT) of sinuses	Opacifications, altered air-fluid levels, and bony changes
Chest x-ray	Chronic changes
Other	
Pulmonary function tests	Results vary with age and sequelae; restrictive or obstructive pattern may be identified

MEDICAL MANAGEMENT

The goals of management are to ensure optimum health and development, prevent infections, and identify and treat infections early to prevent sequelae. Since there is no way to restore B cells and B-cell function, treatment focuses on providing pooled immunoglobulins.

GENERAL MANAGEMENT

Rest: Encourage rest during periods of infection; other times normal activities are recommended

Nutrition: Encourage an age-appropriate diet, which may need to be modified with gastrointestinal infections and/or diarrhea.

Vital signs: Monitor temperature at home as an indicator of infection.

Fluids: Monitor fluids and electrolytes; maintain fluid intake either PO or IV, according to body weight, particularly during infections with febrile episodes and diarrhea.

Regular hearing test: To monitor hearing loss secondary to otitis media.

Physical activity: Encourage participation in physical activity as tolerated.

Routine evaluation of clinical and serum immunoglobulin status

Dental care: Every 6 months to prevent and treat caries.

Pulmonary function test: To monitor respiratory status.

Health maintenance: Ensure that no live oral polio vaccine is given to patient or household members (virus is shed in the stool); no measles, mumps, and rubella (MMR) vaccine for patient (these are live viruses); no vaccines are needed while patient is receiving gamma globulins, because the pooled immunoglobulin contains antibodies to many pathogens (e.g., polio, measles, and diphtheria).

DRUG THERAPY

Intravenous immunoglobulin (IVIG): Used for immunoglobulin replacement therapy; pretreatment medications may include Benadryl and Tylenol; serum IgG trough level is evaluated q 3-6 mo to determine therapeu-

MEDICAL MANAGEMENT—cont'd

tic dose of IVIG; if serum IgG is less than 500 mg/dl, dose or frequency may be increased; may also be given IM when vascular access is problematic (IM is not optimum treatment).

Antibiotics: Continuous use of antibiotics may be necessary: with a history of *Pneumocystis* pneumonia prophylaxis with Septra (e.g., 5-10 mg/kg 3 times a week); positive cultures of the sinopulmonary tract; and acute and chronic otitis media and sinusitis; appropriate antibiotics are given for other infections that develop.

Antipyretics: Tylenol for fever management.

SURGERY

Sinus drainage for advanced sinusitis; polyethylene (PE) tubes for chronic otitis media.

Selective IgA Deficiency

Selective IgA deficiency (SIgAD) is characterized by a low serum level of the immunoglobulin IgA. The disease is associated with normal cellular immunity, allergies, recurrent infection, gastrointestinal disorders, autoimmunity, and cancer.

Secretory IgA provides local defense against antigens by preventing foreign substances from entering the body. IgA immunoglobulin is found in the saliva, tears, nasal mucosa, and bronchial, vaginal, and prostatic secretions, as well as in the mucosa of the small intestine. When IgA is not available, the individual is at increased risk of microbial invasion.

SIgAD is the most common immunodeficiency disorder reported. The incidence in the normal population is approximately 1 in 700 individuals. A genetic predisposition has been implicated, with both autosomal recessive and autosomal dominant modes of inheritance. Although studies have been inconsistent regarding HLA associations, HLA-A1, HLA-B8, and HLA-D$_3$ appear to be the most common HLA associations. There is also a greater prevalence of selective IgA deficiency in families with other immunodeficiency disorders.

PATHOPHYSIOLOGY

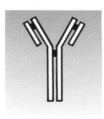

The exact cause of SIgAD is unknown. It has been suggested that the development of B cells somehow is arrested, or the synthesis or release of IgA from B lymphocytes is decreased. However, since the number of circulating B cells with surface IgA appears to be normal, this disorder may be related to impaired B-lymphocyte differentiation. Lymphocyte culture studies have demonstrated that IgA B lymphocytes synthesize but do not secrete immunoglobulin. Therefore the underlying defect probably occurs in the transformation of the IgA B lymphocyte into the immunoglobulin-secreting plasma cells. Some patients also have an associated IgG2 subclass deficiency, which may be related to the numerous clinical manifestations of this disorder, particularly recurrent infections.

SIgAD may be a primary or secondary disorder. Secondary SIgAD generally arises from administration of certain drugs such as phenytoin or other anticonvulsant agents. Withdrawal of these medications does not consistently return IgA levels to normal.

CLINICAL MANIFESTATIONS

The onset of SIgAD generally occurs during the first decade of life. However, many patients remain asymptomatic and survive into the sixth or seventh decade without severe disease or complications. These patients may lack symptoms because they are able to manufacture sufficient amounts of IgG and IgM antibody.

A number of disorders are commonly associated with SIgAD, and these may develop independently or concomitantly. It has been proposed that repetitive irritation by microbial agents and other antigens on the compromised mucosa could predispose the individual with SIgAD to an increased risk of infection, autoimmune disorders, allergies, gastrointestinal disorders, autoantibodies, and cancer. The most common clinical features of SIgAD are recurrent viral or bacterial sinopulmonary infections that may develop into chronic or recurrent pneumonia.

Allergies are also common in SIgAD. It has been suggested that because of the decreased amount of antibody competing for antigens, and/or as a result of increased allergenic protein absorption, antigen binding to IgE immunoglobulin is enhanced, subsequently triggering an allergic response. Allergies in SIgAD are more difficult to manage and appear to be stimulated by infection and environmental substances.

Some patients develop antibodies against IgA, putting them at risk of an anaphylactic reaction if exposed to blood products containing IgA. It is thought that these antibodies are autoantibodies that develop from passive transfer of maternal IgA via the placenta, or as a result of sensitized breast milk.

A number of autoimmune and gastrointestinal disorders also have been associated with SIgAD. Autoimmune disorders include systemic lupus erythematosus (SLE), rheumatoid arthritis, juvenile rheumatoid arthritis, Sjögren's syndrome, pernicious anemia, dermatomyositis, Coombs-positive hemolytic anemia, chronic active hepatitis, ankylosing spondylitis, and dermatomyositis. Associated gastrointestinal disorders frequently observed with SIgAD include celiac disease (defective bowel absorption), ulcerative colitis, regional enteritis, and primary sclerosing cholangitis. Patients generally have autoantibodies characteristic of the specific autoimmune disorder that they develop.

Immunodeficiency diseases frequently seen in conjunction with SIgAD are ataxia-telangiectasia, chronic mucocutaneous candidiasis, and Nezelof syndrome.

IgA deficiency has also been reported in association with some cancers, including thymoma, reticulum cell sarcoma, carcinoma of the esophagus, and lymphoblastic leukemia.

The prognosis in IgA deficiency often is good, and morbidity generally is associated with recurrent sinopulmonary infections, autoimmune disorders, and, less frequently, malignancies.

COMPLICATIONS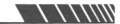

Cancer
Pneumonia
Uncontrolled allergies
Complications from related disorders

NURSING CARE

See pages 125 to 138.

DIAGNOSTIC STUDIES AND FINDINGS

Diagnostic Test	Findings
Serum IgA level	Decreased (usually <5 mg/dl)
Serum immunoglobulins IgG, IgM, IgE, and IgD	Normal or elevated
IgG2 subclass	May be decreased
Autoantibodies	Associated with specific autoimmune disorder (e.g., antinuclear Ab, anti-DNA Ab); may have autoantibodies against IgG, IgM, and/or IgA
B lymphocytes	Normal number of B cells, including IgA-bearing lymphocytes
Immunizations	Normal response
Delayed hypersensitivity skin testing	Normal response
T-lymphocyte function (response to phytohemagglutinin [PHA] and allogenic cells)	Normal
Circulating T cells	Generally normal, although may be low; may have increased suppressor T cells
Hematocrit, hemoglobin, red blood cells	May be decreased (anemic)
Coombs' test	May be positive with hemolytic anemia
Sinus x-rays	May show sinusitis
Chest x-ray	May show pneumonia
Pulmonary function test	May be abnormal, depending on degree of pulmonary involvement
Gastrointestinal biopsy	Abnormal; varies with type and severity of involvement (e.g., abnormal D-xylose absorption in malabsorption); may show antibody directed at basement membrane

MEDICAL MANAGEMENT

No IgA replacement therapy currently is available. Therefore treatment is aimed at managing infections and serial assessment for autoimmune disorders and malignancies.

GENERAL MANAGEMENT

Monitor for infections: Assess for fever, elevated WBC, positive cultures, and clinical manifestations (e.g., purulent nasal drainage, pain, cough).

Packed RBCs: Administer to treat anemia; they should be washed before administration to reduce the risk of a transfusion reaction.

Activity and diet: Encourage a routine of activity and rest and a well-balanced diet with adequate fluids to support the immune system; gluten-free diet is used for patients with celiac disease.

Environmental control: Minimize exposure to allergens and individuals who are ill.

Treat chronic pulmonary disease: Institute chest physical therapy, breathing exercises, postural drainage, and oxygen therapy as prophylaxis or treatment.

Perform serial screening: Observe for autoimmune disorders and malignancies.

Autoimmune disorders: Treat in the same manner as for a patient without SIgAD.

DRUG THERAPY

Antibiotics: Treatment should be specific to the microbial agent, and prompt and aggressive, to prevent compromising pulmonary complications and systemic infections.

Do not treat with gamma globulin: Gamma globulin contains only a small amount of IgA; with IV administration it does not reach the local secretory areas where normal IgA is located; also, it may enhance the development of anti-IgA antibodies, causing subsequent anaphylaxis during administration of blood products.

Antihistamines or cromolyn: These drugs may be used to control allergies.

Phenytoin and other anticonvulsant agents: Administration of these drugs should be minimized to prevent secondary SIgAD.

ADJUNCTIVE THERAPY

Sinus drainage for recurrent or advanced sinusitis.

Common Variable Immunodeficiency

Common variable immunodeficiency (CVID), also known as acquired hypogammaglobulinemia, is a general category of immunodeficiency involving B-cell immunity that may subsequently result in abnormalities in T-cell immunity. CVID is not thought to be a single defect; however, common to all with this form of immunodeficiency is the absence of antibody production and/or function.

EPIDEMIOLOGY

Next to IgA deficiency, hypogammaglobulinemia is the most common type of primary immunodeficiency. It can occur at any age. Frequently the diagnosis of immunodeficiency is not made until after 4 years of age and often not until the individual is a teenager or young adult; in the latter case the disease has been referred to as "late-onset hypogammaglobulinemia." CVID occurs in males and females equally. In some cases an autosomal recessive mode of transmission has been identified. The disease generally develops sporadically, with no apparent inheritance pattern. However, family members of those affected may have a higher incidence of IgA and/or IgG subclass deficiency and autoimmune disease.

PATHOPHYSIOLOGY

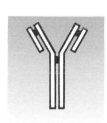

The pathogenesis varies in individuals with CVID. This primary B-cell immunodeficiency is characterized by total serum immunoglobulins of less than 300 mg/dl and IgG usually less than 250 mg/dl. Immunoglobulins may be low in one or more classes. Unlike X-linked agammaglobulinemia (X-LA), in which B cells are absent, hypogammaglobulinemia may manifest a low, normal, or high number of B cells. However, these mature B cells (plasma cells) may be unable to secrete immunoglobulin or respond to antigen stimulation. Because the number of B cells is normal, it is thought that the defect may arise from a problem in the synthesis or release of immunoglobulin. It has been suggested that this defect is the result of increased suppressor T-cell activity or failure of T-cell cooperation. The number and function of T cells often are normal, but may deteriorate over time.

Although the exact cause of hypogammaglobulinemia is unknown, a number of factors have been proposed to explain the pathogenesis of the disease and the alteration in B-cell function, including an intrinsic B-cell defect; failure of T cells to adequately stimulate B cells to terminally differentiate; an autoimmune defect, whereby autoantibodies are made and directed against B and T cells; enzymatic abnormalities; and associated hypogammaglobulinemia following infection with the Epstein-Barr virus (EBV).

CLINICAL MANIFESTATIONS

Hypogammaglobulinemia is suspected when an individual has a history of chronic infections, primarily the sinopulmonary type, and is found to have significantly decreased levels of immunoglobulins with normal numbers of B cells. When tested, antibody production is consistently abnormal. When an infant has reduced immunoglobulins for his age, only time and serial testing of immunoglobulin will determine if this is a transient hypogammaglobulinemia of infancy or CVID. More commonly, individuals manifest the disease later in childhood and adulthood.

Clinical findings may include fever, cough, abnormal sputum, rhinorrhea, sinus tenderness, tachypnea, shortness of breath (particularly with exercise), otitis media, and lymphadenopathy. Chest x-rays may reveal chronic changes from repeated infections, and pulmonary function tests often are abnormal. Recurrent pulmonary infections and chronic lung disease are more common in this form of hypogammaglobulinemia than in other types of hypogammaglobulinemia. The incidence of pulmonary manifestations increases with age.

As seen in X-LA, infections are not easily treated, and often little time elapses between illnesses. The organisms most commonly responsible for the infections are *Staphylococcus* sp., *Streptococcus pneumoniae*, *Escherichia coli*, and *Haemophilus influenzae*. Also, individuals with hypogammaglobulinemia are at risk for protozoal and enteroviral infections, despite normal T-cell function.

Individuals with CVID often develop lymphadenopathy, splenomegaly, and hepatomegaly. Gastrointestinal problems, including infections (e.g., giardiasis) and protein-losing and malabsorptive gastroenteropathies, are commonly reported and are manifested by diarrhea, weight loss, and abdominal pain.

Autoimmune disorders also have been associated with hypogammaglobulinemia, such as systemic lupus erythematosus (SLE), idiopathic thrombocytopenic purpura, hemolytic anemia, dermatomyositis, Graves' disease, and a disorder resembling rheumatoid arthritis. Accompanying signs and symptoms may include rash, fatigue, arthralgia, myalgia, proximal muscle weakness, arthritis, bruising, and bleeding.

Although hypogammaglobulinemia is predominantly a B-cell defect, in time it may involve T cells. When T-cell defects develop, cellular immunity is impaired and the potential for other types of infection and complications increases. The individual also becomes more susceptible to viral and opportunistic infections and to malignancies, primarily lymphomas and gastric cancers.

As with X-LA, it has been postulated that before intravenous gamma globulin was available, persons with CVID had a higher incidence of problems and complications. It is believed that this treatment, as well as early identification and treatment of infections, will improve the prognosis for individuals with CVID.

COMPLICATIONS

Conjunctivitis
Dental caries
Chronic otitis media (may lead to hearing loss)

Chronic sinusitis
Pulmonary infections (bronchiectasis)
Restrictive and obstructive lung disease
Failure to thrive
Gastrointestinal infections
Protein-losing enteropathies
Encephalitis, meningitis
Live virus–induced infections
Malignancies (lymphomas and gastric cancers)
Granulomas
Thrombocytopenia
Coombs-positive hemolytic anemia
Oligoarthritis
Dermatomyositis
Lupus-like disease

NURSING CARE

See pages 125 to 138.

DIAGNOSTIC STUDIES AND FINDINGS

Diagnostic Test	Findings
Laboratory tests	
Complete blood count with differential	Decreased Hb and Hct may be present, related to associated disorders (e.g., hemolytic anemia, pernicious anemia)
Immunoglobulins	Serum immunoglobulins <300 mg/dl; IgG usually <250 mg/dl
Quantitative T- and B-cell studies	Number of B cells may be low, normal, or high; number of T cells usually is normal early on but may decrease over time
Qualitative B-cell function studies (titers before and after immunization)	No antibody formation after stimulation with specific antigen
Qualitative T-cell studies (PHA)	Normal, but may deteriorate over time
Cultures	
Sinopulmonary drainage	*Staphylococcus* organisms, *S. pneumoniae, H. influenzae, Branhamella catarrhalis*
Stool	*Giardia lamblia*
Spinal fluid	Echovirus (meningitis/encephalitis)
Radiologic studies	
Computed tomography (CT) scan of sinuses	Opacifications with altered air-fluid levels and bony changes
Chest x-ray	Chronic changes
Pulmonary function tests	Findings vary with age; may show restrictive or obstructive lung disease
Lymphoid tissue biopsy	Decreased plasma cells
Antinuclear antibodies (ANA)	To detect autoimmune disease

MEDICAL MANAGEMENT

The goal of treatment is to ensure optimum health and development. Management is directed at preventing infections and treating them early if they develop.

GENERAL MANAGEMENT

Rest: Encourage rest during periods of infection.

Monitor vital signs: Observe closely for evidence of fever and possible infection.

Nutrition: Encourage age-appropriate diet; adapt diet for gastrointestinal infections or malabsorption problems.

Fluids and electrolytes: Monitor for dehydration and electrolyte disturbances secondary to fever and/or gastrointestinal disorders (e.g., diarrhea).

Regular hearing test: To monitor hearing loss secondary to otitis media..

Monitor pulmonary status: At routine intervals, check chest x-ray, pulmonary function tests, and tolerance for physical activity with individuals who have developed chronic lung disease.

Regular dental visits: To prevent and treat dental caries.

Health maintenance: Ensure that no live oral polio vaccine is given to the patient or a household member (the virus is shed in the stool); no measles, mumps, and rubella (MMR) vaccine is given to the patient (these are live viruses); no vaccines are needed while the patient is receiving gamma globulin, because the pooled immunoglobulins contain antibodies to many pathogens including polio, measles, and diphtheria.

DRUG THERAPY

Gamma globulin: IV gamma globulin (IVIG) is given q 3-4 wk (100-400 mg/kg); during an acute illness, may be given weekly or daily; premedication may include Benadryl and Tylenol; first infusion is given in the hospital to allow monitoring for potential reactions (may be given IM though not as effective).

Antibiotics: Prophylaxis achieved with Septra for a history of *Pneumocystis* or poor T cell numbers and/or function (usually 3 consecutive days a week); all infections and positive cultures require treatment with the appropriate antibiotics.

Antipyretics: Tylenol is given for fever while patient is taking antibiotics.

SURGERY

Sinus drainage for chronic and recurrent infection; polyethylene (PE) tubes for chronic otitis; splenectomy has been performed for hemolytic anemia and hypogammaglobulinemia, but the mortality rate from disseminating infection is very high.

Wiskott-Aldrich Syndrome

Wiskott-Aldrich syndrome (WAS) is an X-linked, recessive immunodeficiency disorder in males characterized by thrombocytopenia, eczema, and recurrent pyogenic infections.

PATHOPHYSIOLOGY

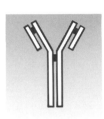

Wiskott-Aldrich syndrome is a rare disorder first described by Wiskott in 1937. There are approximately 4 cases per 1 million live male births. WAS is associated with thrombocytopenia, eczema, and recurrent infections. Although the underlying defect is unknown, it has been established that WAS involves both cellular and humoral immunity.

Several explanations have been postulated about the pathogenesis of WAS, including: (1) the absence of a specific surface glycoprotein, which normally is present in lymphocytes, monocytes, and platelets; its absence causes a decrease in the size of lymphocytes; (2) patients with WAS are known to be unable to respond to polysaccharide antigens; and (3) abnormal granules in platelets and macrophages render them ineffective against infectious invasion.

CLINICAL MANIFESTATIONS

Although the severity of the immunodeficiency varies, the affected child typically manifests recurrent infections, petechiae, and/or bleeding episodes within the first 6 months. The most common bacterial infections result in meningitis, otitis media, skin abscesses, pneumonia, and sepsis. As these children grow older, they become increasingly susceptible to other types of organisms and may have recurrent infections caused by viruses (e.g., herpes or cytomegalovirus [CMV]), protozoa (e.g., *Pneumocystis carinii*), or fungi (e.g., *Candida* sp.).

Eczema generally is present by 1 year of age in patients with WAS. It frequently is associated with thrombocytopenia and is often secondarily infected. Thrombocytopenia, in association with bleeding, typically is present at birth and often is worse during infectious episodes. Bleeding, which may be life threatening, may occur anywhere, as demonstrated by epistaxis, hematuria, or intracranial or conjunctival hemorrhage.

Patients with WAS who survive into their teens become susceptible to malignancies. Approximately 10% of patients develop cancer. Acute leukemia and lymphomas are the most common malignances reported.

COMPLICATIONS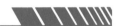

Recurrent or persistent infection
Life-threatening sepsis
Acute hemorrhage
Exsanguination and death
Acute leukemia
Lymphomas
Lymphoreticular cancers of the central nervous system
Chronic keratitis
Chronic renal failure

NURSING CARE

See pages 125 to 138.

DIAGNOSTIC STUDIES AND FINDINGS

Diagnostic Test	Findings
Platelet count	Markedly decreased; also, platelets are very small
Isohemagglutinins	Low or absent
T-cell function	Normal but decreases with age
Circulating lymphocytes	Normal numbers
Immunoglobulins	Normal or increased IgG, decreased IgM, increased IgA and IgE

DIAGNOSTIC STUDIES AND FINDINGS—cont'd

Diagnostic Test	Findings
Immunization with polysaccharide antigen	Impaired response
Monocytes and macrophages	Abnormal
Hematocrit and hemoglobin	Decreased (anemia)
Coombs' test	May be positive
Urinalysis	Hematuria

MEDICAL MANAGEMENT

GENERAL MANAGEMENT

Monitor platelet count: Institute bleeding precautions for levels <25,000/mm^3 or standard set in specific facility.

Monitor for bleeding: Assess for clinical manifestations of bleeding (e.g., ecchymosis, petechia, active bleeding); test all body secretions for blood (e.g., stool, urine, emesis, sputum); severe epistaxis may require nasal packing.

Monitor for infection: Observe for fever, positive cultures, and clinical manifestations (e.g., productive cough, oozing rash).

Activity: Encourage patient to avoid contact sports to minimize risk of bleeding.

Health maintenance: Encourage parent to maintain a safe environment (e.g., no sharp toys, pad crib or bed); immunizations with live attenuated viruses should be avoided; all blood products should be CMV negative and irradiated with 1500 rad before administration; breast milk should be avoided (may contain competent lymphocytes).

DRUG THERAPY

Platelet transfusions: Transfusions are given to treat or prevent bleeding.

Intravenous immunoglobulin (IVIG): IVIG is used to minimize the risk of infection; should be given only IV; IM injection may cause unnecessary bleeding.

Antibiotics: Infections should be treated promptly and aggressively with the appropriate antibiotics; prophylactic therapy may be used with frequent recurrent infections or for *P. carinii* infection, using trimethoprim-sulfamethoxazole (e.g., Septra); in many cases oral penicillin is administered daily to patients who have undergone a splenectomy.

Corticosteroids: Corticosteroids should be avoided in treating thrombocytopenia, because they increase the risk of infection.

ADJUNCTIVE THERAPY

Bone marrow transplant (80% survival rate with a matched sibling donor); splenectomy for uncontrollable bleeding or for increased risk of intracranial bleeding.

Severe Combined Immunodeficiency Disease

Severe combined immunodeficiency disease (SCID) is characterized by the complete absence of normal cell-mediated (T-cell) and antibody-mediated (B-cell) immunity. Unless diagnosed and treated promptly, infants with this disorder develop life-threatening infections and frequently die before 1 year of age.

EPIDEMIOLOGY

The exact incidence of SCID is unknown, and many infants die before the diagnosis is made. It is the most serious of all the primary immunodeficiency diseases, with a variety of different identifiable forms. Most SCID cases are inherited either in an autosomal recessive or in an X-linked manner; however, there are a number of sporadic forms as well.

It is now well recognized that there are many variants of this condition. For example, some cases involve only a partial loss of T-cell function, whereas others manifest almost complete T-cell loss. In approximately 60% of autosomal recessive cases, enzyme abnormalities in purine metabolism may be identified. The most common is adenosine deaminase (ADA) deficiency. ADA is an essential enzyme for normal lymphocyte function. Another enzyme deficiency associated with SCID is purine nucleotide phosphorylase (PNP) deficiency. Similar variations may be observed in B-cell immunity with regard to immunoglobulin patterns.

PATHOPHYSIOLOGY

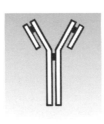

Infants with SCID have an immunodeficiency of both T and B cells. The causative defect is unknown, but the most popular explanation is the absence of a stem cell population. It has also been proposed that SCID results from the failure of stem cells to differentiate into T and B lymphocytes. Another theory is that the thymus or bursa equivalent (the bursa of Fabricius is the anatomic location of B-cell differentiation in birds) fails to develop normally, not allowing for an environment conducive to effective lymphocyte differentiation. A final explanation is that a defect exists in the thymus and bone marrow, the organs primarily responsible for T- and B-cell development.

CLINICAL MANIFESTATIONS

Infants with SCID often have life-threatening bacterial, fungal, protozoal, and/or viral infections and frequently die before 1 year of age. Organisms most commonly responsible for these infections include respiratory syncytial virus (RSV), parainfluenza virus, *Escherichia coli*, and *Haemophilus influenzae*, with particular susceptibility to candidal infections, *Pneumocystis carinii* pneumonia, and cytomegalovirus (CMV). During the first few months after birth, infants may be protected from bacterial infections by the passive transplacental delivery of maternal IgG antibodies. This passive transfer of immunoglobulin may protect them from being symptomatic from the disease for a couple of months after birth. However, they generally develop susceptibility to a variety of gram-positive and gram-negative organisms.

Clinical signs and symptoms typically start soon after birth. The specific features of SCID are primarily reflected in the recurrent nature, type, location, and severity of infection. Common findings include pneumonia, oral candidiasis, and chronic otitis media. Other frequent findings include oral ulcers, failure to thrive, chronic diarrhea, and dermatitis. Although rarely seen, an infant with SCID can develop viral infections and progressive poliomyelitis following immunization with a live virus vaccine such as oral polio.

Patients with SCID are also at risk for developing graft-versus-host disease (GVHD). This is the result of maternal infusion of immunocompetent lymphocytes that have crossed the placenta and entered the fetal circulation. Administration of nonirradiated blood may also result in GVHD.

COMPLICATIONS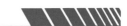

Chronic, recurrent, and fulminant infections
Anemia
Progressive poliomyelitis
Graft-versus-host disease
Death

NURSING CARE

See pages 125 to 138.

DIAGNOSTIC STUDIES AND FINDINGS

Diagnostic Test	Findings
Total lymphocyte count	Decreased absolute lymphocyte count, usually <1,000/μl; in newborns <2,500/μl is abnormal
T cells	Lymphopenia; depressed T-cell numbers
CD3	Low or absent
CD4	Absent
CD8	Absent
Immunoglobulins	Decreased; loss of antibody response following immunization
B cells	Absent (may be present in purine nucleotide phosphorylase [PNP]); few or absent circulating B cells
Lymphocyte function (response to PHA, PWM, allogeneic cells, and antigens)	Markedly diminished or absent
Skin testing	Absent delayed hypersensitivity response
Adenosine deaminase enzyme	Activity may be absent
Chest x-ray	Thymus shadow absent
Skin biopsy	Demonstrates invasion of foreign cells into the skin to establish GVHD (e.g., maternal immunocompetent T cells)
Open lung biopsy	To confirm *P. carinii* infection if suspected
Fetal blood sampling	Decreased levels of lymphocytes

MEDICAL MANAGEMENT

GENERAL MANAGEMENT

Prenatal: Family counseling should be offered following test results to assist parents in making a decision to abort or maintain the pregnancy. If the parents decide to maintain the pregnancy, a cesarean section delivery into a sterile environment is recommended.

Neonatal: The diagnosis of SCID is confirmed, and arrangements for a bone marrow transplant (BMT) are made as soon as possible while the infant is not infected. Keep the infant in a protected environment until after the BMT and adequate recovery of the immune system.

Routinely monitor for infections: Observe for fevers, cultures, and clinical manifestations.

General health: Avoid immunizations with live attenuated viruses; housemates (e.g., siblings) should not receive oral polio, because it is shed in the stool; avoid blood products containing immunocompetent lymphocytes; all blood products should be CMV negative and irradiated with 1500 rad before administration; avoid breast milk, because it may contain competent lymphocytes, resulting in GVHD.

DRUG THERAPY

Immunoglobulin: May be given IV (100-400 mg/kg q 1-4 wk) or IM (0.2-0.4 ml/kg every month); dosage varies according to the severity of the illness and patient response.

Specific antibiotic therapy: Should be used to treat infections; prophylaxis is encouraged for patients with chronic or recurrent infections (e.g., trimethoprim-sulfamethoxazole [Septra, Bactrim] to prevent pneumocystosis).

ADJUNCTIVE THERAPY

Bone marrow transplantation (BMT).

Disorders of Complement

Complement components participate in host defense by killing bacteria, through opsonization and chemotaxis, and possibly by eliminating antigen-antibody complexes. Thus complement deficiencies may result in a number of defects, ranging from recurrent bacterial infections to an increased risk of autoimmune disorders. In particular, systemic lupus erythematosus (SLE) and glomerulonephritis have been associated with deficiencies in complement components C1, C4, and C2.

Disorders of complement have also been associated with genetic defects that are inherited primarily as autosomal recessive traits. Affected individuals are those with no gene product, who have two heterozygous-deficient parents. When an individual is totally deficient in one of the classic pathway proteins or one of the terminal components, the lytic function and complement titer (CH_{50}) are absent. This is also true for the alternative pathway.

When there is a deficiency in one of the classic complement components, normal activation of the complement cascade can occur only to the point of the deficient component. Theoretically, activation of the remainder of the cascade should not occur. However, because the classic and alternative pathways share the same terminal components, activation through another point in the cascade compensates for the deficiency.

Deficiencies in C1, C4, and C2 proteins are the most common. Generally individuals with these deficiencies are in good health and do not develop recurrent infections. However, when infections do occur, they usually are bacterial. C2 is also often associated with autoimmune diseases, particularly SLE and juvenile rheumatoid arthritis.

C3 is vital to both the classic and alternative complement pathways. Individuals with C3 deficiencies experience frequent recurrent bacterial infections and run a greater risk of developing chronic glomerulonephritis. Individuals with deficiencies in C5 through C8 also have an increased risk of infection, primarily with recurrent *Neisseria* disorders.

Hereditary angioedema is an autosomal dominant disorder associated with C1 inhibitor deficiency. Without this inhibitor the action of C1 on C4 or C2 is left uncontrolled, resulting in the release of large amounts of vasoactive peptides, which increase vascular permeability. This disorder is characterized by recurrent episodes of subcutaneous and submucosal local edema that lasts 1 to 4 days. It primarily affects the extremities and gastrointestinal mucosa but can be life threatening when the upper airway is involved. Treatment includes avoiding precipitating factors (e.g., trauma and emotional stress) and using drug therapy, primarily plasmin inhibitors and anabolic steroids.

Secondary complement deficiencies arise when a disease decreases synthesis or triggers increased consumption of complement proteins. With increased activation, as occurs in immune-complex disorders, increased tissue damage results because of the inflammatory mechanisms modulated by complement. Some disorders associated with secondary deficiencies of complement are asplenia, sickle cell anemia, protein-deficient states (e.g., burns, cirrhosis), acute nephritis, immune-complex disease (e.g., SLE), and bacteremia.

DIAGNOSTIC STUDIES AND FINDINGS

Studies and findings vary, depending on disease involved and laboratory reading the test (see box).

NURSING CARE

See pages 125 to 138.

MEDICAL MANAGEMENT

Currently no treatment is available for complement disorders. Management consists primarily of antibiotic prophylaxis and aggressive antibiotic therapy for infection (e.g., Septra).

PROTEINS OF THE COMPLEMENT SYSTEM

Complement	Normal serum concentration (μg/ml)	Associated disorders
Classical pathway		
C1q	65-150	Glomerulonephritis, SLE
C1r	35-50	SLE-like syndrome, glomerulonephritis
C1s	30-50	SLE-like syndrome
C4	350-400	SLE-like syndrome, Sjögren's syndrome
C2	15-25	SLE, discoid lupus, polymyositis, Henoch-Schönlein purpura, Hodgkin's disease, vasculitis, glomerulonephritis, rheumatoid arthritis, common variable hypogammaglobulinemia
C3	1250-1400	Glomerulonephritis, recurrent pyogenic infections, vasculitis, SLE
Alternative pathway		
C3	1250-1400	See above
Factor B	240	None known
Factor D	1	Recurrent pyogenic infections
Factor P properdin	25	None known
Membrane lysis		
C5	65-80	Recurrent neisserial infections, SLE
C6	55-60	Recurrent neisserial infections
C7	55	Recurrent neisserial infections, Raynaud's phenomenon and sclerodactyly, vasculitis, SLE, rheumatoid arthritis
C8	55	SLE, recurrent neisserial infections
C9	60	Neisserial infections
Regulatory proteins		
C1 inhibitor (C1 INH)	100-180	Hereditary angioedema, increased incidence of autoimmune disorders
C4 binding protein	250	None known
Factor I	25	Recurrent pyogenic infections, vasculitis, glomerulonephritis
Factor H	500	Glomerulonephritis, disseminated pyogenic infections
S protein	500	None known

PRIMARY IMMUNODEFICIENCY DISORDERS

Disorder	Proposed etiology	Clinical features	Serum immunoglobulins	Circulating lymphocytes B cells	Circulating lymphocytes T cells	Treatment
Antibody (B-cell) mediated						
X-linked hypogammaglobulinemia (Bruton's disease)	Defect in pre-B and B-cell differentiation; X-linked	Recurrent infections, particularly pneumonia, sinusitis, otitis media, meningitis, sepsis; panhypogammaglobulinemia; arthritis of large joints	All decreased	Absent	Normal	Replacement gamma globulin IM or IV; antibiotic therapy; pulmonary postural drainage; symptomatic and prophylactic care; no live virus vaccines
Transient hypogammaglobulinemia of infancy	Unknown; maturation defect	Recurrent bacterial infections primarily the first 6 mo of life; recovery at 1-2 yr	Decreased IgG and IgA	Normal	Decreased helper T cells	Gamma globulin; patients often recover spontaneously
Common, variable immunodeficiency (acquired hypogammaglobulinemia)	Unknown; intrinsic B-cell defect; altered T helper cell function; autosomal dominant or recessive; most unclassifiable	Aquired predisposition to recurrent pyogenic infections (e.g., sinus, pulmonary); lymphadenopathy; splenomegaly; malabsorption; diarrhea; giardiasis; increased incidence of autoimmune disorders; lymphoreticular malignancy	Decreased; poor function	Normal or decreased	Normal; may have progressive decreased numbers and function	Gamma globulin IV; antibiotic therapy; no live virus vaccine, irradiated blood products
Immunodeficiency Hyper IgM	Unknown	Recurrent pyrogenic infections (e.g., otitis media, pneumonia, septicemia); neutropenia, hemolytic anemia	IgM and IgD normal or increased; low IgA and IgG	Increased or normal IgM; absent or decreased IgG and IgA	Normal	Gamma globulin IV; antibiotic therapy

PRIMARY IMMUNODEFICIENCY DISORDERS—cont'd

Disorder	Proposed etiology	Clinical features	Serum immunoglobulins	Circulating lymphocytes		Treatment
				B cells	**T cells**	
Selective IgA deficiency	Unknown; may be a decreased synthesis of IgA or altered terminal differentiation failure to IgA	Recurrent sinusitis, pulmonary infections; increased incidence of atopic allergy; celiac disease, autoimmune disorders (e.g., SLE, RA, chronic active hepatitis); may develop antibody against IgA	IgA decreased or absent	Normal	Normal	Should not be treated with gamma globulin (contains small amounts of IgA); antibiotic therapy; IgA-deficient donors should be used for blood transfusions
X-linked lymphoproliferative syndrome (Duncan's syndrome)	Genetic defect associated with Epstein-Barr virus; switch defect from IgM to IgG specific antibody	Hypogammaglobulinemia, susceptible to fatal EBV and mononucleosis infections, lymphoma	Decreased	Normal	Altered helper/suppressor ratio	No effective treatment; gamma globulin
Cell (T-cell) mediated						
DiGeorge syndrome	Abnormal thymic development with T-cell defects	Thymic aplasia or hypoplasia, hypocalcemia, abnormal facial appearance, hypoparathyroidism, congenital cardiac defects	Normal or decreased	Normal	Decreased	Calcium and vitamin D supplements; fetal thymus transplant; repair of congenital cardiac defects; no live virus vaccines
Chronic mucocutaneous candidiasis	Possible autoimmune origin, suggesting that the thymus also functions as an endocrine organ	Lifelong chronic candidal infections of skin, nails, and mucous membranes with or without endocrinopathy; hypoparathyroidism associated with hypocalcemia; Addison's disease	Normal	Normal	Normal altered function	No treatment to prevent idiopathic endocrinopathy; topical, PO, or IV antifungal therapy

PRIMARY IMMUNODEFICIENCY DISORDERS—cont'd

Disorder	Proposed etiology	Clinical features	Serum immunoglobulins	Circulating lymphocytes		Treatment
				B cells	T cells	
Combined antibody mediated (B cell) and cell mediated (T cell)						
Severe combined immunodeficiency disease (SCID)	Inheritance unclear; defect in stem cell differentiation and maturation of T and B cells	Pancytopenia; severe infections (viral, bacterial, fungal, protozoal); failure to thrive, chronic diarrhea, persistent thrush (oral candidiasis), otitis media, *P. carinii* pneumonia, and sepsis; GVHD secondary to maternal infusion of cells during delivery or blood transfusion	Absent or decreased	Absent or decreased	Absent or decreased	Antibiotic therapy; no live viral vaccines; irradiated blood products; pulmonary postural drainage; histocompatible BMT
Immunodeficiency with ataxia-telangiectasia	Defect in T-cell maturation; T-cell immunity is depressed or absent; autosomal recessive	Progressive cerebellar ataxia, with additional neurologic symptoms developing over time; telangiectasia, recurrent sinusitis, pulmonary infections, increased risk of viral and bacterial infections; may have lack of secondary sexual characteristics, variable developmental problems	Varies: decreased IgA (40%), IgE, and IgG (IgG_2); increased IgM	Normal	Decreased or normal	Antibiotic therapy, postural drainage, gamma globulin if indicated, no live attenuated virus vaccines, irradiated blood products, fetal thymus transplantation

PRIMARY IMMUNODEFICIENCY DISORDERS—cont'd

Disorder	Proposed etiology	Clinical features	Serum immunoglobulins	Circulating lymphocytes B cells	Circulating lymphocytes T cells	Treatment
Nezelof's syndrome	Unknown: possible thymic hypoplasia; cellular immunodeficiency with abnormal immunoglobulin synthesis	Susceptible to recurrent and persistent infections (viral, bacterial, fungal, protozoal); lymphadenopathy, hepatosplenomegaly	Varies	Normal	Marked decrease	Antibiotic therapy; gamma globulin; pulmonary postural drainage; no live virus vaccines; irradiated blood products; fetal thymus transplantation; histocompatible BMT
Wiskott-Aldrich syndrome	X-linked; defect in stem cell membrane	Thrombocytopenia (characterized by small platelets) with bleeding (e.g., petechiae, GI, intracranial), eczema, recurrent pyrogenic infection (e.g., otitis media, pneumonia, meningitis, and sepsis); malignancy	Decreased IgM; often elevated IgA and IgE	Normal	Decreased	Antibiotic therapy; *no* corticosteroids to treat thrombocytopenia due to increased risk of infection; IV gamma globulin; histocompatible BMT
Adenosine deaminase deficiency (ADA)	Enzyme deficiency or absence; autosomal recessive defect	Severe recurrent viral, bacterial, fungal, protozoal infections; radiologic bone abnormalities	Progressive decrease	Varies	Varies	Antibiotic therapy; no live virus vaccines; irradiated blood products (monthly infusions of erythrocytes to provide a source of enzyme); BMT; thymus transplant; bovine adenosine deaminase and polyethylene glycol to prolong enzyme half-life
Purine nucleotide phosphorylase (PNP) deficiency	PNP enzyme deficiency; autosomal recessive	Recurrent pneumonia, otitis media, and pharyngitis; progressive disorder	Normal but progressive decrease	Normal	Decreased	Irradiated red cell and plasma infusions; antibiotic therapy, BMT
Acquired immunodeficiency syndrome (AIDS)	Human immunodeficiency virus (HIV)	Acquired predisposition to severe, recurrent, and persistent opportunistic infections (protozoal, fungal, viral, bacterial) and malignancies; Kaposi's sarcoma; *P. carinii* pneumonia; oral candidiasis, hairy leukoplakia; intestinal problems; neurologic changes	Normal or increased	Normal or increased	Decreased	Antibiotic therapy; azidothymidine (AZT); interferon research protocols available

PRIMARY PHAGOCYTIC DYSFUNCTION DISORDERS

Disorder	Proposed pathogenesis	Clinical features	Treatment
Chronic granulomatous disease	X-linked inheritance; enzyme deficiency; 50% are autosomal recessive (component of NADPH oxidase); impaired respiratory burst; altered neutrophil function; inability to kill certain microorganisms (antimicrobial defect)	Lymphadenopathy; chronic lymph node drainage; hepatosplenomegaly; chronic infected ulcerations and abscesses; recurrent pneumonias; diarrhea; associated with *Staphylococcus, Serratia, Pseudomonas, Aspergillus*	Prophylactic antibiotics; obtain specific bacterial diagnosis and treat with appropriate antibiotics; gamma interferon has been used to enhance the respiratory burst activity of neutrophils and monocytes
Chédiak-Higashi syndrome	Autosomal recessive; abnormal granule formation, neutrophil chemotactic responsiveness, and intracellular killing of microorganisms	Recurrent pyrogenic infections, hepatosplenomegaly; partial albinism; progressive CNS alterations; lymphoreticular malignancy	No specific treatment; antibiotic therapy; anticholinergic drugs to improve granulocyte function; histocompatible BMT
Job syndrome/hyper-IgE immunodeficiency syndrome	Not only phagocytic disorder; abnormal chemotaxis; alteration in T-cell function; suggested suppressor T-cell deficiency	Eczema; recurrent "cold" staphylococcal infections of the skin, lymph nodes, subcutaneous tissues, lungs, and eyes; eosinophilia; extreme elevation in IgE	Antibiotic therapy
Lazy leukocyte syndrome	Defective chemotaxis of neutrophils associated with neutropenia; impaired migration of peripheral neutrophils	Neutropenia; recurrent bacterial infections	Antibiotic therapy
Tuftsin deficiency	Familial deficiency of a phagocytosis-stimulating substance	Recurrent local and systemic infections	No treatment; gamma globulin may be effective
Glucose-6-phosphate dehydrogenase deficiency (G6PD)	X-linked inheritance; complete absence of leukocyte G6PD activity; decreased hydrogen peroxide production; inability of neutrophils to kill bacteria	Recurrent bacterial infections; hemolytic anemia	Specific microorganism is identified and treated with appropriate antibiotic
Myeloperoxidase deficiency	Complete deficiency of leukocyte myeloperoxidase, altering and delaying the killing of microorganisms	Susceptibility to candidal and staphylococcal infections	Antibiotic therapy

1 ASSESS

ASSESS-MENT	OBSERVATIONS	DiGeorge syndrome (DGS)	Chronic mucocutaneous candidiasis (CMC)	X-linked agammaglobulinemia (X-LA)	Selective IgA deficiency (SIgAD)	Common variable immunodeficiency (CVID)	Wiskott-Aldrich syndrome (WAS)	Severe combined immunodeficiency disease (SCID)
General		May be developmentally delayed with signs of mental retardation; recurrent opportunistic infections with fever. At birth, or in the following year, hypocalcemia unresponsive to standard calcium replacement therapy	Diagnosed in other family members; recurrent candidal infections	Onset 5-6 mo of age; recurrent bacterial infections with fever	Recurrent viral or bacterial infections with fever	Recurrent infections with fever, often caused by pneumococci or *H. influenzae*	Recurrent bacterial infections with fever	Recurrent viral, fungal, bacterial, and protozoal infections with fever
Head, eyes, ears, neck, throat		Low-set, externally rotated, malformed ears with notched pinnae; unusually small jaw; wide-set eyes; blunted nose, fish-shaped mouth, and antimongoloid slant to the eyes	White curdlike substance at the corners of mouth and on oral mucosa (thrush); withdrawn appearance	Pulling at ears; decreased hearing; upper airway congestion; ocular erythema and drainage; nasal drainage; sinus tenderness; no lymph nodes or tonsils; significant dental decay	Nasal drainage; sinus tenderness; nasal mucosa swollen, pale, boggy, and usually gray secondary to allergies	Twisting head and pulling at ears; may have altered hearing; upper airway congestion and nasal drainage; ocular erythema and drainage; lymphadenopathy	Epistaxis; bleeding gums; reddened conjunctivae; pulling at ears with impaired hearing	White curdlike substance on tongue and oral mucosa (thrush); pulling at ears; impaired hearing; purulent nasal drainage; tender sinuses

→ › ›

ASSESS-MENT	OBSERVATIONS						
Gastroin-testinal, renal, and nu-tritional	May be poor feeder; de-creased weight and height for age; poor growth	Hepatitis may precede onset of endocrinopa-thy	Malab-sorption sec-ondary to *Giar-dia lam-blia* infesta-tion; de-creased weight and height	Malab-sorption (celiac dis-ease); de-creased weight	Increased bowel sounds, diar-rhea, hepato-spleno-megaly; de-creased weight and height; malab-sorption; abdom-inal pain	De-creased weight and height; diar-rhea, heme-positive stools; hema-turia	De-creased weight and height; chronic diar-rhea; malab-sorption
Mucous mem-branes (mouth, vagina, perianal areas)	White curdlike substance on mucosa (thrush), espe-cially mouth and perianal areas (indicat-ing candidal infection)	White curdlike substance cov-ering mucous membrane, in-dicating can-didal infection, vulvovaginal erythema and odor, scratch-ing	Herpetic lesions; oral thrush	Unre-mark-able; oral thrush; herpetic lesions; bacterial infec-tions	Oral thrush; herpetic lesions	Oral thrush; herpetic lesions; pete-chiae; ecchy-motic, bleeding gums	Oral ul-cers; oral thrush; herpetic lesions
Skin and nails	Skin may be pale or cyan-otic (varies de-pending on cardiac abnor-mality); clubbed nails; nail beds may be yellow-ish from fungal infection	Interdigital white or yellow ero-sions around nail beds and fingers; superfi-cial beefy-red areas in body folds (e.g., groin, under breasts) with small vesico-pustules and white curdlike patches on sur-face of lesion; skin may be obliterated by serous exu-date, crust, and granulomatous formation; itch-ing, "gloved" hands	Recurrent bacterial derma-titis	Generally unre-mark-able	Recurrent skin in-fections; general-ized edema if malab-sorption is se-vere enough to cause protein losses	Eczema-toid skin with ar-eas of redness and drainage; skin ab-scesses; areas of pete-chiae and ec-chy-moses	Recurrent infec-tions; maculo-papular rash as-sociated with GVHD

ASSESS-MENT	OBSERVATIONS						
Cardio-vascular	Findings vary, depending on the cardiac anomaly (e.g., truncus arterio-sus: dyspnea, cyanosis, re-current respira-tory infections, heart failure, systolic ejection murmur often preceded by ejection click, S_2 split, ECG changes indica-tive of cardiac hypertrophy)	Normal rate and rhythm, no murmur, palpable peripheral pulses; no indication of cardiac anomaly; tachycardia with severe infections					
Respira-tory	Unremarkable unless pneumonia is present (e.g., dyspnea, tachypnea, use of accessory muscles, grunting, nasal flaring, retractions, decreased breath sounds, crackles, yellow or green sputum, indi-cating pulmonary infection)						
Neuro-muscular	Tetany, car-popedal spasms, sei-zure activity secondary to hypocalcemia; altered muscle tone, de-pressed re-flexes, increased excit-ability	Tetany and sei-zures in the presence of hypoparathy-roidism sec-ondary to hypocalcemia	Nuchal rigidity with menin-gitis	Unre-mark-able	Unre-mark-able	Delayed develop-ment	Delayed develop-ment
Psycho-social	Loss of develop-mental mile-stones; less alert, de-creased activ-ity; failure to thrive; may have develop-mental delay	Behavioral changes (e.g., irritable, anx-ious, de-pressed)	Varies de-pending on med-ical course, re-sources, and coping strate-gies of patient and family	Varies de-pending on se-verity	Varies de-pending on med-ical course, re-sources, and coping strate-gies of patient and family	Irritability, loss of develop-mental mile-stones; failure to thrive	Irritability, loss of develop-mental mile-stones; failure to thrive

2 DIAGNOSE

NURSING DIAGNOSIS	SUBJECTIVE FINDINGS	OBJECTIVE FINDINGS
Altered protection related to immunodeficiency	Patient or parent reports frequent recurrent infections; unable to receive routine immunizations; malaise; itchy skin; feeling hot; pulling at ears; shortness of breath; frequently exposed to children with contagious diseases	Fever; lethargy; eczema; inflamed tympanic membrane; adventitious breath sounds; nasal drainage; yellow or green sputum; low to absent T cells (DGS, CMC); low to absent B cells (X-LA); low immunoglobulins (X-LA, CVID); both B and T cells low or absent (WAS, SCID); absolute neutrophils less than 500 with IVIG
High risk for infection related to inadequate immunity	Reports increased dyspnea and irritability (infant is crying); increased white coating over tongue, mouth, and other mucous membranes; skin tenderness and itching	History of T-cell or B-cell inadequacy, rendering an increased susceptibility to infections; oral thrush; upper airway congestion with decreased breath sounds, crackles, productive or nonproductive cough; fever; lymphadenopathy; splenomegaly; absolute neutrophils less than 500
Hyperthermia (fever) related to infection	Reports fevers, chills, malaise, weakness, irritability, and poor feeding	Fever; diaphoresis; dyspnea; tachycardia; skin warm; positive cultures; leukocytosis
Impaired skin and mucous membrane related to chronic infection	Complains of "cotton" feeling to mouth; vaginal itching; tender nail beds; dry, itching skin	Skin folds have erythematous areas covered with white patches; mucous membranes coated with white curdlike substance (candidal infection); ridged, discolored, yellow-tinged nails; eczema, pustules, rash; lymphadenopathy
High risk for injury related to seizures secondary to hypocalcemia (DGS, CMC)	Parent reports history of injuries related to seizure activity	Bruises and other noticeable signs of immediate or past injury; seizures may lead to aspiration or other types of neuromuscular injury; decreased calcium
Altered nutrition: less than body requirements due to chronic infections and anorexia	Complains of decreased appetite, nausea, and abdominal discomfort; infants are irritable and will not take formula	Decrease in food and fluid intake, vomiting; decreased weight; children are not within normal growth curve for height and weight; anemia, pallor; hyperactive bowel sounds; abdominal tenderness; low albumin
Diarrhea related to giardiasis or other intestinal infection	Reports frequent liquid stools; complains of abdominal tenderness and cramping	Hyperactive bowel sounds, up to 10 stools/day; incontinence of stool; laboratory and diagnostic findings indicating intestinal infections; dry mucous membranes; tarry stools
Impaired gas exchange related to alveolar-capillary membrane changes, secondary to inflammation caused by pneumonia	Complains of shortness of breath	Hypoxic (Pao_2 <80 mm Hg); pallor; irritability; restlessness; diminished breath sounds with crackles; fever; tachypnea, retractions, grunting, flaring, cyanosis

NURSING DIAGNOSIS	SUBJECTIVE FINDINGS	OBJECTIVE FINDINGS
Impaired home management related to overcrowding and poor sanitation	Family reports living in a single-dwelling home with three other families; lack of cleanliness	Overcrowding; lack of a clean environment; lack of support and information about community resources
High risk for altered growth and development related to prolonged illness and hospitalization	Parent or child reports decreased interest in playing; increased need to be held; irritability; infant with unpredictable temperament	Child is developmentally delayed for age (based on the Denver Developmental Screen); flat affect; inappropriate behavior; infant with unconsolable crying and irritability; decreased physical growth for age; missed school or work

Other Related Nursing Diagnoses: Alteration in cardiac output related to the mechanical factors of a congenital abnormal heart (preload, afterload, and contractility) and electrical instability (dysrhythmias) (DGS); **Diarrhea** related to malabsorption or infection; **High risk for injury** related to thrombocytopenia (WAS); **Body image disturbance** related to overwhelming candidal infections of the skin and/or vitiligo; **Ineffective breathing pattern** related to inflammatory process and pleuritic pain caused by pneumonia; **Potential for activity intolerance** related to weakness, myalgia, and arthralgia; **Potential for fluid and electrolyte abnormalities** related to the development of Addison's disease; **Ineffective airway clearance** related to excessive sputum caused by pulmonary disease or infection; **Family coping: high risk for altered growth** related to self-actualization needs; **High risk for ineffective family coping** related to severity of diagnosis

3 PLAN

Patient goals

1. The patient will maintain protection from possible infection within the limits of the immunodeficiency.
2. The patient will be free of opportunistic infections and their complications.
3. Chronic infections will be managed effectively by the patient or family.
4. The patient's temperature will be within normal limits.
5. The patient will regain and maintain intact skin and mucous membranes.
6. The patient will not experience seizures as a result of hypocalcemia.
7. The patient's nutrition will improve and remain adequate for individual growth and development.
8. The patient will not have diarrhea.
9. The patient's gas exchange will improve.
10. The patient and family will be knowledgeable about community resources and will use them appropriately.
11. The patient or family will maintain a clean and sanitary home environment.
12. The patient will demonstrate "catch-up" growth and attain appropriate development for age.

4 IMPLEMENT

NURSING DIAGNOSIS	NURSING INTERVENTIONS	RATIONALE
Altered protection related to immunodeficiency	Encourage good handwashing for patient and anyone coming in contact with patient (e.g., before meals, after using toilet; for small children, periodic handwashing is helpful); disposable hand wipes are useful for outings, school, or work.	To decrease risk of microorganisms entering host and possibly causing an infection.

→ ❯ ❯

NURSING DIAGNOSIS	NURSING INTERVENTIONS	RATIONALE
	Screen all visitors for colds or infections; check temperature of all visitors up to 12 yr.	To minimize exposure to infectious agents.
	Provide meticulous skin and perineal care with mild, antiseptic soap and water; provide oral care daily, and encourage routine dental visits.	To protect immunocompromised patient from infection.
	Encourage clean environment for all activities; toys and items used often should be cleaned routinely; keep patient's room clean and free of excess dust and equipment.	To minimize risk of contamination and infection.
	Clean all cuts and scrapes immediately with antiseptic soap; report any unusual redness or drainage.	To prevent infection and ensure prompt treatment with antibiotics.
	Identify patients at risk for inadequate nutrition, and monitor closely (weight, height [infants and children], intake and output, caloric intake).	Adequate diet supports immune functioning.
	Monitor CBC.	As an indicator of adequate protection: Hb $\geq$12 g/dl, WBCs $\geq$5,000/cm^3, PMNs $\geq$50%, B lymphocytes >20%, T lymphocytes >70%.
	Central lines should be managed with sterile technique according to hospital policy.	To prevent infection.
	Administer only CMV-negative or leucopor-filtered blood products.	To prevent CMV infection.
	Administer only irradiated blood products.	Blood products may contain competent lymphocytes capable of causing GVHD.
	Infants should not be given breast milk.	Breast milk may contain competent lymphocytes that could cause GVHD.
	No live viral vaccinations (e.g., measles, mumps, and rubella) should be given to the patient; oral polio should not be given to the patient or housemate.	To prevent risk of viral infection through these vaccinations; polio is shed in the stool
	Prevent exposure to varicella and to individuals who have been recently vaccinated with a live vaccine (e.g., oral polio) or exposed to other infectious diseases (e.g., herpes simplex, herpes zoster [shingles]).	These individuals are capable of shedding the virus, which puts the patient at risk.
	In collaboration with physician, administer prophylactic antibiotics and monitor response (prophylactic antibiotics should be administered before dental work is done).	To prevent the development of specific infections (e.g., acyclovir against viruses; Septra or pentamidine against *P. carinii* pneumonia).

NURSING DIAGNOSIS	NURSING INTERVENTIONS	RATIONALE
	Avoid unnecessary manipulative and invasive procedures (e.g., dental manipulation, biopsy, barium enema, arteriogram, surgery); when such procedures are necessary, institute prophylaxis with antibiotics as ordered.	An immunodeficient individual is susceptible to local or systemic infections when tissues are invaded.
	Provide protective isolation (in some cases this will require a laminar airflow hood or room, or a room with a HEPA filter [e.g. SCID]).	To minimize exposure to infections that could be life threatening.
High risk for infection related to inadequate immunity	Monitor for signs and symptoms of infection (e.g., fever, changes in vital signs, pain, irritability, cough).	To provide prompt intervention with antibiotics and appropriate treatment (e.g., postural drainage).
	Provide frequent, vigorous oral care as ordered (e.g., mouthwash rinse; sodium bicarbonate and nystatin).	To prevent oral lesions and prevent or treat thrush candidiasis.
	When indicated, provide and teach sinus, bronchial, and pulmonary postural drainage.	To promote drainage of nasal, bronchial, and pulmonary secretions and to decrease congestion, thus minimizing risk of infection.
	Encourage a balance of rest and activity and an adequate diet.	To support the immune system and minimize the risk of infection.
	Obtain cultures as ordered, and report results.	To detect any infection, allowing prompt treatment.
	Encourage ambulation; if patient is unable, reposition frequently.	To help prevent pulmonary compromise and increased susceptibility to respiratory infections, and to maximize circulation.
	In patients who are severely immunodeficient, neutrophil count <500 and immunocompromised, avoid fresh fruit, vegetables, and tap water (use sterile water, especially with infant).	Fruits, vegetables, and water may harbor bacteria that could cause an infection.
	If a fever is present, administer antipyretics (e.g., acetaminophen or aspirin) as ordered, and monitor response.	To decrease fever and promote comfort. Antipyretics can hide an infection; only give as ordered.
	Provide patient with waste receptacle for used tissues, and instruct him to cover his nose and mouth when coughing; encourage frequent handwashing.	To prevent the spread of an existing infection to other organs and individuals.
	Ensure that staff members caring for patient do not have an infectious disease.	To minimize risk of infection in an immunocompromised patient.
	Monitor chest x-rays in collaboration with the physician.	To assess extent and location of pulmonary involvement.

→ › ›

NURSING DIAGNOSIS	NURSING INTERVENTIONS	RATIONALE
	Infuse immunoglobulin per hospital protocol as ordered, and monitor response (e.g., X-LA; SCID).	To provide antibodies to fight potential infections.
Hyperthermia (fever) related to infection	Assess for signs of infection (e.g., redness, purulent drainage; yellow or green sputum).	Infection is the most common cause of a fever.
	Monitor temperature q 2 h or more often as indicated.	To detect changes in temperature; decrease in temperature is associated with resolution of infection; secondary increase is associated with complications; waxing and waning of temperature may be associated with CMV.
	Monitor for signs of dehydration (e.g., decreased weight, disorientation, decreased urine output, increased specific gravity, poor skin turgor, hyperventilation).	Significant fluid loss accompanies each degree of temperature increase; hyperventilation can result in respiratory alkalosis.
	Administer antipyretics, and monitor response; in children, acetaminophen should be used rather than aspirin.	To lower the set point in the hypothalamus; aspirin has been implicated in Reye's syndrome in children with viral infections and should not be given.
	Apply hypothermic blanket, or tepid sponge baths; use ice packs in areas of high blood flow (e.g., back of neck, behind knees, under arms and breasts); adjust environment with fan or air conditioning.	To promote heat loss by convection and conduction; tepid water is preferred to alcohol because water evaporates at a higher temperature; discontinue cooling blankets when temperature is ≥38.33° C (101° F).
	Monitor fluids and electrolytes and hourly intake and output; administer fluids as ordered, or encourage oral fluids	Fluids, sodium, and potassium are lost through sweating, diarrhea, and vomiting; lost fluids and electrolytes must be replaced.
	Encourage a high-calorie diet, and ensure adequate rest.	Metabolic rate increases with each degree of a fever; adequate nutritional support and rest are necessary to meet metabolic rate.
Impaired skin and mucous membranes related to chronic infection	Monitor mucous membranes and skin for changes.	To guide therapeutic interventions and identify treatable conditions.
	Refer to dentist, and encourage regular visits.	To provide routine periodontal care.
	Provide and teach oral hygiene (soft toothbrush, nonabrasive toothpaste); encourage frequent rinsing of mouth with saline or half strength hydrogen peroxide; apply lip balm.	To provide comfort and assist in preventing spread of infection.

NURSING DIAGNOSIS	NURSING INTERVENTIONS	RATIONALE
	Administer topical or systemic antibiotics as ordered, and monitor response.	To control opportunistic infections and reduce factors that contribute to skin impairment.
	Caution patient to avoid spicy and salty foods and foods of extreme temperature.	To prevent further irritation of the oral mucosa.
	Encourage fluid intake appropriate to weight of patient and adapted to other organ system involvement (i.e., kidney, neurologic disease).	To maintain hydration of mucous membranes.
	Bathe or encourage routine bathing with mild antiseptic soap and water; blot dry.	To remove excess exudate and keep skin clean and dry.
	Administer antipyretics as ordered, and monitor response.	To relieve itching.
	Caution patient against scratching; use mitts on infants or soft restraints if patient is confused to prevent scratching (check circulation and fingers qh if mitts are used).	To prevent spread of infection, potential scarring, and introduction of bacteria into lesions; to monitor circulatory compromise.
	Keep body dry and exposed to air; encourage patient to avoid heat, moisture, and occlusive clothing; encourage him to use natural fabrics (e.g., cotton).	To prevent further risk of skin breakdown and infection.
	In collaboration with physician and nutritionist, monitor nutritional intake and albumin level; weigh daily (bid for infants).	To optimize nutritional status and promote healing of skin.
	Apply warm soaks to feet and hands.	To promote suppuration and drainage from nail beds.
	Encourage routine meticulous nail care (clean nails with mild antiseptic soap and water, trim cuticles, clip nails short).	Prevent spread of infection, reduce existing pathogens, and provide comfort.
High risk for injury related to seizures secondary to hypocalcemia (DGS, CMC)	Monitor calcium and phosphorus levels.	To prevent hypocalcemia, tetany, and seizures; normal total calcium, 9-10.5 mg/dl; phosphorus, 2.5-4.5 mg/dl.
	Monitor for tetany.	May be an indicator of hypocalcemia and impending seizure.
	Administer calcium and vitamin D supplements as ordered, and monitor response.	To achieve and maintain normal calcium levels and prevent seizure.
	Maintain bed in low position at all times, and keep side rails padded and up.	To minimize risk of injury in the event of a seizure and if the patient falls out of bed.
	Keep call light within reach at all times.	To enable patient or family to summon help if needed.

→ > >

NURSING DIAGNOSIS	NURSING INTERVENTIONS	RATIONALE
	Maintain seizure precautions; keep oral airway (right size), suction equipment, and oxygen at bedside.	To facilitate a prompt response if a seizure occurs.
	During a seizure: maintain airway patency (administer oxygen as ordered), and monitor for respiratory or cardiopulmonary arrest; support and protect head; turn patient onto side; ease patient to floor if in a chair; place pillows along side rails; loosen constrictive clothing; provide privacy; stay with patient (family of infant)	To prevent hypoxia, aspiration, and musculoskeletal trauma; monitor for potential arrest to allow rapid intervention; ensure safety and patient's privacy; these measures minimize fear and anxiety when patient resumes consciousness and provide support to patient and family.
	After seizure: maintain airway patency; suction as indicated; monitor vital signs and neurologic status; administer oxygen as ordered and monitor response; reorient patient; keep patient on his side in a comfortable position; provide oral hygiene.	To prevent hypoxia and aspiration, to remove secretions, and to check for blood from possible tongue lacerations; monitor physiologic changes and response to seizure; reorient patient and provide support and comfort.
Altered nutrition: less than body requirements due to chronic infections and anorexia	Assess food likes and dislikes; monitor food and fluid intake q 24 h.	To guide therapeutic plan and identify nutritional adequacy and any changes in nutritional intake.
	Consult with nutritionist to make a complete assessment, particularly with infants and small children.	To guide therapeutic interventions, using the special expertise of a health team member.
	Routinely monitor Hct, Hb, total protein, and albumin.	To determine protein balance and adequate nutrition.
	Routinely monitor weight and height.	To establish baseline and note any changes.
	Provide small, frequent meals that include foods or formula the patient likes.	To reduce fatigue during eating, and provide patient with desirable foods.
	Provide a high-protein diet.	To support the immune system.
	Monitor for nausea, vomiting, and diarrhea.	These may decrease intake of adequate nutrition or may suggest an ongoing infectious process.
	Provide oral care before eating.	To enhance the taste of food and minimize taste from candidal infection or other infectious processes.
	Encourage parents to use bottles and nipples brought from home; encourage parents to feed infant.	To make mealtime a pleasant experience and to enhance dietary intake.
	Serve food at room temperature; provide a comfortable environment (e.g., hold infants in a rocking chair); allow time to eat.	To encourage adequate nutritional intake; room-temperature food decreases the risk of irritating oral mucous membranes.

NURSING DIAGNOSIS	NURSING INTERVENTIONS	RATIONALE
	Evaluate the need for dietary changes, enteral feeding, or parenteral nutrition; tube feedings are initiated only when necessary via a nasogastric (N/G) tube (common in infants and small children).	To meet patient's daily caloric and dietary needs.
	Aspirate gastric contents via N/G tube, to determine amount of food remaining in stomach.	To prevent overdistention of stomach, minimize risk of aspiration, and determine amount of feeding actually absorbed.
Diarrhea related to giardiasis or other intestinal infection	Assess consistency, frequency, and quantity of stools, and for presence of blood.	To establish baseline and to guide therapeutic interventions.
	Auscultate bowel sounds.	Hypermotility is common in diarrhea.
	Monitor weight daily and intake and output.	To evaluate sharp changes in fluid status and monitor for dehydration.
	Monitor for signs and symptoms of fluid and electrolyte imbalances (e.g., disorientation, irritability, weakness, nausea).	To prevent complications from large amounts of fluid, sodium, and potassium, lost with persistent diarrhea.
	Administer prescribed antibiotic, antimotility agents, and psyllium (Metamucil), and monitor response and effectiveness	To slow intestinal motility; psyllium acts to absorb fluid and form a more solid mass; antibiotic treats infection.
	Monitor perianal area for excoriation; cleanse with soap and water; rinse completely after every stool; apply A & D ointment, zinc oxide, or skin barrier as indicated.	To decrease risk of skin breakdown and minimize discomfort; heavy ointments and skin barrier protect skin from excessive moisture.
Impaired gas exchange related to alveolar-capillary membrane changes, secondary to inflammation caused by pneumonia	Auscultate lungs for crackles, consolidation, and pleural friction rub.	To help determine adequacy of gas exchange and to detect areas of consolidation and pleural friction rub.
	Assess level of consciousness, lethargy, anxiety, and irritability.	These may indicate hypoxia.
	Monitor ABGs.	To determine need for oxygen therapy.
	Monitor CBC.	To detect amount of hemoglobin available to carry oxygen.
	Monitor skin color and capillary refill.	To determine circulatory adequacy, necessary for gas exchange.
	Administer antibiotics as ordered, and monitor response.	To halt microbial growth and support adequate gas exchange.
	Administer oxygen as ordered, and monitor response.	To improve gas exchange and decrease work of breathing.
	Balance activities with rest periods.	To decrease oxygen demand and prevent hypoxia.

→ 〉 〉

NURSING DIAGNOSIS	NURSING INTERVENTIONS	RATIONALE
	Suction as needed.	To remove excessive secretions and improve gas exchange.
Impaired home management related to overcrowding and poor sanitation	In collaboration with social worker, investigate community resources for long-term maintenance and possible alternative housing; initiate referrals for assistance in home maintenance.	To use expertise of social services and community resources appropriately and efficiently.
	Discuss specific life-style changes and alterations in home environment that will promote health (e.g., decrease crowding, routine cleaning and washing, removal of waste products [e.g., old food]).	To facilitate a life-style that promotes maximum health and safety.
	Problem solve with family to develop a plan for improving home environment that is consistent with family values.	To promote family involvement and commitment and to realistically identify what can be improved or altered.
High risk for altered growth and development related to prolonged illness and hospitalization	Perform an initial age-appropriate developmental screening assessment.	To establish baseline and guide therapeutic interventions.
	Involve child life specialist in planning developmental program.	Health team member's expertise in child development will enhance individual patient program.
	Encourage parents to take an active role in maintaining their child's developmental growth.	To ensure that developmental milestones are accomplished in a supportive and encouraging environment.
	Provide parents with information about community resources and organizations that can help them adjust.	To help families with children who are developmentally delayed (e.g., support groups).
	Help parents understand and learn to predict child's day-to-day behaviors.	To help parents attain maximum level of coping and adaptation to their child's behavior.

5   EVALUATE

PATIENT OUTCOME	DATA INDICATING THAT OUTCOME IS REACHED
Patient and family engage in activities to prevent recurrent infections.	The patient conducts all activities in a clean environment and participates in daily hygiene; he avoids individuals who are ill; patient and family can identify the signs of an infection and seek appropriate health care.

PATIENT OUTCOME	DATA INDICATING THAT OUTCOME IS REACHED
Patient has fewer recurrent infections and complications, and chronic infections are effectively managed by patient or family.	There are no new signs of infection; laboratory findings indicate all cultures to be negative; patient is afebrile; vital signs are normal; there are no infectious lesions.
Patient's temperature is within normal range; comfort and safety are maintained if patient has a fever.	Temperature is between 37° C (98.6° F) and 38° C (100.4° F) orally; pulse and respiratory rate are normal for age; skin is cool and without excess perspiration; patient has no complaints of headache; fluids and electrolyes are within normal limits; Reye's syndrome has been prevented.
Patient's skin and mucous membranes are intact.	Patient has no lesions; patient and/or family uses appropriate skin care techniques and topical medications.
Patient is free of injury from seizures caused by hypocalcemia.	Patient has not fallen during seizure, and he has no evidence of musculoskeletal injury; there is no hypoxia or aspiration; patient and family can discuss first aid strategies for decreasing injury at home; patient understands the importance of calcium and anticonvulsant therapy monitoring.
Patient has adequate calorie and protein intake to meet metabolic and growth and development needs.	Documented intake indicates adequate nutritional calories and protein; serum albumin is within normal limits ($\geq$3.4-4.5 g/dl); weight remains stable or improves appropriately for age.
Patient experiences maximum comfort, and diarrhea has been controlled; complications have been minimized.	Stools are soft, well formed, and of normal color and occur normally for individual; cramps and abdominal tenderness have been relieved; perianal skin is intact and causes no discomfort.
Patient maintains adequate gas exchange.	ABGs are normal: pH 7.35-7.45, Pao_2 80-95 mm Hg, Pco_2 35-45 mm Hg, O_2 saturation 95%-100%; there is no use of accessory muscles and no sternal retraction; respiratory rate is 12-20/min (25-30/min in infants); patient has no complaints of dyspnea; breath sounds are clear to auscultation.
Patient and family are knowledgeable about community resources.	Patient and family can describe and use appropriate resources and services available to provide assistance with living conditions.
Patient or family has adapted home and life-style to promote maximum health and safety.	Home environment is free of excessive dirt and waste; changes have been made consistent with family values.

→ → ›

PATIENT OUTCOME	DATA INDICATING THAT OUTCOME IS REACHED
Patient is meeting developmental milestones.	Child is making strides toward achieving normal growth and development; parents are able to maintain child at home; parents understand laws and resources related to the individual education programs for children with chronic illness

PATIENT TEACHING

1. Teach the patient and family the disease trajectory and long-term management strategies.
2. Teach the patient and family the purpose of all tests and procedure.
3. Teach the patient and family about all medications: their purpose, dosage, side effects, and how to administer them at home.
4. Teach the patient and family the importance of routine dental care and of using prophylactic antibiotics during dental procedures.
5. Educate the family about isolation precautions (e.g., SCID).
6. Teach the patient and family problem-solving strategies for coping with impaired health (e.g., handwashing, clean environment, avoiding ill individuals, routine hygiene [mouth care, bathing]).
7. In collaboration with the nutritionist, instruct the patient and family in a diet adequate for obtaining and maintaining ideal body weight (for children to promote growth and development).
8. Teach the patient and family skin and nail care techniques; stress the importance of routine hygiene and of keeping nails and cuticles trimmed.
9. Teach the patient relaxation exercises for coping with chronic discomfort and itching.
10. Teach the patient and family the signs and symptoms of an infection; instruct them to notify their health care provider when these occur (e.g., fever, redness, pain, cough, purulent drainage, anorexia, fatigue, irritability).
11. Teach the patient and family bronchial and postural drainage to be performed at home if frequent respiratory infections occur.
12. Teach the patient and family the importance of wearing a medical alert bracelet.
13. Teach the patient and family that the patient is not to receive live viral vaccines and that family members should not receive oral polio vaccine (shed in the stool).
14. Teach the patient and family to call their health care provider if the patient has been exposed to a contagious disease (e.g., chickenpox).
15. Teach the patient and family good handwashing technique.
16. Teach the patient and family about the seizure disorder.
17. Teach the family first aid for seizures and airway maintenance; encourage the patient and family to share this information with friends, teachers, co-workers, and others.
18. Encourage the family to seek genetic prenatal counseling in anticipation of future pregnancies.
19. Encourage routine follow-up with primary health care provider.
20. Instruct family about the laws and resources regarding Individual Education Programs (IEP) for chronically ill children.

CHAPTER 6

Rheumatoid Disorders

Systemic Lupus Erythematosus

Lupus is the Latin word for wolf. This term has been used since 1230 to describe the cutaneous skin changes that resemble the malar erythremia of a red wolf. **Systemic lupus erythematosus (SLE)** is a chronic, multisystem, autoimmune disorder characterized by the development of autoantibodies directed against autologous tissue and serum factors, particularly nucleic acids, erythrocytes, coagulation proteins, phospholipids, lymphocytes, platelets, and a number of other host components. SLE is distinguished by an inflammatory lesion that affects several organ systems, specifically the skin, joints, kidneys, and serous membranes. It may present as a fulminant illness or more often as a chronic, recurrent disorder.

EPIDEMIOLOGY

Commonly called lupus, SLE has no known cure. It affects approximately 500,000 individuals in the United States, and thousands more have the discoid form of the disease. More than 16,000 Americans develop SLE every year. Although the origin of the disease remains a mystery, increasing evidence suggests that several factors—genetic, hormonal, immunologic, and viral—may play a role in the onset and perpetuation of SLE.

Virtually anyone may be affected. However, SLE predominantly affects women during their childbearing years by a ratio of about 9:1; approximately 1 in every 700 women between 15 and 64 years of age develops the disorder. Of the women diagnosed with SLE, it is three times more common in black women than in white women. Women who are diagnosed with the disease in their sixth decade account for approximately 12% of the total cases.[195]

Once considered a fatal illness of young women, SLE now has an approximate 15-year survival rate of 85%. This improved prognosis reflects advances in the diagnosis and treatment of the disease. However, patients with central nervous system involvement and renal failure have poorer prognoses. Complications, especially infections associated with long-term use of steroids to control the disease, also significantly contribute to early mortality.

Despite the significant improvements in treating SLE, it can be a serious and potentially life-threatening illness. Because of this, and also because it has been recognized as an autoimmune disease prototype, SLE has become the subject of worldwide research.

PATHOPHYSIOLOGY

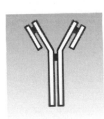 SLE is considered an autoimmune disease that occurs when antibodies intended to destroy invading antigens turn on the host and attack normal healthy tissue. These antibodies that develop against the host are called *autoantibodies*. The presence of autoantibodies reflects a loss of tolerance, or autoimmunity, and constitutes a serious defect in the regulatory components of the immune system.

Patients with SLE produce antibodies against several components of the host. The primary autoantibodies produced are directed at the cell nuclei and are called **antinuclear antibodies, or ANA.** Of particular interest are the antibodies produced against native double-stranded DNA (ds-DNA); these antibodies are considered a typical feature of SLE. Antibodies are also produced against denatured single-stranded DNA (ss-DNA) and to nucleohistones (complex nucleoprotein).[19]

The cause of autoantibody formation is not clear. It

is not certain what triggers the host to produce antibodies against ds-DNA; it may be viral or host DNA that is the immunogen for the anti-DNA antibody formation.[64]

Antinuclear antibodies generally do not cause significant cellular destruction alone, primarily because it is difficult for them to come into direct contact with the nuclei of living cells. However, when the cells die, the antinuclear antibodies form immune complexes with the nuclear antigens in the bloodstream. This triggers the inflammatory response, the primary mechanism by which tissue destruction and subsequent clinical disease occur.

The deposition of circulating immune complexes containing autoantibodies against host DNA can cause massive tissue damage. As immune complex aggregates become deposited in various tissues and organs, they form the characteristic SLE lesion. Immune complexes also activate the complement cascade, thereby attracting granulocytes and perpetuating the inflammatory reaction. Chronic deposition of immune complexes leads to continual destruction of host tissue. The intensity and location of the inflammatory process dictate the severity of the clinical response and organ involvement.

Immune complexes may circulate or may be deposited within capillary plexuses, near basement membranes, and in other tissues such as the glomeruli; the renal interstitia; the serosal pleural, pericardial, or peritoneal membranes; the choroid plexus; and the vasculature of the lungs. The most common targets of tissue destruction are the kidneys, skin, joints, and central nervous system. In the kidneys, for example, this manifests as glomerulonephritis.

As autoantibodies are produced against the host, antigen-antibody immune complexes are formed. These complexes localize in small vessels throughout the body, causing vasculitis.

By some unknown mechanism, regulatory T lymphocytes (suppressor T cells) normally prevent autoantibody formation. In SLE a defect in suppressor T-cell function inhibits this protective action. It is not clear whether this is the result of anti-T-cell antibody function or a primary suppressor T-cell deficiency. Polyclonal hypergammaglobulinemia occurs as a result, since B cells tend to proliferate unrestrained by normal suppressor mechanisms. Natural killer (NK) cell activity is also reduced, a development that is not related to the number of NK cells or to their ability to recognize and bind to a target, but rather to their inability to kill. NK cells may be depressed because of their continuous exposure to elevated levels of interferon. In addition, interleukin-1 (IL-1) and IL-2 production and IL-2 responsiveness are decreased in SLE.

Lymphocytotoxic antibodies with T-cell specificity often occur in patients with SLE. These antibodies can destroy T lymphocytes in the presence of complement. They have a particular specificity for T-cell surface antigens and can be released from the lymphocyte cell surface in the form of specific antigen-antibody complexes. These complexes block the function of other lymphocytes and contribute to immune complex deposition, which can cause vasculitis and nephritis. These autoantibodies can also coat peripheral blood T cells in order to interfere with HLA typing. This autoantibody formation has been identified in part as being genetically linked.[64]

Genetic Predisposition

Family studies have shown a genetic link to the development of SLE, with increased susceptibility in identical twins of over 65%.[154] A subset of SLE patients have also shown an inherited deficiency in complement factors C4a and cell surface C3b receptors and tend to share a common B-cell alloantigen. The role these alloantigens play in the pathogenesis of SLE is not yet certain. However, the C4A and C3b receptor deficiency may impair the antibodies' ability to clear circulating immune complexes, thus amplifying the autoimmune process. In addition, a large number of patients with SLE do not have the HLA-DR2 and HLA-DR3 haplotypes. Patients who have HLA-DR2 more often tend to produce anti-ds-DNA antibodies (Sjögren's syndrome antigen A; SS-A/Ro).[9,59,64,154]

Types of Systemic Lupus Erythematosus

Lupus is divided into two types, systemic lupus erythematosus (SLE) and cutaneous lupus erythematosus, also known as *discoid lupus erythematosus* (DLE). DLE is a milder form of the disease and usually affects only the skin. It predominates on the face, neck, and occasionally the upper chest. Telangiectasia may be noted in conjunction with erythema and is distributed primarily over the palms and fingers. The skin may become raised or scaly, or irregular bald spots may develop on the scalp. DLE usually is characterized by discoid skin lesions, called plaques. These plaques can be very disfiguring and can cause severe and stigmatizing scarring. In some cases joint pain, mild anemia, and leukopenia may be seen. Approximately 10% of patients with discoid lesions eventually develop the clinical and laboratory abnormalities of SLE.

SLE is considered a more severe form of the disorder; however, if well controlled, it may also be mild. SLE more often causes severe damage to internal organs, targeting primarily the kidneys, brain, heart, and lungs. SLE may also cause death and secondary severe complications.

MEDICATIONS THAT MAY CAUSE DRUG-INDUCED LUPUS

Aminosalicylic acid	Phenytoin
Chlorpromazine*	Primidone
Chlorthalidone	Procainamide*
Dephentoin	Quinidine
Hydralazine*	Reserpine
Isoniazid*	Streptomycin
Methyldopa*	Sulfonamides
D-Penicillamine	Tetracycline
	Trimethadione

*Strong correlation.

Reduced serum complement and antibodies to double-stranded DNA have become routine correlates of active SLE, which is distinguishable from other lupus variants.

Drug-Induced Lupus

In the past 10 years many drugs have been implicated in the development of a reversible lupus-like syndrome. The clinical features of drug-induced lupus generally are mild and often include arthralgias, arthritis, skin rash, fever, and pleurisy. Nephrosis and central nervous system involvement do not typically occur. Serologic test results often are similar to those for SLE; most patients have a positive ANA but do not have antibodies against ds-DNA. Although most clinical symptoms resolve when the drug is discontinued, it is not unusual for serologic abnormalities to persist. Perhaps certain drugs alter tissues to such a degree that they act as immunogenic stimuli. The most common drugs that cause this disorder are hydralazine and procainamide. Both drugs can bind to and alter the physical properties of DNA, possibly enhancing its immunogenicity. There also may be some correlation between an individual's ability to metabolize certain drugs and a predisposition to SLE.[153]

CLINICAL MANIFESTATIONS

SLE is a syndrome and not a specific disease; therefore the presentation and course can vary considerably, affecting one or more organs. During the illness a number of symptoms may develop that may be either intermittent or prolonged. Frequently these symptoms are totally independent of one another and may or may not occur simultaneously or serially. It is possible that eventually every organ system may become involved.

The course of the illness may include periods of exacerbations, called *flare-ups,* and periods when the disease is in control, called *remission.* Precipitating factors associated with flare-ups are thought to include sunlight, varying types of stress, infection, injury, surgery, pregnancy, exhaustion, nervous tension, and emotional upsets.

There is no specific clinical pattern; the onset may be acute and fulminant, affecting many organ systems simultaneously, or insidious, evolving over months to years. Although the initial signs and symptoms vary, the classic symptoms are fever, weight loss, malaise, and lethargy. The following sections discuss the more common clinical findings, which may appear independently or in combination.

General Manifestations

Nonspecific general complaints of SLE usually include fatigue, decreased appetite, weight loss, chronic or recurrent low-grade fevers (85%), and myalgias; 5% to 10% of patients with SLE will develop the sicca complex associated with Sjögren's syndrome (see p. 196).

Vascular Manifestations

Small vessel vasculitis is characteristic of SLE. The pathologic changes that develop are the result of an inflammatory process and include thickening of the intimal cell lining, fibrinoid degeneration, sclerosis, and thrombosis. These changes subsequently result in damage to vessel walls, leading to ischemia and infarction.

Skin Lesions and Mucous Membrane Involvement

Skin lesions and mucous membrane involvement occur in approximately 85% of patients with SLE. A wide variety of skin lesions may appear, and the classic characteristics include the erythema butterfly rash over the bridge of the nose and on the cheeks and the linear erythema along the eyelids. Lesions may become scaly and pruritic over the neck, upper chest, and extremities. The rash may resolve without permanent disfigurement, or it may cause atrophy to the area, and/or cause hypopigmentation or hyperpigmentation. Photosensitivity is very common and occurs in almost one third of cases, contributing to further skin eruptions and sensitivity.

Other clinical features of the skin may include bullae, patchy areas of purpura, urticaria, angioneurotic edema, patches of vitiligo, subcutaneous nodules, and thickening of the epidermis. An underlying hemorrhagic tendency or vasculitis is demonstrated primarily by palpable purpura; mucocutaneous lesions such as purpura, petechiae, and ecchymosis; and small, punctate, ulcerative lesions on the fingers and palms.

Other lesions that may occur less often but are still related to SLE include dermal atrophy, mucosal ulceration that involves both oral and genital mucosa, and gangrene secondary to vascular insufficiency that may progress in conjunction with Raynaud's phenomenon.

The erythematous, scaling, disclike plaques that are characteristic of DLE may also be seen on SLE skin biopsies. Immunofluorescent studies of patients with DLE reveal the presence of immune complexes, specifically the lumpy deposits of IgM that are diagnostic of this disorder.

Alopecia is particularly common, with frontal alopecia seen more frequently in women.

Musculoskeletal Manifestations

Polyarthralgias and polyartheritis occur in approximately 90% to 95% of patients with SLE at some time during the course of their illness. The dominant problem is articular movement. The arthritis that develops may resemble rheumatoid arthritis, but bony erosions and severe deformities are unusual. In SLE, articular involvement tends to be a symmetric, nondeforming arthritis that affects the small joints of the hands, wrists, knees, and metatarsophalangeal joints. Mild deformities may develop in the digits, but it is unusual to find contractures and joint erosion on x-rays. Half of patients with SLE have morning stiffness, 7% develop rheumatoid nodules, and approximately 30% demonstrate rheumatoid factor. SLE may also manifest pain and/or swelling with redness over the joint.

Synovial fluid is clear yellow with a low viscosity when tapped. Generally it has a white count that does not exceed 4,000/μl, most of which are lymphocytes. Avascular necrosis of the bone is common, with the femoral head being the most frequently involved. Steroids, which are commonly administered in SLE, may contribute to avascular bone necrosis.

Polyserositis

Polyserositis is the inflammation of the serosal surfaces of the pericardium, thorax, and abdomen. It often results in pericarditis, pleuritis, and, less frequently, peritonitis. The most common symptom is pain.

Pericarditis is the most common cardiac manifestation of SLE. It often is the first clinical problem the patient manifests. Pericardial friction rub, commonly associated with pericarditis, can lead to arrhythmias. However, severe myocardial ischemia in SLE rarely results in tamponade.

Pleurisy and pleural effusions resulting from inflammation of the pleura are relatively common. Although 75% of patients with SLE demonstrate pleural fluid, massive pleural effusions are rare. Involvement of the pleura often produces pleuritic chest pain and shortness of breath.

Although peritonitis is extremely rare, it typically gives rise to diffuse abdominal pain, nausea, vomiting, anorexia, and ascites, indicating inflammation of the abdominal peritoneal membrane. These patients must also be evaluated for other causes of abdominal pain (e.g., hepatosplenomegaly and systemic adenopathy). Liver function studies should be evaluated for chronic active hepatitis and lupoid hepatitis.

Patients with pericarditis and pleuritis may also have concomitant peritonitis.

Pulmonary Manifestations

Lupus pneumonitis is as common as pleuritic pain with or without evidence of a rub or pleuritis in patients with SLE. Resistive interstitial lung disease is the most common pulmonary problem in lupus. However, whenever a pulmonary infiltrate develops in patients with SLE, particularly those taking corticosteroids, infection must be the first consideration. Chest x-rays usually are normal but may demonstrate atelectasis or interstitial fibrosis. Other pulmonary symptoms may include pulmonary hypertension, alveolar hemorrhage, pneumothorax, hemothorax, and vasculitis.

Pleural effusions that occur in SLE are the transudate type, with a total white cell count of approximately 3,000/μl. These white cells usually are lymphocytes. A hemorrhagic pleural effusion is extremely rare.

Cardiovascular Manifestations

As previously mentioned, pericarditis is the most common cardiac manifestation of SLE, occurring in approximately 50% of all patients. It causes chest pain, cardiac friction rub, dyspnea, and fever. Large-volume pericardial effusions and tamponade are rare.

Myocarditis occurs in fewer than 10% of patients. In those who have it, congestive heart failure with tachycardia, gallop rhythm, and cardiomegaly is common. Arrhythmias are unusual and are considered an ominous preterminal event.

Valvular involvement often is seen on postmortem pathologic examinations. It is characterized by vegetative lesions, called *Libman-Sacks lesions*, which generally are found in the mitral valve leaflets. These lesions rarely cause functional defects.

Vasculitis in the small vessels is frequently observed in patients with active SLE. Cutaneous manifestations include splinter hemorrhages, periungual occlusions, fingertip infarction, and atrophic ulcers. Peripheral neuropathy and arteritis are also common. It is possible that patients may experience a cerebral vascular accident as a result of this SLE vasculitis.

Renal Manifestations

Renal involvement is the most common complication in SLE and usually develops within the first 2 years after the diagnosis of SLE is made. DNA-containing immune complexes are the major cause of lupus glomerulonephritis, or **lupus nephritis.** Four characteristic renal lesions can be identified by light microscopy, immunofluorescence, and electron microscopy (see box). Diffuse proliferative glomerulonephritis and membranous glomerulonephritis often are associated with progression to chronic renal failure.

Clinically lupus nephritis is characterized by proteinuria, abnormal urinary sediment (including red and white cell casts), hematuria, cylinduria, and pyuria, and is followed by the typical symptoms of impending renal failure. Hypertension is frequently seen in patients with SLE who have renal involvement. In addition, a high sedimentation rate and an increase in serum levels of anti-ds-DNA antibodies often occur before the onset of lupus glomerulonephritis.[64,154]

Generally, patients with an identified focal glomerular nephritis on renal biopsy have a better renal prognosis than those with diffuse proliferative or membranous glomerulonephritis. Patients who develop end-stage renal failure requiring dialysis have been shown to go into a state of remission. The exact mechanism for this is not known, but the uremic state has been suggested; or it may be that SLE affected primarily the kidneys, which have failed.

Gastrointestinal Manifestations

Gastrointestinal manifestations include abdominal pain, diarrhea, hemorrhage, pancreatitis, cholecystitis, and bowel infarction. Abdominal pain is very difficult to diagnose in patients taking steroids. Pain may be the result of medications, other therapy, or the disease itself. Generally abdominal pain in patients with SLE is uncommon, and if it occurs, it usually is the result of serositis or vasculitis.

Hepatomegaly is present in about one third of patients, and hepatic dysfunction is typically rare. Splenomegaly is an infrequent finding.[166,167]

Neuropsychiatric Manifestations

Mental and neurologic symptoms occur in approximately 35% to 40% of all patients with SLE. Symptoms usually relate to the central nervous system and not the peripheral nerves. One of the primary explanations for neuropsychiatric manifestations in SLE is that the choroid plexus is a major filtration site for immune complexes and their deposition. On postmortem examination, patients who showed neurologic disorders tended to have an accumulation of immunoglobulin and DNA throughout the choroid plexus.[145] Cerebrospinal fluid

---

RENAL LESIONS IN LUPUS NEPHRITIS*

Mesangial glomerulonephritis: hypercellularity and deposition of immune complexes in the mesangium

Focal glomerulonephritis: segmental proliferation and immune complex deposition in the mesangium and subendothelium of the glomerular capillaries

Diffuse proliferative glomerulonephritis: profuse cellular proliferation; immune complexes are deposited in the subendothelial layer

Membranous glomerulonephritis: normal glomerular cellularity with a thickened capillary basement membrane; immune complexes are deposited primarily in the subepithelial and intramembranous layer

*Listed in order of increasing severity.

---

often has an elevated protein concentration with a mild lymphocytosis and depressed complement C4 level. In patients with nonfocal central nervous system involvement, antineural antibodies may be present in the cerebrospinal fluid.

Neuropsychiatric manifestations vary considerably, ranging from a number of behavioral disturbances (e.g., mild anxiety, depression, minor memory defects) to major psychosis. Primary disturbances initially identified usually are changes in mentation, progressing from mild to severe aberrant behaviors.

Organic symptoms can include focal vascular lesions, which may result in seizures or multifocal neurologic defects. Other manifestations might include convulsions, cranial nerve palsies, aseptic meningitis, migraine headaches, seizures, peripheral neuritis, and cerebrovascular accidents.

Ocular Manifestations

Ocular manifestations of SLE occur in 20% to 25% of all patients. The characteristic lesion is located in the retina and is called a cytoid body. It is a small, oval, white, fluffy opacity that is caused by a focal ischemic degeneration of the nerve fiber layer in the retina. It generally occurs secondary to retinal vasculitis. Other nonspecific manifestations include conjunctivitis, retinal hemorrhage, and exudates. Corneal ulceration may be seen; however, this usually occurs in conjunction with Sjögren's syndrome.

Hematologic Manifestations

In 80% of all patients with SLE, a normochromic anemia is present. With renal insufficiency or failure, the anemic state becomes progressively worse. Occasionally a hemolytic anemia develops that may be an antibody-mediated autoimmune phenomena.

Mild leukopenia is seen in approximately half of all patients at some time in the course of the disease. It often is seen in conjunction with lymphopenia. Thrombocytopenia is also common, occurring in about 30% of patients. The erythrocyte sedimentation rate may also be elevated, particularly in patients with active disease.

Pregnancy and SLE

Pregnant patients with SLE have a 25% increased risk of exacerbation of their disease, spontaneous abortion, stillbirth, and premature labor and delivery. In contrast, 25% will go into remission and another 25% will remain the same.

DIAGNOSTIC STUDIES AND FINDINGS

Diagnostic test	Findings
Antinuclear antibody (ANA)	Positive in titers >1:80; present in approximately 95% of patients
Anti–double-stranded DNA (ds-DNA) antibody	Positive in titers >1:80
Anti–single-stranded DNA (ss-DNA) antibody	May be present in patients with SLE who are ANA negative
Anti-ribosomal (anti-RNA) antibody	Present in 25%-50% of patients
LE cell prep (lupus erythematosus cell prep)	Positive in 70%-80% of patients; may decrease with steroid therapy
Rheumatoid factor (RF) (anti-IgG antibody)	Positive in titers >40% in 30% of patients
Serum immunoglobulins	Hypergammaglobulinemia
Circulating immune complexes	Present during flare-ups, with deposition along basement membranes
Complete blood count (CBC)	Pancytopenia or selective deficits; mild lymphopenia, worse during flare-ups; 80% of patients have normochromic, normocytic anemia
Complement	C3 and C4 decreased during flare-ups, indicating acute inflammation; C5-9 often increased during flare-ups, otherwise within normal limits (these changes are present in approximately 80% of patients)
C-reactive protein	Elevated during flare-ups, indicating acute inflammation
Erythrocyte sedimentation rate (ESR)	Elevated during flare-ups, indicating acute inflammation
Direct Coombs' test	Positive in approximately 10%-65% of patients; positive with hemolytic anemia because of autoantibody production against erythrocytes
Coagulation profile	Prolonged prothrombin time and thromboplastin time if circulating anticoagulant antibodies are present; occurs in approximately 10%-15% of patients
Rapid plasma reagin (RPR) test	Falsely positive in approximately 10%-20% of patients
Urinalysis	Abnormal WBC/RBC casts and sediment and protein associated with renal damage
Renal biopsy	Frequently an accumulation of irregular or granular immunoglobulin and complement is observed with immunofluorescence along the glomerular basement membrane and in the mesangium, causing focal, diffuse, membranous, or interstitial nephritis
Skin biopsy	Approximately 90% of patients demonstrate immunoglobulin (Ig) (IgG and IgM) and complement deposition in the dermal-epidermal junction on biopsy; usually not associated with "lupus rash"; patients with only DLE generally demonstrate only deposition of Ig and complement in involved skin areas
Chest x-ray	May demonstrate cardiomegaly, pleural effusions, or plate-like atelectasis
Joint x-rays	May demonstrate soft tissue swelling and mild osteopenia without erosions
Lumbar puncture to evaluate cerebrospinal fluid	Often elevated protein concentration; mild lymphocytosis; decreased complement C4

DIAGNOSIS OF SLE

Diagnosis of SLE can be made only through a comprehensive history and physical examination and in-depth evaluation of laboratory data. No single test is diagnostic for SLE, and clinical manifestations may in some cases make it difficult to differentiate from rheumatoid arthritis. In addition, the onset of the disorder can be insidious and the symptoms vague, which may present an initial diagnostic problem.

Since the symptoms of SLE can affect almost every organ, eleven clinical findings have been developed to assist in the diagnosis. The presence of four or more of these symptoms, either simultaneously or serially, in conjunction with positive laboratory data generally confirms the diagnosis of SLE.[93,153,168]

1. **Malar rash:** fixed erythema, flat or raised, over malar eminence, tending to spare nasolabial folds
2. **Discoid rash:** erythematous, raised patches with adherent keratotic scaling and follicular plugging; atrophic scarring
3. **Photosensitivity:** skin rash as a result of unusual reaction to sunlight; based on patient history or observation
4. **Oral or nasopharyngeal ulcers:** usually painless
5. **Arthritis:** nonerosive, minimum two joint involvement, characterized by tenderness, swelling, or effusion
6. **Serositis:** pleuritis, convincing history of pleuritic pain or rub that is ausculated; evidence of pleural effusion or pericarditis documented by electrocardiogram, rub, or evidence of pericardial effusion
7. **Renal disorders:** persistent proteinuria of 500 mg/day or 3+ if quantitative; no preformed or cellular casts; may be red cell, hemoglobin, granular, tubular, or mixed
8. **Neurologic disorders:** seizures in the absence of offending drugs or known metabolic derangements (e.g., uremia, ketoacidosis, electrolyte imbalance) or psychosis in the absence of offending drugs or known metabolic derangements
9. **Hematologic disorders:** hemolytic anemia with reticulocytosis or leukopenia with a WBC $<4,000/\mu L$ total on two or more occasions, or thrombocytopenia less with a platelet count of $<100,000/\mu L$ in the absence of offending drugs or lymphopenia
10. **Immunologic disorders:** manifested by positive LE-cell preparation, anti-DNA antibodies directed against the genetic material in host cells, or a false positive serologic test for syphilis (VDRL). Known to be positive for at least 6 months and confirmed by *Treponema pallidum* immobilization or fluorescent treponemal antibody absorption test
11. **Antinuclear antibody (ANA):** abnormal titer of antinuclear antibody by immunofluorescence or equivalent assay at any point in time in the absence of drugs known to be associated with drug-induced lupus syndrome

ANTINUCLEAR ANTIBODIES

A number of antinuclear and anticytoplasmic antibodies have been identified in patients with SLE. The method most commonly used to detect these antinuclear factors is immunofluorescence. The immunofluorescent assay for ANA can detect several autoantibodies (including LE-cell factor) to nuclear components. Almost all patients with SLE have a positive ANA titer; however, titers may vary with disease activity. Four clinically significant patterns of immunofluorescent staining have been described in patients with SLE:

1. A homogeneous or diffuse pattern, found in patients with drug-induced or systemic SLE
2. A peripheral or outline pattern, seen in patients with active SLE
3. A "speckled" pattern, which demonstrates the presence of antibodies against non-DNA nuclear constituents
4. A "nucleolar" pattern, seen in patients with scleroderma

COMPLICATIONS

Chronic renal failure
Hemolytic anemia
Central nervous system disease
Pulmonary hemorrhage
Pneumonitis
Myocarditis
Pericarditis
Severe thrombocytopenia or granulocytopenia
Mesenteric vasculitis

POSTMORTEM PATHOLOGIC FINDINGS

Libman-Sacks vegetations in the heart are found on postmortem examination of patients with SLE. These lesions cause a verrucous (nonbacterial) endocarditis. They appear as necrotic debris, fibrinoid material, and trapped, disintegrating, fibroblastic and inflammatory cells. They most often are found along the base of the valves and less commonly on the chordae tendineae and papillary muscles.

Other postmortem findings may include a periarterial fibrosis (called an "onion skin" lesion) in the spleen and hematoxylin lesions. Hematoxylin lesions occur as homogeneous, nuclear, globular masses that stain blue-purple with hematoxylin. They have been seen in the heart, lungs, kidneys, spleen, lymph nodes, and serous and synovial membranes.

AUTOANTIBODIES IN SYSTEMIC LUPUS ERYTHEMATOSUS

Autoantibody	Possible clinical manifestations
Antinuclear anti–double-stranded DNA (ds-DNA)	Nephritis, vasculitis, pleuritis, pericarditis, synovitis, peritonitis
Antineuronal	Cerebritis, organic brain syndromes, peripheral neuropathies
Anticoagulant	Coagulopathies
Anti–red blood cell (RBC)	Anemia
Anti–white blood cell (WBC)	Leukopenia, lymphopenia, infection
Antiplatelet	Thrombocytopenia
Anti–basement membrane	Nephritis, dermatitis

MEDICAL MANAGEMENT

There is no known cure for SLE. Management of the disorder depends on the nature and severity of the manifestations and the organs affected. The goals of treatment include therapeutic management of the signs and symptoms of the syndrome, early recognition of flare-ups, suppression of inflammation, induction of remission, and prevention of untoward complications of the illness and required therapy.

GENERAL MANAGEMENT

Physical activity: Encourage a balance between rest and exercise; flare-ups warrant temporary rest, otherwise a regular exercise program should be implemented; walking, swimming, and bicycling are recommended.

Protection from the environment: Instruct patient to avoid sun (ultraviolet) and fluorescent light exposure; to use sunscreen.

Stress management: Encourage patient to use strategies to minimize stress in daily life routines.

Nutrition/diet: No added salt (if taking steroids), daily multivitamin with minerals; encourage foods high in protein and complex carbohydrates, moderately low in saturated fat and cholesterol.

Birth control: Instruct patient to avoid birth control pills or intrauterine device (IUDs); preferred method of contraception is a diaphragm and foam.

Renal function: Monitor for elevated BUN and creatinine, rising anti-DNA ANA titers, falling complement, and urinary sediment, which indicate active kidney disease.

Preventing infection: Monitor closely for any signs or symptoms of infection, with immediate follow-up on patient's complaints of clinical symptoms of infection.

Routine physical and follow-up: Patients should be seen biyearly (more frequently with active disease or multisystem involvement) to monitor for disease manifestation in specific organs and side effects of medications.

DRUG THERAPY

Indications for drug therapy depend largely on the severity of the disease. Drug requirements range from no medication to aspirin or antimalarial drugs to corticosteroids and cytotoxic drugs for severe forms of the disease. The primary purposes of drug therapy in SLE are to suppress the disease process, decrease inflammation, alter the immune system, and maintain functioning of other body organs and systems.

Salicylates (aspirin) and nonsteroidal antiinflammatory drugs (to control inflammation and suppress the disease process)

Aspirin is used as an antiinflammatory agent to control musculoskeletal pain—it is important to keep blood levels constant; often used when arthritis is the predominate symptom and other organs are not involved; daily oral dose is 3-6 g for adults.

Nonsteroidal antiinflammatory drugs (e.g. indomethacin [Indocin]) are also used but given with caution in the presence of renal dysfunction; adult dosage is 25-50 mg PO 3-4 times/day.

Patients taking these medications should be monitored for gastrointestinal bleeding.

Antimalarial drugs (hydroxychloroquine or chloroquine) (to control skin lesions and joint pain): Hydroxychloroquine (Plaquenil) is used to control discoid and other skin lesions and rheumatic manifestations; adult dosage is 200-400 mg bid PO. Because retinal toxicity may occur at higher doses, patients should receive pretreatment and annual ophthalmic examinations.

Continued.

MEDICAL MANAGEMENT—cont'd

Corticosteroids (antiinflammatory agents)

Prednisone oral or IV (e.g., Orasone, Deltasone, Meticorten): Indications for steroid use are renal, skeletal muscle, myocardium, and central nervous system involvement, hemolytic anemia, thrombocytopenic purpura, and sometimes to control progressive skin lesions and fever.

The dosage varies with the intensity of the disease. General guidelines for prednisone administration are:
   Mild: 5-10 mg daily
   Moderate: 20-30 mg daily with a gradual taper once the disease is under control
   Major organ involvement and polymyositis: 50-100 mg daily (taper)

On rare occasions a patient may be prescribed 100-150 mg daily in divided doses with a taper. Any amount of prednisone given as a single oral dose in the morning has less adrenal-suppressing activity than the same amount given in divided doses throughout the day. Therefore, if taken in divided doses, prednisone has greater lupus-suppressing activity than does the same amount of drug given as a single morning dose.

Intraarticular steroid injections may prove useful in alleviating synovitis and joint pain.

Methylprednisolone IV (Solu-Medrol):

SLE crisis is rare, but the therapy for it is 1 g or 15 mg/kg/day in divided doses IV for 3 consecutive days. This generally is considered a "steroid pulse" and is a lifesaving measure. (Cytotoxic agents are also given at the same time.) Daily oral prednisone dose usually is continued through the treatment episode.

Topical steroids are used for skin eruptions and flare-ups: hydrocortisone (Cortaid), fluocinonide (Lidex), betamethasone dipropionate (Diprosone), flurandrenolide (Cordran), betamethasone valerate (Valisone), and fluocinolone acetonide (Synalar).

Cytotoxic agents (when steroids are not effective):   Chlorambucil (Leukeran); azathioprine (Imuran); cyclophosphamide (Cytoxan, Neosar). These drugs are reserved for patients who do not respond to corticosteroids. They have serious complications and side effects (secondary malignancies, bone marrow suppression, infection, and liver toxicity), and they must be used with caution. Although they are used to suppress the clinical manifestations of SLE, long-term effectiveness and resulting toxicity must be considered.

Dosing guidelines for adults: azathioprine, 25 mg 3 times/wk to 150 mg qd PO; cyclophosphamide, 25 mg 3 times/wk to 150 mg qd PO; chlorambucil, 2 mg twice a week to 10 mg qd PO.

Other medications:

Antibiotics; antihypertensive agents; sympatholytic drugs (to treat Raynaud's syndrome).

ADJUNCTIVE THERAPY

Plasmapheresis

Total lymphoid irradiation (TLI)

Renal replacement therapy: short-term—dialysis or hemofiltration; long-term—peritoneal dialysis, hemodialysis, or kidney transplant

SURGERY

Joint replacement may be indicated if chronic synovitis and pain are problematic.

<u>1</u> ASSESS

ASSESSMENT	OBSERVATIONS
History	Recent infection, frequent sun exposure, stressful life-style or recent stressful event, familial prevalence
Medications	Review current medications (prescribed, over the counter, herbal therapy, and illicit drugs)
General complaints	Recurrent low-grade fever 37.2°-38° C (99°-100.4° F), anorexia, weight loss, malaise, fatigue, lethargy, sicca complex (see Sjögren's syndrome)
Skin and mucous membranes	Facial erythema with butterfly dermatitis over bridge of nose and on cheeks; types of skin lesions: diffuse, transient rashes; urticarial lesions; bullae; patches of vitiligo; subcutaneous nodes; thickening of epidermis; livedo reticularis; "discoid lesions"; demarcated, annular, erythematous plaques with or without atrophy, scaling, and telangiectasia; photosensitivity, with classic distribution of skin lesions over sun-exposed areas of the skin; pruritus may or may not be present; generalized purpura and petechiae; ulcers: oral, nasal, genital, legs, and digital pads, with potential for gangrene
Hair	"Lupus hair": thin, unruly, fractures easily; alopecia, particularly around frontal hairline
Musculoskeletal	Polyarthralgias, arthritis, diffuse myalgias, steroid-induced osteoporosis, aseptic bone necrosis or myopathy that may result in episodic joint and muscle pain with or without changes, immobility, or joint deformities
Pulmonary	Dyspnea related to pleurisy, pleural effusion, pneumonitis, interstitial fibrosis, pulmonary emboli; decreased pulmonary function; pulmonary hypertension
Cardiovascular	Chest pain, pericardial friction rub, tachycardia, or orthopnea that may be related to pericarditis, endocarditis, or myocarditis; redness and pain in an extremity related to thrombophlebitis; diffuse vasculitis; Raynaud's syndrome
Renal	Peripheral edema, hypertension, anemia, electrolyte imbalances, nausea, decrease in urination related to lupus nephritis
Gastrointestinal	Abdominal pain related to gastric and duodenal ulcers (may be steroid induced), diarrhea, dysphagia, peritonitis, "acute abdomen"
Hematologic	Anemia with pallor and fatigue; thrombocytopenia with prolonged bleeding, easy bruising; increased risk of infection related to lymphocytopenia, lymphadenopathy, leukocytosis, granulocytopenia
Ocular	Visual impairment generally related to cytoid bodies or retinal vasculitis; periorbital edema
Neuropsychiatric	Lupus cerebritis seizures, cranial neuropathies, visual disturbances, vertigo, nystagmus, cranial nerve palsies, aphasia, headaches, peripheral neuropathies, anxiety, depression, mania, insomnia, confusion, hallucinations, disorientation, emotional lability, psychosis
Immunologic	Increased ANA titers, LE prep cell, decreased complement

2 DIAGNOSE

NURSING DIAGNOSIS	SUBJECTIVE FINDINGS	OBJECTIVE FINDINGS
Impaired skin integrity related to integumentary manifestations resulting from immunologic alterations	Complains of transient rashes, skin irritation and discomfort, and hair loss	Erythematous rash over sun-exposed areas of skin, with butterfly dermatitis on the face; frontal alopecia
Impaired physical mobility related to arthritis and generalized weakness	Complains of weakness and joint and muscle pain with activity	Decreased activity; unable to complete routine daily activities; remains in bed more than usual; joints are stiff and reddened
Ineffective breathing pattern related to pulmonary complications, most commonly pneumonia	Complains of difficulty breathing	Dyspnea, fever, rhonchi, crackles (rales) in posterior lung fields on auscultation, tachypnea, productive cough
Decreased cardiac output related to reduced ventricular filling (most commonly due to pericarditis)	Complains of chest pain and shortness of breath	Dyspnea, tachypnea, tachycardia, jugular venous distention, muffled heart sounds, friction rub, fever, arrhythmias, pale, diaphoresis
Altered renal tissue perfusion related to renal complications secondary to immune complex deposition	Complains of ankle swelling, weight gain, nausea, decreased appetite, fatigue	Peripheral edema, increased fluid weight gain (>2 kg/48 h), elevated blood pressure, elevated BUN and creatinine, hyperkalemia, increased ESR; urinalysis demonstrates proteinuria (>500 mg/24 h) with red and white casts, mild hematuria
Altered nutrition: less than body requirements related to anorexia, electrolyte imbalance, or chemotherapy side effects	Complains of decreased appetite and fatigue	Decreased food and fluid intake, intermittent vomiting, decreased body weight
Ineffective individual coping related to organic brain syndrome associated with SLE and difficulty dealing with the diagnosis and its implications	Complains of inability to concentrate and "losing time"; reports persistent fatigue and depression	Emotionally labile, decreased activity, lethargic, changes in judgment and intellectual function, disoriented, may develop seizures
Potential activity intolerance related to flare-ups, chronic anemia, arthralgias, and myalgias	Reports avoiding activities and a decreased ability to participate in ADLs	Fatigue with minimal exertion; movements are guarded and slow; decreased Hgb and Hct

NURSING DIAGNOSIS	SUBJECTIVE FINDINGS	OBJECTIVE FINDINGS
Body image disturbance and **altered role performance** related to multisystem involvement of SLE, including skin changes	Reports difficulty in adjusting to body changes and fear of rejection by others because of appearance	Seeks treatment alone, without usual companion; hides most of skin under clothing; if hospitalized, does not leave room
Potential for infection related to alteration in immune system or to treatment	Complains of skin rash and difficulty breathing	Currently taking high-dose steroids; poor nutritional status; areas of skin breakdown; decreased lung expansion; decreased breath sounds on auscultation over lower posterior lung fields; thick, purulent sputum with productive cough; fever

3 PLAN

Patient goals

1. The patient's integument will remain intact.
2. The patient will be able to perform routine daily activities.
3. The patient's breathing pattern will be effective, without fatigue or dyspnea.
4. The patient's cardiac output will remain stable.
5. The patient's renal function will have stabilized.
6. The patient will consume adequate calories and fluid and maintain an adequate nutritional state.
7. The patient will demonstrate effective coping skills.
8. The patient will maintain her activity level.
9. The patient will have a positive, accepting, and realistic body image.
10. The patient will have no signs or symptoms of infection.

4 IMPLEMENT

NURSING DIAGNOSIS	NURSING INTERVENTIONS	RATIONALE
Impaired skin integrity related to integumentary manifestations resulting from immunologic alterations	Assess and monitor skin and mucous membranes daily: inspect and palpate, noting color; vascularity; lesion size, configuration, and distribution; edema; moisture; temperature; texture; thickness; mobility; and turgor.	To detect site of skin breakdown or disruption in mucous membranes and to monitor for infection.
	Measure intake and output; provide adequate nutrition.	To ensure adequate hydration and nutrition, to maintain an intact skin, and to ensure sufficient nutrients for healing.
	Encourage patient to perform oral hygiene (brushing, flossing, mouthwash); irrigate lesions as ordered.	To promote comfort and decrease risk of infection; commercial mouthwashes contain alcohol and are not recommended; use normal saline, water, or 1:2 or 1:4 hydrogen peroxide.

→ 〉 〉

NURSING DIAGNOSIS	NURSING INTERVENTIONS	RATIONALE
	Provide hypoallergenic, nondrying soaps and mild shampoos; no hair dryers.	To prevent skin breakdown, promote healing, and minimize damage to already thin, fragile hair.
	Keep skin clean and dry.	To maintain an intact skin and prevent breakdown.
	Encourage patient to keep sun exposure minimal by wearing long-sleeved blouses or shirts and wide-brim hats and by using sunscreens with a sun protection factor (SPF) of 15; recommend ultraviolet shields for protection from indoor lighting if patient is very sensitive.	Most patients are photosensitive, and ultraviolet light can cause episodes of exacerbation; SPF is related to the amount of paraaminobenzoic acid, or PABA, in the sunscreen.
	Encourage patient to ambulate three or four times during the day; if patient is unable, change her position q 1-2 h.	To maintain circulation to skin and prevent skin breakdown.
	Administer topical steroidal or antiinfective creams and ointments as ordered; assess response.	To protect from further damage and promote healing.
	Monitor drugs patient is taking.	High-dose steroids can increase skin's susceptibility to impairment.
	Provide active and passive ROM exercises.	To maintain circulation and oxygenation to tissues and to assist in preventing skin impairment and breakdown.
	Do not use adhesive tapes directly on skin.	To avoid stripping epidermis when removing tape.
	Use natural sheepskin pad.	To reduce friction and irritation and provide comfort and resistance to pressure distribution.
Impaired physical mobility related to arthritis and generalized weakness	Assess degree of limitation: ROM, joint integrity, presence of pain (location, duration, quality, severity, and precipitating or alleviating factors), deformity, and muscular atrophy.	To detect degree of limitation and to assist in developing a plan of activity.
	Perform ROM exercises routinely in collaboration with physical therapist.	To maintain joint mobility and muscle strength.
	Administer thermal therapy to muscles and joints.	Heat may improve mobility and relieve pain.
	Provide a balanced regimen of activity and rest.	To promote mobilization and increase strength, yet avoid fatigue and exhaustion.
	Consult with occupational therapist, physical therapist, and exercise physiologist to develop an exercise plan.	Expert team members can provide an individualized activity plan.

NURSING DIAGNOSIS	NURSING INTERVENTIONS	RATIONALE
	Encourage patient to participate in routine exercise and rest schedule.	To maintain muscle strength and ability to participate in routine activities.
	Help patient use mobility aids (e.g., splints), particularly during flare-ups.	To provide support to the affected joint and to maintain mobility and function.
	Encourage patient to participate in self-care activities.	To maintain function and promote well-being and self-esteem.
Ineffective breathing pattern related to pulmonary complications, most commonly pneumonia	Assess pulmonary status: auscultate lungs for decreased breath sounds, rhonchi, or crackles (rales).	To detect or prevent respiratory compromise and to determine adequacy of gas exchange, effectiveness of breathing, and areas of congestion and atelectasis.
	Monitor respiratory rate and rhythm.	To determine the work of breathing.
	Monitor chest x-ray and ABGs.	To determine the extent of pulmonary involvement and the acid-base balance, adequacy of gas exchange, and need for oxygen.
	Monitor changes in activity tolerance.	Activity may induce dyspnea.
	Teach patient deep-breathing exercises, and encourage her to perform them as often as needed; encourage her to use blow bottles.	To facilitate deep breathing and assist in the management or prevention of pulmonary complications.
	Monitor for changes in behavior, increased apprehension, irritation, and alteration in orientation.	May indicate hypoxia.
	Administer oxygen, analgesics, inhalants, bronchodilators, antibiotics, and steroids as ordered; monitor response.	To promote gas exchange and flow to and from the alveoli and to assist in the resolution of pulmonary complications.
	Measure tidal volume and vital capacity.	To monitor volume of air moving in and out of lungs.
	Provide chest physiotherapy and postural drainage as necessary.	To facilitate mobilization of secretions.
	Position the patient in optimum body alignment (high Fowler's) for breathing.	To optimize diaphragmatic contractions.
Decreased cardiac output related to reduced ventricular filling (most commonly due to pericarditis)	Auscultate apical pulse for cardiac rate and rhythm, and monitor q 2 h.	To identify irregularities.
	Auscultate for heart sounds q 2 h for pericardial friction rub (may be distant or intermittent); heard best at left midsternal border during expiration.	Friction rub reflects friction between roughened pericardial and epicardial surfaces; friction rub may indicate an effusion or pericarditis.

NURSING DIAGNOSIS	NURSING INTERVENTIONS	RATIONALE
	Monitor vital signs q 2-4 h as indicated or ordered.	To detect pericardial restriction, decrease in blood pressure, and tachycardia.
	Assess for subjective syncope or palpitations.	These may reflect a sudden decrease in cardiac output in response to antiarrhythmic agents.
	Assess for pulsus paradoxus, narrowing pulse pressure, and respiratory filling of neck veins.	To detect early signs of increasing intrapericardial pressure and possible impending tamponade.
	Monitor ECG, and document changes.	To obtain a baseline for evaluation and to differentiate pericarditis from other cardiac complications.
	Assess for subjective complaints of chest pain; have patient sit up, lean forward, and breathe out.	Pericarditis characteristically appears with a sharp pain radiating from the left anterior precordia to the left shoulder; a change in position may minimize pain; if progressive, pain may be related to ischemic changes and require urgent medical intervention.
	Administer antibiotics, analgesics, and steroids, and monitor patient's response.	To reduce pain and enhance cardiac function.
Altered renal tissue perfusion related to renal complications secondary to immune complex deposition	Monitor fluid status, intake and output, daily weight, and blood pressure; check for peripheral edema and shortness of breath; administer diuretics as ordered, and monitor patient's response.	Increased fluid volume may indicate that kidneys are unable to handle excess fluid as a result of decreased renal function; diuretics may help remove excess fluid.
	Monitor blood pressure for hypertension; administer diuretics and/or antihypertensive agents as ordered, and monitor response.	Hypertension may be the result of volume overload or disruption of the renin-angiotensin mechanism.
	Assess for nausea and anorexia; administer zinc as ordered.	Increased urea levels cause anorexia and nausea; zinc may improve appetite in patients with renal insufficiency.
	Modify diet as indicated (decrease foods high in potassium and protein).	To prevent hyperkalemia and azotemia; protein breaks down into urea.
	Monitor urinalysis and 24-h creatinine clearance (Crcl); normal Crcl is 80-120 ml/min.	Proteinuria >500 mg/day and Crcl <50 ml/min are indicators of decreasing renal function and require further evaluation.
	Monitor serum laboratory values, specifically elevations in BUN, creatinine (Scr), potassium, and phosphorus (alterations in calcium-phosphorus balance) and decreased Hct, Hgb, and carbon dioxide.	To detect early signs of renal insufficiency; normal BUN is 8-20 mg/dl, normal Scr is 0.5-1.2 mg/dl, potassium 3.5-5 mEq/L, calcium 8.5-10.5 mg/dl, phosphorus 2.5-4.5 mg/dl, carbon dioxide 24-32 mEq/L.

NURSING DIAGNOSIS	NURSING INTERVENTIONS	RATIONALE
	Administer antihypertensive agents, bicarbonate, aluminum hydroxide and/or calcium, and erythropoietin as ordered, and monitor patient's response.	To prolong renal function and maintain acid-base balance, calcium-phosphorus balance, and Hct.
	In collaboration with nephrology nurse, educate patient and family about renal insufficiency and replacement therapy when appropriate.	To provide patient and family with accurate information about renal insufficiency and failure and to obtain informed consent for treatment options when appropriate.
Altered nutrition: less than body requirements related to anorexia, electrolyte imbalance, or chemotherapy side effects	Weigh patient daily while hospitalized and every week after discharge; include a height for pediatric and adolescent patients.	To obtain baseline and ongoing data on adequacy of nutritional intake and to guide therapeutic interventions.
	Measure fluid intake and output.	To determine fluid balance and whether weight gain is true weight gain or fluid.
	Monitor albumin, transferrin, and serum protein.	These indicate whether protein intake is adequate.
	Measure midarm circumference and triceps skin fold.	These indicate protein and fat stores, respectively.
	Encourage patient to eat small, frequent meals and to take vitamin supplements.	To promote adequate nutritional intake.
	Consult dietitian to develop a nutritional plan.	To provide expertise in assisting patient with individual diet plan, taking into consideration caloric needs, protein, carbohydrate, and fat requirements, and renal function.
	Encourage family and friends to participate in meals.	To provide comfort and support and to create a positive attitude toward meals.
	Provide oral hygiene before eating.	To improve taste of food, encourage adequate caloric intake, and prevent infection.
	Monitor electrolytes.	Alterations in electrolytes can cause fatigue, weakness, and anorexia.
	Administer antiemetics as ordered, and monitor patient's response.	Nausea is a main side effect of chemotherapy; renal insufficiency may also cause nausea, as a result of uremia.
	Provide diet instruction in collaboration with the dietitian.	To provide accurate information and improve adherence to an adequate diet.

NURSING DIAGNOSIS	NURSING INTERVENTIONS	RATIONALE
Ineffective individual coping related to organic brain syndrome associated with SLE and difficulty dealing with the diagnosis and its implications	Assess and monitor changes in neurologic status: orientation, judgment, and intellectual function.	To obtain baseline data, monitor changes, and guide therapeutic interventions.
	Assess patient's coping mechanisms and behavior.	SLE is a chronic, progressive disorder that requires life-style adjustments; depression is common, and dementia is symptom of advanced disease.
	Make sure patient receives accurate information about SLE.	To minimize any misconceptions and to promote adjustment.
	Teach patient exercises in visualization and relaxation.	To alter patient's mental appraisal of the situation and to make it more manageable.
	Provide emotional support, and work with patient to identify resources for support and coping mechanisms that have proved helpful in the past.	To give patient control over her situation.
	Encourage visits by family and friends at home and in the hospital.	Social support can assist in generating coping skills.
	Encourage participation in local chapter of Lupus Foundation of America.	To provide support and assistance in gaining new insights into the management of SLE.
	Help patient identify coping tactics that have been successful in the past when dealing with difficult situations.	To encourage patient's participation and independence; recollecting previous strategies may help identify methods of coping.
	If orientation is a problem, provide patient with a clock, calendar, and familiar articles; frequently orient to place and time.	To maintain orientation and a sense of control over environment.
	Provide seizure precautions, and maintain environmental safety.	To protect patient.
Potential activity intolerance related to flare-ups, chronic anemia, arthralgias, and myalgias	Observe response to activity.	To determine extent of activity tolerance.
	Minimize factors that contribute to flare-up (e.g., sun exposure, stress, infection).	To minimize risk of flare-ups and to maintain activity tolerance.
	Encourage a balance of rest and activity.	To minimize fatigue.
	Administer analgesics as ordered, and monitor response.	To decrease discomfort of arthralgia and myalgia.
	During flare-ups, perform activities for patient until she can perform them.	To meet patient's needs without causing fatigue.

NURSING DIAGNOSIS	NURSING INTERVENTIONS	RATIONALE
	During quiescent periods, encourage patient to participate in regular aerobic exercise that does not stress joints (e.g., swimming, walking, stair climber).	To promote optimum well-being.
	Consult exercise physiologist to develop individualized exercise plan, and encourage patient to participate.	Expert team member will promote development of an individualized exercise routine in collaboration with patient; this promotes active involvement and aderence to the program and encourages independence.
	Explore with patient what activities are therapeutic, enjoyable, and within her capabilities.	Patients are more likely to participate in activities that they can perform and find enjoyable.
	Assess sleep and nutritional status.	Sleep deprivation may contribute to potential inactivity.
	Assess and monitor Hgb and Hct.	A marked decrease in Hct and Hgb may indicate poor nutrition, renal insufficiency, or a GI complication that may contribute to inactivity and requires further evaluation.
Body image disturbance and **altered role performance** related to multisystem involvement of SLE, including skin changes	Assess patient's perception of body image; investigate what aspects are not pleasing and how changes are perceived as deviating from social norms; determine what personal, social, or community resources are available.	To adequately assess the disturbance to body image and the specific threat, and to guide therapeutic interventions.
	Help patient explore and express feelings about changes in body image.	To help patient realize what changes in body image imply for her.
	Teach patient ways to improve body image (e.g., improved personal hygiene, wearing makeup, change in clothes, protecting skin from sun).	To help patient create a better feeling about her appearance by trying new looks.
	Offer opportunities for social contact, and encourage participation in self-help groups.	Introducing different contacts and services can help patient gain new skills and confidence.
	Acknowledge and give positive reinforcement whenever patient attempts to improve body image.	To demonstrate support and acceptance and to assist in developing patient's self-confidence and a positive body image.
	Encourage patient to participate actively in usual roles and responsibilities.	To maintain an active role within the family, independence, and a positive outlook.
	Encourage family members to maintain open communication with patient.	Open communication may minimize stress of role performance, assist family in modifying roles, and identify and support strengths related to adequate role performance.

➜ ❯ ❯

NURSING DIAGNOSIS	NURSING INTERVENTIONS	RATIONALE
Potential for infection related to alteration in immune system or to treatment	Assess and monitor temperature, vital signs, and WBC.	Fever, tachycardia, tachypnea, and an elevated WBC are indicators of infection.
	Assess breakdown in integument, including mucosa.	Infection is resisted through the body's defense mechanisms, the skin being the prime mechanical barrier; disruption in wound healing and oral candidal infections are common with high-dose steroids.
	Monitor CBC with differential.	Leukopenia and neutropenia increase risk of infection.
	Maintain adequate nutritional balance.	Adequate nutrition supports the immune system.
	Restrict contact with individuals with infectious diseases; advise patient to avoid crowds, particularly when taking high-dose steroids.	To decrease risk of infection.
	Assess all systems, with close attention to neurologic, pulmonary, heart, musculoskeletal, skin, and renal systems and IV line or tube insertion sites.	To detect and prevent infections.
	Help patient establish normal rest and sleep patterns.	Adequate sleep supports the immune system.
	Encourage sanitation and hygiene practices (e.g., routine mouth care, daily bath, good handwashing).	To help keep skin and mucous membranes intact and to decrease risk of proliferation and transmission of infectious organisms.
	Use aseptic technique when providing care; wash hands thoroughly before and after contact with patient.	To prevent introduction of microorganisms.
	Monitor urinalysis, cultures, and chest x-rays.	To detect and prevent infections.
	Promote physical activity as tolerated.	To assist in preventing pulmonary infections and venous stasis.
	Maintain a clean environment.	To minimize risk of microorganisms coming into contact with patient.
	Place patient in protective isolation according to hospital policy (absolute neutrophil count <500 μL generally requires isolation).	To protect patient from risk of infection.
	Administer appropriate antibiotics, antipyretics, and analgesics as ordered, and monitor patient's response.	Prophylactic medication may be necessary when patient is severely immunocompromised.
	Protect patient from injury.	Injury may promote entry of microorganisms that could cause infection.

5 EVALUATE

PATIENT OUTCOME	DATA INDICATING THAT OUTCOME IS REACHED
Integument remains intact.	There is no rash or skin breakdown; mucous membranes are pink and intact; skin is warm and dry; there is no sign of infection; patient knows appropriate skin care.
Patient can perform routine daily activities.	Patient participates in a routine exercise program and regular activities.
Breathing pattern is effective.	Patient is breathing without difficulty; ABGs are normal; vital capacity measurements are optimum for patient.
Cardiac output is maintained.	Patient is hemodynamically stable and normotensive; COP is 4-5 L/min; skin is warm and dry; patient is resting quietly; heart and breath sounds are normal; chest x-ray is normal, and ECG demonstrates normal sinus rhythm.
Renal function has stabilized.	Euvolemia, weight stable; appetite is adequate; urine/plasma ratio is normal; BUN and creatinine, Hct, and electrolytes are normal, and patient is normotensive.
Nutritional status has improved.	Patient can identify factors causing nutritional deficits and maintains food intake to meet metabolic demands; weight has increased; albumin is 3.2-4.5 g/dl; triceps skin fold is 12 mm in men, 23 mm in women; midarm circumference is 32.7 cm in men, 29.2 cm in women.
Patient can cope effectively with SLE.	Patient demonstrates accurate appraisal of illness, expresses feelings appropriately, and develops strategies to assist with coping.
Patient can perform ADLs without pain or fatigue.	Patient demonstrates increased interest in participating in activities and does not complain of pain or fatigue.
Patient has a positive, accepting, and realistic body image.	Patient expresses constructive integration of body image, demonstrates an understanding of changes and strategies to improve body image, and reports feeling much better about herself.
There are no signs or symptoms of infection.	Patient remains afebrile; vital signs, WBCs, and urinalysis are normal; cultures are negative, and chest x-ray is clear; patient does not have a productive cough; skin remains intact; and line and tube insertion sites are free of redness, swelling, or drainage.

PATIENT TEACHING

1. Provide patient and family with information about lupus as a syndrome, and encourage contacting the local chapter of the Lupus Foundation of America.
2. Teach patient and family side effects of all medications and how to manage these side effects. For example, it is best to eat first when taking aspirin or steroids. Specific issues to review regarding steroids include (a) diet: low salt, high protein, long-chain carbohydrates, and monitor caloric intake; (b) monitoring for hyperglycemia when on high doses; (c) monitoring for hypertension; (d) checking weight daily for excessive gain; (e) good mouth hygiene; (f) tapering drug.
3. Teach patient and family the importance of avoiding contact with person who may have contagious infections. Avoid crowds when on high-dose steroids.
4. Teach patient and family the importance of fre-

→ > >

quent assessment for signs and symptoms associated with infection. While steroids are being given, many of these findings are masked, so the slightest change in temperature (>38° C 100.4° F), wound characteristics, pain, or shortness of breath, or other parameters should be reported immediately.

5. Teach the importance of skin care. Instruct patient to avoid dryness and the use of irritating soaps, shampoos, hair dryers, and chemical coloring or permanent waving of hair. Encourage use of hypoallergenic makeup and wearing a wig, scarf, or turban if there is significant hair loss. Teach photosensitive patients to avoid sun exposure; this includes other forms of ultraviolet light, such as tanning salons, as well; limit outdoor activities between 10 AM and 4 PM, wear long sleeves, pants, and wide-brimmed hats, and use sunscreen products with a sun protection factor (SPF) of at least 15.

6. Teach methods of maintaining activity level and coping with arthralgias and myalgias: (a) encourage routine aerobic activity, preferably swimming, walking, or bicycling, and instruct avoidance of activities like jogging that put stress on the joints; (b) range-of-motion exercises; (c) balance between rest and exercise; (d) use of analgesics and nonsteroidal antiinflammatory agents; (e) joint supports at night; (f) participation in physical therapy classes; and (g) contacting the Lupus Foundation of America and the Arthritis Foundation.

7. Teach the importance of regular follow-up by health care provider for a physical exam and blood tests.

8. Teach the importance of recognizing factors that lead to a flare-up: psychologic, emotional, and physical stress; abrupt cessation of medications; photosensitivity; and pregnancy.

9. Teach warning signs of a flare-up: fever (>38° C or 100.4° F), chills, excessive fatigue and malaise, nausea, muscle weakness, increased joint pain, chest pain, oliguria, and dysuria, essentially an exacerbation of *any* old symptom or the development of a new one. Instruct to contact health care provider if this occurs.

10. Teach family planning. Pregnancy is usually allowed during remissions, with close monitoring. Barrier contraceptives such as condoms or a diaphragm with spermicidal jelly are recommended over an intrauterine device (IUD) or birth control pills.

11. Teach the importance of a balanced diet; include restrictions associated with medications.

12. Instruct patient with renal involvement about end-stage renal failure and available treatment options.

13. Teach the importance of keeping a log of the disease course, treatments, and other disease-related information.

14. Teach the importance of obtaining up-to-date information about SLE.

15. Teach patient to carry a medical alert identification at all times.

16. Direct patient and family to appropriate and available resources.

Rheumatoid Arthritis

Rheumatoid arthritis (RA) is classified as an autoimmune disease. It is a chronic, systemic, inflammatory disorder of unknown etiology; it has a predilection for the synovial membranes of several joints and leads to proliferative and degenerative changes.

EPIDEMIOLOGY AND ETIOLOGY

Rheumatoid arthritis affects 1% to 3% of individuals in the United States, with 100,000 to 200,000 new cases

Arthritis means joint inflammation
arth = joint
itis = inflammation

diagnosed each year.[93] RA has a higher incidence among blacks and Caucasians than among Orientals and Hispanics. The onset usually occurs between 20 and 50 years of age, and the disease develops more often in women by a ratio of 3:1.[170]

The clinical pattern of RA demonstrates that 10 to 15 years after diagnosis, 50% of patients have remained the same or improved and 70% continue with full-time employment. However, RA remains one of the major causes of disability, with 10% of these patients having severe, crippling consequences.[93,170]

Although the etiology of RA is unknown, exacerbations may be linked to stressful events. In addition, 35% to 70% of patients with RA carry the HLA-D4 and HLA-DR4 genes, supporting a possible genetic predisposition.[152] It has been postulated that RA develops in genetically susceptible individuals who have an altered response to an environmental antigen. The antigens suspected of initiating the cascade of events that occur in RA have been primarily infectious, including bacteria and viruses (e.g., Epstein-Barr virus [EBV] and rubella). Regardless of the initial stimulus, altered B cell regulation leads to a nonspecific polyclonal Ig response. This response leads to lymphocyte production of antibodies that recognize the host as foreign and attack its own tissues. These altered antibodies are called **rheumatoid factors,** which can develop in high titers as part of this response, form immune complexes (with target Ig and complement) in the serum, and then deposit in synovial membranes where a secondary inflammatory reaction may occur. Importantly, many normal people without RA can have significant titers of RF, and approximately 10% of RA patients test negative for RF. Altered immune cell function, however, is not limited to B cells only; T-cell subsets also can be shown to behave abnormally in patients with RA.[152]

PATHOPHYSIOLOGY

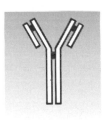 When circulating immune complexes deposit in tissues (in RA, e.g., joints, glomerulus, and pleura), then complement is activated. Activation of complement attracts leukocytes to the synovial membrane, stimulates the release of kinin and prostaglandin, increases vascular permeability, and causes membrane damage by cell lysis. A number of the leukocytes attracted to the synovial membrane perpetuate the inflammatory process by destroying synovial tissue and articular cartilage. Neutrophils and macrophages are leukocytes that phagocytize immune complexes and release very potent lysosomes and enzymes into the synovial space. Synovial and circulating lymphocytes are also activated. B lymphocytes are activated to plasma cells and are stimulated to produce more immunoglobulins and rheumatoid factors. T lymphocytes produce potent mediators that augment and perpetuate the inflammatory response. The immunologic interaction of all these cells results in the release of cytokines, which promote inflammation within the synovial membrane and continue antibody (IgG and IgM) production, including RF.

As the synovial membrane becomes edematous from the infiltration of leukocytes, it protrudes into the joint cavity, causing further inflammation and pain. As the cells of the synovial membrane proliferate and enlarge abnormally, marked hypertrophy of the joint cavity develops. Further, thickening of the synovial membrane, caused by the infiltration of granulation tissue (pannus), tends to cover the surface of the articular cartilage, representing scarlike areas. With progressive inflammation of the synovial membrane, blood vessels subsequently become involved. Occlusion of small venules by hypertrophied synovial endothelial cells, fibrin, platelets, and other inflammatory cells results in decreased blood flow to the tissues, hypoxia, and metabolic acidosis. The onset of acidosis causes the release of hydrolytic enzymes from synovial cells into the surrounding tissues, resulting in erosion of articular cartilage (and later bone) and inflammation in the supporting tissue.

CLINICAL MANIFESTATIONS

The onset of RA may be acute or insidious and generally is marked by joint manifestations. However, extraarticular manifestations are not uncommon and may include fatigue, weakness, a low-grade fever, anorexia, weight loss, and generalized aching and stiffness.

Articular Manifestations

Although RA is considered a systemic disease, joint pain and stiffness often are the initial symptoms, because the synovial linings of the joints are the major sites of tissue inflammation. Generally more than one joint becomes inflamed, and typically joints are symmetrically inflamed bilaterally. The most frequently affected joints are the small joints of the hands, wrists, feet, ankles, and knees, although large joints usually become involved later in the course of the disease. The cervical spine may be involved, but the thoracic and lumbosacral spines generally are not affected.

With inflammation the joint typically is characterized as painful, swollen, tender, and stiff, particularly in the morning, and improves during the day. At the onset of the disease, joint pain generally is attributed to pressure from edema. As the disease progresses, pain may be caused by edema, inflammation, sclerosis of subchondral bone and new bone formation, and grating of unprotected bone surfaces that rub against each other with movement and weight bearing. Joint pain may cause muscle spasms, decreased range of motion, and, in severe cases, muscle contractions and ankylosis with permanent joint deformity.

Joint edema usually is symmetric and is caused by increasing inflammatory exudate within the synovial membrane, hyperplasia of inflamed tissue, and formation of new bone. The joints may feel warm and the synovial membrane "boggy." The skin over the joint may be erythematous and may appear thin and shiny.

As joint inflammation progresses, periarticular tis-

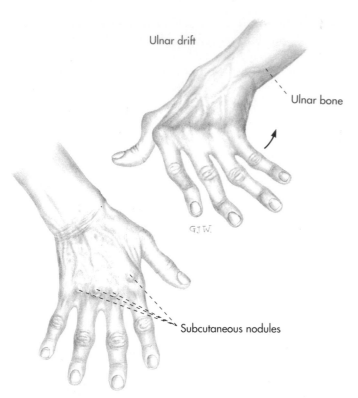

Ulnar drift

Ulnar bone

G.J.W.

Subcutaneous nodules

FIGURE 6-1
Rheumatoid arthritis. A severely affected hand that is wasted, with subcutaneous nodules over the knuckles, swan-neck deformity of middle finger, and ulnar drift of fingers. (From Mourad L: Orthopedic Disorders, St Louis, 1991, Mosby–Year Book.)

Extraarticular Manifestations

Approximately 25% of patients develop extraarticular manifestations such as rheumatoid nodules (which may affect many systems) and vasculitis.[93]

Rheumatoid nodules are made up of a central core of fibrinoid and cellular debris surrounded by mononuclear cells and have an outer margin of granulation tissue containing plasma cells and lymphocytes. They generally are firm, nontender, round or oval masses that may be movable or fixed to tendons or bone. Nodules most often are found in the subcutaneous tissue over bony prominences. Nodules are commonly found on the extensor surfaces of the elbows and fingers. Less involved areas are the back, hands, feet, and knees. These nodules may also invade the skin, pleurae, lung parenchyma, spleen, sclera, dura mater, and larynx and less often cardiac valves and pericardium. Rheumatoid nodules are often associated with active disease and high circulating titers of RF.

Vasculitis that develops in RA frequently is a small-vessel, obliterative vasculitis. It may be accompanied by ischemic skin ulcerations, infarctions of the finger pads and nails, or peripheral neuropathy. Thrombosis of such vessels rarely results in cerebrovascular occlusion, renal insufficiency, and myocardial infarction. Vasculitis has been associated with high titers of circulating immune complexes.

sues become secondarily involved, particularly the cartilage. Chronic inflammatory changes lead to the deterioration of the cartilage, which can result in the development of bone fissures, or cysts. Ligaments and tendons close to the inflamed joints may also become inflamed, causing tendonitis and tenosynovitis that may progress to shortening and fibrosis. Consequently, persistent inflammation can progress to loss of joint range of motion, contractures, and partial dislocation of the joints (subluxation). Permanent deformities noted in advanced RA include ulnar deviation of the hands, boutonnière and swan-neck deformities of the finger joints, plantar subluxation (dislocation) of the metatarsal joints of the foot, and hallux valgus, a deviation of the great toe toward the other toes. Flexion contractures can also develop and are common in the hips and knees.

Joint deformities can cause mild to severe physical limitations. Loss of joint motion is rapidly followed by secondary atrophy of local muscles as a result of lack of use. As muscle atrophy increases, the joint becomes progressively unstable, contributing to further joint problems.

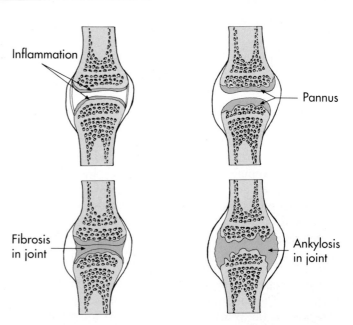

Inflammation

Pannus

Fibrosis in joint

Ankylosis in joint

FIGURE 6-2
Pathologic changes of the joint in rheumatoid arthritis.

Two other syndromes that occur in RA are Sjögren's syndrome and Felty's syndrome. **Sjögren's syndrome** occurs in approximately 25% to 30% of patients with RA (see section on Sjögren's syndrome, page 196). **Felty's syndrome** is RA in association with splenomegaly, neutropenia, and anemia. It may be the result of a hematologic abnormality seen in patients with RA and generally is associated with high RF titers and rheumatic nodules. Other manifestations of Felty's syndrome may include hypersplenism and lymphadenopathy. This syndrome puts these patients at additional risk for developing bacterial infections.

Pulmonary involvement with rheumatoid arthritis may include diffuse pleuritis, interstitial pneumonitis or fibrosis, or multiple intraparenchymal nodules. An example is **Caplan's syndrome** (the development of large lung parenchymal nodules in the presence of pneumoconiosis in patients with RA). **Cardiac abnormalities** in RA are less common and include pericarditis, myocarditis, and conduction disorders. Rheumatoid nodules may also cause valvular deformities in the heart. Nodules in the spleen often cause splenomegaly and when located in the sclera can cause acute glaucoma.

COMPLICATIONS

Permanent joint deformities
Muscle wasting and atrophy
Loss of range of motion
Subluxations (partial dislocation), particularly of C1-C2 that may lead to brainstem infarction
Ankylosis of joints
Carpal tunnel syndrome
Rupture of extensor tendon in fingers
Popliteal cyst (Baker's cyst) and pseudothrombophlebitis
Osteoporosis
Vasculitis
Felty's syndrome, Sjögren's syndrome
Amyloidosis
Avascular necrosis
Recurrent infections (sepsis)
Anemia
Avascular necrosis of the hip joint
Degenerative cardiac conditions
Chronic restrictive pulmonary disorders
Renal insufficiency
Gastrointestinal disturbances and bleeding
Pleural effusion

DIAGNOSTIC STUDIES AND FINDINGS

Diagnostic test	Findings
Rheumatoid factor (RF) (an immunoglobulin)	Elevated titer in 75% to 95% of patients with RA
Serum complement (CH_{50})	May be normal or low; often decreased during active disease or with active vasculitis
Hematocrit, hemoglobin, red blood cell count (RBC)	Normochromic, normocytic anemia common during active disease
White blood count (WBC)	Elevated, indicating inflammation (neutropenia is associated with Felty's syndrome)
Erythrocyte sedimentation rate (ESR)	Elevated (degree of elevation often correlates with disease activity)
C-reactive protein	Elevated during active disease
Synovial fluid analysis	Fluid is clear or cloudy; synovial fluid protein concentration >2.5-3.5 g/dl; leukocyte count often 5,000-20,000/μl (75% are PMNs); glucose level may be low or normal; complement is decreased; RF may be present
Synovial membrane biopsy	Positive for pannus formation and inflammatory changes
X-rays	*Early findings:* soft tissue swelling and articular demineralization; with progressive damage to articular cartilage, the joint space narrows *Later findings:* bone erosion, spondylitis with osteoporosis (mainly the cervical spine), bone cysts, and subluxation of involved articulations
Magnetic resonance imaging (MRI)	May assist in detecting early signs of avascular necrosis of hip and carpal tunnel inflammation
Computed tomography (CT)	May assist in determining presence of synovial cysts

MEDICAL MANAGEMENT

GENERAL MANAGEMENT

The goals of medical management are to relieve pain, prevent joint destruction, and maintain or improve function.

Physical therapy: Includes a balance of rest and exercise adapted to the individual. The program should include active range of motion (ROM) exercises to maintain strength and mobility. Use of heat, cold, massage, or ultrasound may be helpful in minimizing muscle spasms, stiffness, and pain. Whirlpool immersion and paraffin "gloves" can also be used. Splints, braces, a cervical collar, or assistive walking devices (crutches, cane, or walker) may be needed to provide rest to certain joints during active disease.

Occupational therapy: To assist the patient in maintaining independence and completing activities of daily living (e.g., the use of specially designed jar openers or large-handled utensils).

Psychologic support and counseling: Should be offered during periods when coping with the illness becomes difficult for the patient and family and for stress management to minimize the risk of an exacerbation.

Sexual counseling: May be needed to identify strategies for minimizing joint pain and discomfort during sexual activity.

Diet: Should be well balanced; obesity should be avoided because of increased joint stress.

DRUG THERAPY

Patients with RA may be taking an antiinflammatory agent, a corticosteroid, an immunosuppressive drug, vitamins, a calcium supplement for osteoporosis, a drug to minimize gastric distress, and an analgesic at varying times during the day.

Nonsteroidal antiinflammatory drugs: Interfere with prostaglandin production, thus reducing inflammation; they also act to reduce joint pain, stiffness, and swelling.

Salicylates (administered PO): acetylsalicylic acid (aspirin), buffered aspirin (Bufferin), enteric-coated aspirin (Ecotrin), and others.

Nonsalicylates (administered PO): ibuprofen (Motrin, Advil, Nuprin), naproxen (Naprosyn), indomethacin (Indocin), and others.

Corticosteroids: Antiinflammatory drugs that act by inhibiting the release of IL-1 from macrophages and decrease antibody production and prevent release of lysosomal enzymes. They act by relieving joint pain and decreasing the swelling.

Prednisone: administered orally and used for maintenance.

Hydrocortisone intraarticular steroid injections: may decrease synovitis and reduce early flexion contractions.

Hydrocortisone sodium succinate (Solu-Cortef) or *methylprednisolone sodium succinate* (Solu-Medrol): given IV or IM in large doses during and after surgery or other stressful invasive procedures.

Disease-modifying drugs

Gold salt therapy: a slow-acting, antiinflammatory agent administered IM. It is thought to act as a lysosomal membrane stabilizer and may interfere with macrophage function. Auranofin, an oral gold salt preparation, is thought to interfere with T-lymphocyte and macrophage interactions. Monitor for skin rashes, renal function (BUN, creatinine, urine protein), and bone marrow function (CBC with differential).

MEDICAL MANAGEMENT—cont'd

Penicillamine (e.g., Cuprimine, Depen): thought to act by inhibiting helper-T lymphocyte activity. It is a slow-acting, antiinflammatory agent that is given orally. Monitor for renal dysfunction, anemia, fever, skin rash, and decreased platelets accompanied by easy bruising.

Antimalarial drugs (e.g., chloroquine hydrochloride [Aralen Hydrochloride] and hydroxychloroquine sulfate [Plaquenil Sulfate]): given orally and are thought to interfere with monocyte function; however, the action is not completely clear. These drugs can cause eye damage, mandating frequent eye examinations.

Immunosuppressive drugs

Methotrexate (Rheumatrex): specific action in RA is unclear. It may be given PO or IV and requires close monitoring of liver function, CBC, and platelets. If pancytopenia develops, it may be reversed with leucovorin calcium.[89]

Azathioprine (Imuran): specific action in RA is unclear. It may be given IV or PO; close monitoring of liver function and WBC is mandatory.

Cyclophosphamide (Cytoxan): reserved for rheumatoid vasculitis and for patients who fail to respond to other forms of treatment; close monitoring of WBC is mandatory.

Other drugs commonly used

Vitamins as a nutritional supplement; calcium supplements to treat or prevent osteoporosis; drugs to minimize gastric irritation secondary to side effects of antiinflammatory agents and corticosteroids (e.g., sucralfate [Carafate], ranitidine hydrochloride [Zantac], or cimetidine [Tagamet]); analgesics for pain relief.

SURGERY

Arthroplasty to maintain or improve joint motion; arthrodesis (joint fusion) to correct deformities or alleviate pain; synovectomy of inflamed synovial membranes to prevent joint damage and tendon rupture and to decrease pain (spinal fusion may be performed to treat subluxation); osteotomy to change weight-bearing surfaces and relieve pain; Silastic joint implant to improve mobility; jaw implant to improve mastication and disfigurement; total joint replacement (specifically hip and knee) to improve mobility and decrease pain.

EXPERIMENTAL THERAPY[88]

Varying combinations of the above drugs; plasmapheresis; lymphapheresis; total lymphoid irradiation; sulfasalazine (Azulfidine); cyclosporine; gamma interferon; botanical and marine lipids; monoclonal antibodies; fish oil supplements.

DIAGNOSTIC CRITERIA

A definite diagnosis of RA can be made if five or more of the following criteria* are met.
1. Morning stiffness that improves during the day.
2. Pain or tenderness in at least one joint.
3. Swelling (soft tissue or fluid) of one joint.
4. Swelling of a second joint.
5. Symmetric joint swelling on either side of the body.
6. Presence of subcutaneous nodules.
7. X-ray changes, bone decalcification near joint margins, typically in the hands or feet.
8. Positive test for rheumatoid factor.
9. Poor mucin precipitate in the synovial fluid.
10. Histologic evidence of synovitis and chronic inflammation.
11. Characteristic histologic changes in the subcutaneous nodules.

*From the American Rheumatism Association.

1 ASSESS

ASSESSMENT	OBSERVATIONS
General	Fatigue, weakness, weight loss, low-grade fever
Joints (bilateral)	Symmetric signs of articular inflammation (swelling, warmth, erythema, tenderness on palpation) typically affecting small joints of hands and feet; may have muscle spasms and joint deformity
Range of joint motion (ROJM)	Impaired movement; stiff, rigid joints; weak hand grip; pain and difficulty with ambulation; morning stiffness
Peripheral sensation	Decreased sensation in fingers and toes with numbness, tingling, and feeling of pins and needles
Psychosocial	Concern about self-concept, body image, and cost of treatments

2 DIAGNOSE

NURSING DIAGNOSIS	SUBJECTIVE FINDINGS	OBJECTIVE FINDINGS
Impaired physical mobility related to joint inflammation, tenderness, deformity, or nodules	Complains that joints are stiff and tender with slight numbness and tingling in fingers and toes	Joints are swollen, red, warm and tender on palpation; joints of the hands (swan-neck, boutonnière, or ulnar deviation) and feet are enlarged and deformed; subcutaneous nodules are present over extensor surface of forearms; ligaments and tendons are shortened and tight; muscle atrophy is noted in arms and legs
Activity intolerance related to fatigue and anemia	States "wakes up tired"; complains of being unable to participate in normal activities without frequent rest periods and naps during the day; feels short of breath with minimal exertion	Shoulders and head are drooped; demonstrates lack of interest in any activity; buccal mucosa, nail beds, skin, and conjunctivae are pale; respirations are deep with slight dyspnea; respirations increase with ambulation and become labored when going up stairs
Pain related to inflammatory process and joint deformity	Complains of persistent, aching joint pain of hands that is only minimally relieved by analgesics; pain increases with activity (e.g., brushing teeth, doing dishes, typing)	Grimaces and withdraws hands when palpated; pain chart of 1-10 indicates continuous pain level of 6-8; documented analgesic use q 4 h
Self-care deficit related to joint deformities and inflammation (pain)	Complains of being unable to hold thin items firmly or to use them (e.g., toothbrush, knife, or pen); reports inability to open jars, fasten hooks, close buttons, or comb hair easily; states has difficulty going up and down stairs without assistance	Deformed hands with ulnar deviation and fingers with swan-neck appearance; joints are swollen, red, and tender to palpation; fingers, hands, and wrists have minimal range of joint motion and are very stiff

NURSING DIAGNOSIS	SUBJECTIVE FINDINGS	OBJECTIVE FINDINGS
Impaired home maintenance management related to immobility and weakness	Reports difficulty in maintaining a "clean" home environment, cooking, doing laundry; describes debts and financial crisis; expresses lack of knowledge about community resources	Movements are slow and calculated; winces if movement is too fast; lacks necessary equipment and aids to assist in ADLs; lacks knowledge about financial and community resources
Body image disturbance related to deformity	Complains of feeling "ugly" and undesirable; reports having difficulty buying shoes and often wears gloves to cover hands	Wears long-sleeved blouses and tennis shoes with toes cut out; holds hands quietly and keeps them hidden in lap; tucks feet under chair

Other Related Nursing Diagnoses: **Altered role performance** related to physical deformities; **Sleep pattern disturbance** related to pain, muscle spasms, or joint stiffness; **Impaired gas exchange** related to pneumonitis and anemia; **Potential for injury** secondary to gastrointestinal bleeding; **Potential for infection** secondary to Felty's syndrome and chronic neutropenia; **Alterations in sexual patterns** related to body image disturbance, joint pain, and stiffness; **Altered tissue perfusion** related to rheumatoid nodules.

3 PLAN

Patient goals

1. The patient will regain and maintain satisfactory range of joint motion.
2. The patient will have sufficient energy to engage in ADLs or will adapt to decreased energy level.
3. The patient will be able to identify strategies that eliminate or control pain.
4. The patient will be able to perform ADLs with the use of modified equipment as needed.
5. The patient will demonstrate an understanding of home care management and follow-up.
6. The patient will develop and maintain a positive self-image.

4 IMPLEMENT

NURSING DIAGNOSIS	NURSING INTERVENTIONS	RATIONALE
Impaired physical mobility related to joint inflammation, tenderness, deformity, or nodules	Assess ROJM, joint deformities or nodules, overall mobility, and signs of inflammation (swelling, redness, heat, and pain).	To guide therapeutic interventions.
	Coordinate consultation with physical and occupational therapists for individualized programs of exercise and home management.	Professional health team members provide expertise in developing an individualized plan of care.
	Provide passive and active ROJM exercises in collaboration with physical therapist; inflamed joints should be moved only to the point of pain.	To promote mobility, prevent stiffness, and ensure continuity of care; joints are most vulnerable to injury during acute disease.
	Establish a balance between rest and activity.	Rest is a component of minimizing pain and assists in resolving inflammatory process.

→ > >

NURSING DIAGNOSIS	NURSING INTERVENTIONS	RATIONALE
	Provide for periods of bed rest (bed should be flat, patient should be supine and straight; no extra pillows used); use splints and ambulatory aids.	To rest inflamed joints and prevent contractures; using extra pillows under knees, hips, and neck promotes the development of contractures.
	Reposition patient frequently, at least q 2 h.	To prevent muscle fatigue, joint stiffness, and contractures.
	Warm compresses (e.g., paraffin gloves) or cold compresses are particularly helpful if applied before ROJM exercise.	Heat may help promote muscle relaxation, mobility, and pain relief, and cold may decrease swelling and improve mobility.
	Encourage patient to assume prone position with ankles 90 degrees dorsiflexed for 20 min bid; keep blankets off feet during this time.	To prevent shortening of heel cord.
	Perform ADLs for patient until she is able.	To meet patient's daily needs.
Activity intolerance related to fatigue and anemia	Observe response to activity.	To guide therapeutic interventions.
	Monitor Hct and Hgb.	To detect anemia.
	Plan rest periods between activities.	To reduce fatigue.
	Provide progressive increase in activity as tolerated.	Increasing activities slowly promotes endurance and minimizes fatigue.
	Keep frequently used objects within reach.	To decrease oxygen consumption and provide convenience for patient.
	Help patient identify methods of conserving energy (e.g., bed bath, slip-on shoes).	To minimize oxygen expenditure and incorporate patient into plan of care, promoting self-esteem and independence.
	Monitor stools and emesis for occult blood.	To detect possible gastrointestinal bleed.
	In collaboration with physician, evaluate need for iron replacement or blood transfusion.	Iron supplements promote red cell production and increase oxygen-carrying capacity; blood transfusion can correct anemia.
	Provide and encourage an adequate diet.	To provide essential nutrients, support body function, and minimize fatigue and anemia.
Pain related to inflammatory process and joint deformity	Assess pain: joint(s) involved, severity (scale of 1-10), character, duration, and aggravating and alleviating factors.	To assist in guiding therapeutic interventions.
	Help patient determine strategies that have relieved pain in the past.	To identify successful pain relief measures.
	Apply resting splints to involved joints; they should be made of lightweight material and removed at least bid for ROJM.	To provide support, minimize pain, and prevent contractures.

NURSING DIAGNOSIS	NURSING INTERVENTIONS	RATIONALE
	Apply cervical traction as ordered and indicated.	This may decrease muscle spasms related to pain and prevent cervical joint deformities.
	In conjunction with dietitian, calculate ideal body weight, and help patient devise strategies to achieve and maintain that weight.	Achieving ideal body weight minimizes wear and tear on weight-bearing joints and helps prevent further joint deformity and pain.
	Apply moist heat to affected joint; provide ambulatory patients with a warm or hot bath.	Heat may have an analgesic effect and relieve pain.
	Provide paraffin baths for hands and/or feet, particularly in the morning.	To help reduce pain and decrease morning stiffness.
	Provide massage.	To ease muscle tightness and provide comfort.
	Administer analgesics and nonsteroidal antiinflammatory agents as ordered, and monitor patient's response.	Analgesic and nonsteroidal antiinflammatory medications may relieve pain by reducing inflammation in the joint.
	Instruct patient in relaxation techniques and visual imagery.	These may help modify pain by providing a diversional activity.
Self-care deficit related to joint deformities and inflammation (pain)	Assess patient's ability to perform ADLs.	To guide therapeutic intervention and development of individualized care plan.
	Provide modified utensils and other equipment of daily living: padded objects (brush, pen, utensils) for easier gripping, jar opener, button fastener, shoe horn with slip-on shoe that uses Velcro, not shoelaces; encourage patient to practice using modified equipment.	To promote skill and facilitate independence and control, to maintain activity, and to promote self-esteem.
	Allow adequate time to complete ADLs with rest periods between activities.	To promote independence and a sense of mastery and control.
	Allow patient to do as much of her own care as possible; encourage her and acknowledge progress.	To promote self-esteem and independence.
	Keep frequently used items within reach.	For convenience and to maintain independence.
	Implement assist devices (cane, crutches, walker, elevated toilet).	To maintain mobility and functional independence.
	Contact local home health organizations to assist patient at home after discharge.	To provide support services and ensure that patient's basic needs are met.

NURSING DIAGNOSIS	NURSING INTERVENTIONS	RATIONALE
Impaired home maintenance management related to immobility and weakness	Assess safety, hygiene, and social and physical stimulation of home environment.	To guide therapeutic intervention and identify home care needs.
	Consult with patient and family to determine home care needs.	To promote a feasible discharge.
	Provide patient with phone numbers of and contact local agencies to assist with home care management and financial crisis.	To ensure efficient use of community resources and promote a safe home environment.
	Help patient obtain necessary home equipment and supplies (e.g., ramp, elevated toilet, door jam cervical traction unit).	To ensure that adequate home maintenance equipment is available.
	Encourage patient to continue therapeutic regimen of exercise and rest.	To promote muscle strength and flexibility, minimize weakness, and prevent joint deformity.
Body image disturbance related to deformity	Assess concerns about body image and joint deformities.	To guide individualized approach to care.
	Explore implications of deformities with patient.	To identify personal meaning of loss and assist in developing a positive body image.
	Teach patient strategies that may help improve body image (e.g., dress [where to purchase attractive therapeutic shoes], makeup, nail care, exercises, weight control).	To promote a positive, accepting, and realistic body image.
	Encourage patient to participate in local support groups.	Support groups can provide valuable and practical information on improving body image.
	Acknowledge patient's attempts to improve personal body image, and offer positive reinforcement.	To provide support and facilitate development of a positive self-image.
	Encourage patient to use rehabilitative services, and facilitate interaction with others who have made similar adjustments.	To encourage acceptance of body changes and incorporate changes into body image and self-concept.
	Help patient realistically accept her present value and physical self; stress strengths unique to her, and list these for future reference.	To promote a positive and accepting self-image.
	Encourage significant others to help patient develop a positive self-image.	To provide consistent support and to help patient achieve a positive self-image.

5   EVALUATE

PATIENT OUTCOME	DATA INDICATING THAT OUTCOME IS REACHED
Patient maintains maximum level of mobility within limitations of disease.	Patient expresses an interest in participating in activities and demonstrates an understanding of exercise regimen and the need for a balance between rest and activity; her level of mobility is appropriate for physical limitations.
Patient has increased her activity tolerance.	Patient has developed a pattern of rest and activity; she participates in an exercise routine using appropriate rest measures and assistive devices (e.g., splints); she uses appropriate measures to facilitate activity (e.g., warm shower in the morning to minimize stiffness).
Patient can participate in activities without complaining of fatigue.	Hct >35% in women, >42% in men; Hgb >12 g/dl in women, >14 g/dl in men; patient participates in daily routine without fatigue.
Patient identifies strategies that eliminate or control pain.	Pain chart indicates consistent pain relief; patient reports absence or control of pain and demonstrates appropriate use of pain relief measures.
Patient can perform own ADLs.	Patient can dress and bathe herself and participate in routine activities by using appropriate, modified equipment and assistive devices.
Patient has integrated home management strategies into daily living activities.	Appropriate supplies and equipment have been installed and are used in the home; patient demonstrates accurate use of all equipment and contacts community agencies for additional support when needed.
Patient has developed a positive and realistic body image.	Patient demonstrates strategies that promote and maintain a positive body image; she resumes usual social interactions and activities, expresses acceptance of limitations, and maximizes strengths.

PATIENT TEACHING

1. Provide the patient and family with information and instruction about rheumatoid arthritis and the disease's trajectory.
2. Teach the patient and family the importance of all medications, their purpose, side effects, dosage, and administration.
3. Teach the patient relaxation and visualization exercises.
4. Teach the patient how to use paraffin foot and hand baths and heat and cold applications, as well as the cautions with each.
5. Explain the purpose and implications of all procedures and surgical interventions.
6. Teach the patient how to limit or modify activity to protect joints.
7. Teach the patient the importance of a routine exercise program.
8. Encourage the patient to balance activity with rest; provide an example of a proposed daily routine.
9. Teach the patient useful modifications to make daily living easier (e.g., pad utensils, keys, toothbrush, and other household appliances; add rails to stairs, entry and exit areas, and bathtub, use elevated toilet seat; obtain cups with adjustable handles).
10. Encourage the patient to use wrist splints (or other immobilizing braces for other joints) for inflamed joints.
11. Teach the patient and family how to use and maintain home maintenance equipment.

12. Teach the patient strategies for decreasing pain and/ or muscle spasms (e.g., warm or hot showers, whirlpool, or heat before exercises).
13. Teach the patient to maintain her ideal body weight to prevent wear and tear on joints of the lower extremities.
14. Teach the patient the importance of inserts or molds in shoes or the use of corrective shoes to minimize skin and joint trauma, to provide adequate support, and to decrease the risk of injury.
15. Refer the patient and family to a peer support group and local organizations.

Juvenile Rheumatoid Arthritis

Juvenile rheumatoid arthritis (JRA) is a chronic inflammatory disease in children that always involves the joints.

Juvenile rheumatoid arthritis is characterized by synovial inflammation with joint effusion, which eventually leads to erosion, destruction, and fibrosis of the articular cartilage. JRA may also produce lesions in the viscera and connective tissue.

The American Rheumatology Association defines JRA as "joint swelling or restriction of motion with pain, tenderness, or heat . . . for at least 6 weeks' duration, in one or more joints, with the exclusion of all other causes of arthritis."

JRA may represent not just a single disease, but a syndrome with different causes; that is, a series of bodily responses characterized by idiopathic peripheral arthritis that have been grouped under the classification term JRA.[35]

Juvenile rheumatoid arthritis is not simply a childhood version of rheumatoid arthritis (RA), since only 5% to 6% of patients with RA are diagnosed before 16 years of age.[59] Rather, JRA is a disease described during childhood with three distinct variations: polyarthritis, pauciarticular JRA, and systemic JRA.

CLASSIFICATION

The onset of clinical signs in the first 6 months of the disease puts JRA into one of three categories (Table 6-1); most children remain in the early pattern of symptomatology and rarely change classifications.[55] These three categories are *polyarthritis* (more than five joints affected [two subtypes]); *pauciarticular JRA* (four or fewer joints affected [three subtypes]); and *systemic JRA* (arthritis affecting several joints with intermittent fever).

EPIDEMIOLOGY

Although described in all races and geographic areas, JRA is diagnosed more often in white children than in black or Asian children. It is seen more frequently in girls than boys and statistically is the fifth most common chronic illness in children, following asthma, congenital heart defects, diabetes mellitus, and cleft lip and palate. There are approximately 13.9 new cases per 100,000 children annually. In the United States, approximately 63,000 to 77,000 children have JRA.[35,131]

PATHOPHYSIOLOGY

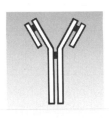

As previously mentioned, JRA is not a child's version of rheumatoid arthritis. Although permanent joint damage is common in RA, 75% to 80% of children with JRA do not demonstrate this problem. However, children with JRA have growth disturbances such as leg length discrepancy, failure to thrive, short stature, and micrognathia. They may have asymmetric growth of the cervical spine and temporomandibular joint (TMJ). Eye inflammation with the potential for blindness is especially noted in children with pauciarticular JRA. Pleuritis and pericarditis with effusions and generalized vasculitis have been noted in some children with systemic JRA.[35]

The etiology of JRA is unknown, although infection, trauma, and stress are possible factors. Autoimmunity may contribute to the etiology and is reflected in the increased rheumatoid factor (RF) and antinuclear antibody (ANA) shown on serum tests. Immunogenetic predisposition, reflected in human lymphocyte antigen (HLA) associations, may also be part of the etiologic puzzle.[5,67,132,189]

The early onset of joint inflammation begins with inflammation and hypertrophy of the synovial membrane. The inflammation causes the synovium to produce more synovial fluid, creating an effusion on the joint. The effusion is rich in lysosomes and enzymes that destroy collagen and cartilage. A vascular membrane, known as pannus, grows over the cartilaginous surface

Table 6-1

CLASSIFICATION AND CHARACTERISTICS OF JUVENILE RHEUMATOID ARTHRITIS

Characteristic	Polyarthritis	Pauciarticular JRA	Systemic JRA
Frequency of cases	40%	50%	10%
Number of joints involved	>5	<4	Varies
Joints involved	Any (usually symmetric; in 50% of patients, hips are involved; in 50%, spine is involved)	Usually lower extremities	Any (only 20% have joint involvement at diagnosis)
Age of onset	Throughout childhood (peak, 1-3 yr)	Early childhood (peak, 1-2 yr)	Throughout childhood (no peak)
Sex ratio (female:male)	3:1	5:1	1:1
Extraarticular manifestations	Minimal; possible low-grade fever, weight loss, rheumatoid nodules, and/or vasculitis	*Type I:* chronic iridocyclitis, mucocutaneous lesion; *type II:* acute iridocyclitis, sacroiliitis	Fever, malaise, myalgia, pleuritis, pericarditis, adenomegaly, splenomegaly, hepatomegaly
Occurrence of uveitis	5%	20%	Rare
Frequency of seropositivity			
Rheumatoid factor	10%	Rare	Rare
Antinuclear antibodies	40%-50%	80% in females with uveitis	10%
Erythrocyte sedimentation rate	Elevated	Elevated	Elevated
Anemia	No	No	Yes
HLA association	*Type I:* DR4; *type II:* none	Male:B27; Female:DR5, DR8	None
Prognosis	Longer duration, more crippling, remission in 25%; *type I:* high incidence of crippling arthritis; *type II:* outlook good	Eventual remission in 60%; *type I:* ocular damage with 10% blindness; *type II:* ankylosing spondylitis; *type III:* best outlook for recovery	Mortality rate is 1%-2% of all JRA patients; joint destruction in 40%

From Whaley and Wong[189]; Cassidy and Petty[35]; Ammann and Wara.[5]

and erodes it. The normal proteoglycan and collagen structures are disrupted and become more vulnerable to stress.[5,55]

A similar inflammatory process can cause pathologic changes in other tissues, such as serositis of the pleura, pericardium, and/or peritoneum. In systemic JRA, vasculitis in the subepithelial tissues causes a rash, and uveitis (inflammation of the iris, ciliary body, and choroid) as seen in pauciarticular JRA.

CLINICAL MANIFESTATIONS
Systemic JRA

1. **Fever,** usually between 39° and 41° C (102.2° to 105.8° F) (rapid onset and return to normal or subnormal daily or twice daily, usually in the afternoon; responds poorly to aspirin).
2. **Morbilliform rash** (macular rash with central clearing, usually located on the central trunk or proximal extremity, may be on palms, soles, and face; comes and goes with fever; migratory and lasts only a few hours).
3. **Hepatosplenomegaly** with transient abnormal liver function tests and liver biopsies (found in one third of children).
4. **Arthritis** within first 6 months of onset (found in only 20% of children and can include any joint; usually symmetric and includes the temporomandibular joint and spine).

Pauciarticular JRA

1. **Arthritis** (usually found in knees, ankles, or both [more than 4 joints] with low-grade inflammatory process; hips are always spared).
2. Patient is **not** systemically ill.
3. **Uveitis** (may be only extraarticular manifestation; eye disease can appear without manifestation or presence of arthritis; other extraarticular manifestations are rare).

Polyarthritis

1. **Arthritis** (in five or more joints; can have acute or insidious onset).
2. **Seropositivity** (RF and ANA).
3. **Low-grade fever** with **rash** (may be present but is not as acute or persistent as in systemic JRA).
4. **Hepatosplenomegaly** (only a slight to moderate finding).
5. **Uveitis** (in 5% of cases).

COMPLICATIONS

See Table 6-1, Prognosis.

DIAGNOSTIC STUDIES AND FINDINGS

Diagnostic test	Findings
Rheumatoid factor (RF)	Present in 10% of patients with polyarthritis
Antinuclear antibodies (ANA)	Present in 40%-50% of patients with polyarthritis and 80% of females with pauciarticular JRA
Erythrocyte sedimentation rate (ESR)	Elevated
Complete blood count (CBC) with differential	Decreased hemoglobin and hematocrit in patients with systemic JRA; mild leukocytosis
Radiographic changes (See Table 6-2)	

Table 6-2

COMMON RADIOLOGIC CHANGES IN CHILDREN WITH JRA

Radiologic changes	Polyarthritis (%)	Pauciarticular JRA (%)	Systemic JRA (%)
Early changes			
Soft tissue swelling or osteoporosis	45	75	45
Periosteal new bone apposition	30	—	50
Advanced changes			
Cartilage destruction	55	25	50
Bone destruction	35	25	20
Bony ankylosis	25	5	15
Large joint subluxation	15	—	20
Epiphyseal fractures	5	—	40
Vertebral compression	20	—	25
Growth abnormalities			
Overgrowth or undergrowth of long bones	30	50	15
Brachydactyly	20	5	30
Micrognathia	15	5	40
Accelerated epiphyseal maturation	5	35	20

Modified from Cassidy and Petty.[35]

MEDICAL MANAGEMENT

GENERAL MANAGEMENT

The goal of management is to suppress and control the inflammatory process; relieve pain and discomfort; maintain joint function and prevent deformities; facilitate good nutrition, physical growth, and motor development; prevent extraarticular complications; correct deformities; provide rehabilitation; prevent psychosocial complications.

Physical and occupational therapy is essential to preserving joint movement by avoiding contracture. By learning positioning and proper alignment, the patient and parents can decrease pain and avoid unnecessary stress on joints. Specific play and sports activities can strengthen musculature and enhance self-esteem by enhancing the patient's capabilities. The patient and parents are taught exercise limitations, range-of-motion (ROM) exercises, and splinting techniques to use during exacerbations to prevent stiffening and pain.

Nutritional therapy is indicated, because many children with JRA are at risk for protein and calorie malnutrition. Anemia is common in all forms of JRA, and iron-containing foods and supplements should be encouraged. Because many of the drugs used to treat JRA affect the absorption and metabolism of specific elements and nutrients of food, nutritional consultation with patient and parents is advisable.

Psychologic or behavioral consultation, or both, are recommended for the reactions and coping problems associated with the diagnosis of chronic diseases. Discipline and compliance problems between parent and child can be diminished by structured systems, including clearly defined expectations, designed for the individual family with the expertise of a child behavior specialist.

DRUG THERAPY

First-line drugs: nonsteroidal antiinflammatory drugs: Most common: aspirin, tolmetin, naproxen, ibuprofen. Most common problem: gastrointestinal (GI) upset.

Second-line drugs: slow-acting antirheumatic drugs: Most common: hydroxychloroquine, gold salts, D-penicillamine, sulfasalazine. Most common problem: bone marrow suppression and other blood dyscrasias.

Corticosteroids: Most common: prednisone, prednisolone ophthalmic drops. Most common problems: GI upset, immunosuppression, cataracts, glaucoma. (Use of prednisolone eye drops mandates quarterly evaluation by an ophthalmologist.)

Cytotoxic drugs (e.g., methotrexate—used only when patient is unresponsive to all other drugs): Most common problems: hepatic damage, bone marrow suppression, immunosuppression.

SURGERY

Surgery may be performed for soft tissue release and tendon lengthening in a child with severe contractures of the knee or hip. Otherwise, surgical intervention is seldom used during the childhood years. However, reconstructive surgery, such as total hip or knee replacement, has been of great benefit to patients with JRA who entered early adulthood with significant disability. Surgical intervention usually is postponed until bone growth has ceased.

---

1 ASSESS

ASSESSMENT	OBSERVATIONS
General complaints	Recurrent temperature elevation *Systemic:* spikes 39°-41° C (102.2°-105.8° F) daily or twice daily with pale red, nonpruritic, macular rash that disappears when afebrile *Polyarthritis:* low-grade, chronic fever (>39° C [102.2° F]); malaise, irritability, poor appetite; fluctuation of signs and symptoms; lymphadenopathy (tender lymph nodes on palpation)

ASSESSMENT	OBSERVATIONS
Musculoskeletal	Pain, stiffness, and decreased ROM often with fever, in morning or after inactivity; walks with shuffling gait and assumes position of comfort (flexion); involved joints may be swollen and warm and tender on palpation; severe myalgias and arthralgias with febrile episodes
Gastrointestinal tract	Nausea and vomiting; pain in epigastric area; blood in emesis, stool, or both; pain that increases after taking therapeutic medications; tarry stools; decreased weight
Growth retardation	Stature often short for age; poor weight gain; growth slowed or stopped with observable symptoms; lower percentile ranking on normal growth curve; delayed appearance of secondary sex characteristics; localized growth retardation such as micrognathia (small mandible) or brachydactyly (small feet and hands) (asymmetric arthritis may result in limb length discrepancy secondary to premature epiphyseal maturation)
Abdomen	Hepatomegaly; splenomegaly; mesenteric lymphadenopathy may cause generalized abdominal pain

2 DIAGNOSE

NURSING DIAGNOSIS	SUBJECTIVE FINDINGS	OBJECTIVE FINDINGS
Altered body temperature related to inflammatory process	Chills, weakness, irritability, myalgia, arthralgia	Elevated temperature with intermittent spikes, tachycardia, elevated ESR, anemia, diaphoresis
Pain related to inflammatory process in joints	Pain in specific joints, decrease in movement and exercise tolerance, irritability, crying, difficult to console, withdrawal from social interaction, guarding of limb or body area, unable to sleep	Swollen joints that are warm to touch; pain increases on palpation
Pain related to gastrointestinal symptoms secondary to medications	Irritability, crying, difficult to console, unable to sleep; has epigastric pain and nausea	GI symptoms increase within 1 h of taking therapeutic drugs; vomiting; blood in stool and/or emesis, blackish stool; anorexia; anemia (Hct <35%)
Altered nutrition: less than body requirements related to anorexia	Decrease in food intake, lack of interest in food, pulling away from bottle, cries when food is presented	Weight loss, lack of weight gain and growth; lack of energy and strength; muscle atrophy; caloric intake is less than body requires
Altered growth and development related to hospitalization	Regression to earlier stages of development, withdrawal from social interaction, outbursts of anger and despair	Return to bottle from cup feeding, return to diapers from continence, not walking alone, will not smile or laugh
Impaired physical mobility related to limited range of motion of limbs	Stiffness after inactivity; pain, weakness	Contractures, extension inability, muscle atrophy, radiographic changes
Potential sensory/perceptual alteration (visual) related to inflammatory process	Usually none until irreversible changes occur	Inflammation in anterior chamber of eye (uveitis), ANA positive

3 | PLAN

Patient goals

1. The patient will have a normal body temperature.
2. The patient will have no pain or will be able to cope with pain.
3. The patient will have no or minimal GI discomfort with therapeutic drugs.
4. The patient will maintain adequate nutrition to optimize growth and energy.
5. The patient's parents will understand the child's regression response to the stress of hospitalization and will be knowledgeable about methods to support their child.
6. The patient will not have any increase in physical immobility.
7. The patient's parents will understand the need for regular ophthalmologic consultation.

4 | IMPLEMENT

NURSING DIAGNOSIS	NURSING INTERVENTIONS	RATIONALE
Altered body temperature related to inflammatory process	Take temperature q 4 h and q 1 h during spikes.	Elevated temperature reflects acute inflammatory process.
	Graph temperature as to time of day of elevations.	To predict times of elevation and begin comfort measures promptly.
	Inspect skin for pale red, nonpruritic, macular rash during elevated temperatures.	To monitor for *systemic* JRA.
	Administer antipyretics as ordered, and monitor patient response.	To reduce temperature.
	Provide tepid baths.	To decrease temperature and provide comfort.
	Assess for dehydration: poor skin turgor, dry mucous membranes, diaphoresis.	As temperature rises, insensible water loss via skin increases; children have greater surface area per body weight compared to adults, making them more prone to dehydration.
	Monitor fluid intake and output q 4 h, noting degree of diaphoresis.	To avoid negative fluid balance from dehydration. Adequate urine output: infant, 1-2 ml/kg/h; toddler/school age, 1 ml/kg/h; adolescent, 0.5-1 ml/kg/h (if fluid intake is adequate).
	Encourage fluid intake as tolerated.	To maintain fluid balance. Adequate intake for child: ≤10 kg, 100 ml/kg/day; next 10 kg, 50 ml/kg/day; next 10 kg, 25 ml/kg/day; then 10 ml/kg/day for every kg over 30 kg.
	In collaboration with physician, consider IV fluids if oral intake inadequate.	To prevent dehydration.

NURSING DIAGNOSIS	NURSING INTERVENTIONS	RATIONALE
Pain related to inflammatory process in joints	Administer antiinflammatory medications (e.g., aspirin, ibuprofen) as ordered and monitor patient response.	To reduce inflammation and associated discomfort.
	Administer analgesics as ordered (e.g., acetaminophen with or without codeine) and monitor patient response.	To reduce discomfort or degree of perceived discomfort.
	Apply heat packs to affected joints (heat wet towel in microwave, cover with plastic, and apply to joints for 20 min); give warm tub baths (38° C [100.4° F] for 10 min) or warm whirlpool baths; soak hands and feet in warm water (for 20 min).	To provide comfort: use with extreme caution in children who cannot talk yet.
	Make sure patient rests during exacerbations; splint and position joint in neutral or extension.	To prevent discomfort from immobilization of affected joints while preventing flexion contractures.
	Encourage parent or significant person to stay with child; if not available, nurse should be with child as much as possible.	To provide psychologic support and to decrease anxiety that can intensify discomfort.
Pain related to gastrointestinal symptoms secondary to medications	Administer therapeutic medications with food if not contraindicated.	To decrease GI erosion, pain, nausea, and burning, which can aggravate anorexia.
	Administer histamine H_2-receptor antagonist medications (ranitidine and cimetidine) as ordered and monitor patient response.	To decrease gastric secretion (which often aggravates GI side effects of therapeutic medications) and thus promote comfort and avoid anorexia.
	Administer antacids as ordered (with therapeutic medication if not contraindicated) and monitor patient response.	To enhance GI comfort and prevent GI bleeding and anorexia.
	Check emesis and stool for blood and occult blood; note characteristics of both.	To monitor GI bleeding and possible cause for sudden drop in Hct and Hgb.
Altered nutrition: less than body requirements related to anorexia	Assess for lack of weight gain or for weight loss; check weight and height with normal growth curve and child's previous growth curve percentile ranking; assess child for muscle atrophy; weigh daily while hospitalized, weekly at home.	Malnourishment impairs the body's ability to grow and develop optimally, reduces the strength and endurance needed to accomplish necessary exercise, and decreases the body's defenses against infection.
	Monitor daily caloric intake, noting appetite and types of foods eaten.	Calories are very important for increased energy needs; sources of vitamins, minerals, protein, fat, and carbohydrates are important for healing and growth. Also, drug regimens can interfere with absorption and metabolism of nutrients.
	Offer supplemental foods; give patient choices; ask nutritionist to assist with assessment and determining direct nutritional requirements.	To provide the most nutritious foods that patient is willing to eat. Use of health care team and expert assists in individualizing and optimizing care.

NURSING DIAGNOSIS	NURSING INTERVENTIONS	RATIONALE
Altered growth and development related to hospitalization	Encourage child to participate in age-appropriate games, activities, and interactions while not acutely ill.	To optimize learning through experience, to help patient learn to recognize her abilities and limitations, and to promote self-esteem, interest, and social skills.
	Teach parents that it is normal for a child to regress during periods of stress; teach them to be accepting and calm and to avoid criticizing the child.	To avoid embarrassment for parent and increased stress on the child, and to maintain a supportive relationship between parents and child.
Impaired physical mobility related to limited range of motion of limbs	Consult physical therapist about methods and schedule for ROM exercises; have therapist teach them to parents in presence of nurse; discuss activities that involve good ROM with minimal joint stress (e.g., swimming, riding a tricycle).	To individualize exercise schedule and methods to patient's needs; parents and patient learn exercises and activities to be continued at home to maintain optimum ROM and prevent further limitation; nurse can help parent with learning exercises when therapist is not present.
	Teach parents how to apply splints and achieve proper alignment during exacerbations.	To continue therapy, avoid contractures, and promote comfort at home.
	Have parents and child talk with occupational therapist in presence of nurse.	To teach parents and child ADLs, with age-appropriate expectations and consideration; limited ROM, nurse can help parents and child practice strategies.
Potential sensory/ perceptual alteration (visual) related to inflammatory process	Teach parents and child (if appropriate) about asymptomatic inflammatory eye disease and need for ophthalmologic consultation every 3 mo.	To enhance knowledge and compliance and to ensure early treatment of inflammatory eye disease in order to avoid vision loss.

5 EVALUATE

PATIENT OUTCOME	DATA INDICATING THAT OUTCOME IS REACHED
Body temperature is normal.	Temperature is within normal limits; no rash is present; joints have returned to baseline size and are no longer warm; patient's well-being has improved, and she is playful and interested in environment; there is no excessive diaphoresis, and intake and output are within normal limits for size and age.
Pain has resolved or is under control.	Patient has fewer complaints of pain; she shows more interaction with environment and a positive affect; spontaneous movement has increased, and patient shows desire to go home.
Patient has no or minimal GI side effects from therapeutic drugs.	Patient's appetite is good; she has no complaints of pain or nausea; there is no trace of blood in stool and no emesis.

→ > >

PATIENT OUTCOME	DATA INDICATING THAT OUTCOME IS REACHED
Patient's nutritional status has improved.	Patient shows interest in food and maintains or gains weight; has energy to play and participate in activities.
Developmental regression has diminished.	Child responds to environment in accordance with normal baseline as evaluated by parent. Parents demonstrate understanding of child's behavior and react by being supportive and nurturing.
Physical mobility has increased.	Patient wants to be active and can move with little or tolerable discomfort; ROM of joints has improved or returned to baseline, noted by improved posture and extension of limbs; child is spontaneously, actively, and appropriately playful for age.
Patient's vision is stable, and parents understand need for regular ophthalmologic visits.	There is no change in patient's visual ability, and ophthalmologic checkups are done every 3 months.

PATIENT TEACHING

1. Teach the patient and parents about the disease and necessary treatments.
2. Explain the various medication therapies and the side effects of the drugs selected for treatment; emphasize the importance of complying with the specified regimen, and explain ways to prevent gastrointestinal side effects and anorexia.
3. Teach the patient and parents the signs and symptoms of exacerbations, and stress the need to notify their pediatrician of these symptoms.
4. Review the comfort measures to be used during exacerbation (e.g., drugs, splinting, heat applications, baths, and proper alignment).
5. Explain the need for proper nutrition and calorie consumption; discuss methods of appetite enhancement for the child's age group.
6. Review instruction in range-of-motion exercises; provide lists of activities in which the child is encouraged to participate.
7. Teach the parents how to assist the child with activities of daily living in ways appropriate to the child's developmental age.
8. Explain the need for regular ophthalmologic checkups.
9. Give the parents the names and addresses of various organizations centered on the needs of children with JRA.
10. Explain the need to discuss the child's special needs with her teachers and principal (e.g., medications, exercise and movement, splints, psychosocial issues).

Progressive Systemic Sclerosis (Scleroderma)

Scleroderma means "hard skin." **Progressive systemic sclerosis (PSS),** or **scleroderma,** is a chronic, inflammatory, connective tissue disorder characterized by fibrotic and degenerative changes in the skin, joints, capillaries, arterial vessels, and visceral organs.

EPIDEMIOLOGY

Progressive systemic scleroderma is a rare and devastating disease of unknown etiology. It is primarily a disorder of connective tissue, and its hallmark feature is excessive fibrosis of the skin and viscera. Cytotoxic factors or toxins have been suggested as possible causes, but the exact cause has yet to be determined. The incidence is approximately 4 to 12.5 new cases per million in the population, with children being least affected. It is observed in women three times more often than in men, and there is no racial predisposition. Scleroderma does not appear to have a strong familial association, and there are no conclusive studies identifying a specific human leukocyte antigen (HLA) haplotype.

Scleroderma is often seen in association with Raynaud's phenomenon and, less frequently, Sjögren's syndrome and primary biliary cirrhosis. The onset of the disease usually begins between the third and fourth decade of life and follows a progressive and highly variable course. The disease trajectory tends to be slow and disabling; however, if the internal organs are involved, it can be rapidly fatal. Although many individuals adjust fairly well to this disorder, 40% die within 5 years, often as a result of pulmonary or esophageal dysfunction.

PATHOPHYSIOLOGY

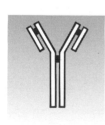

The exact mechanism that causes scleroderma remains unclear. Factors that have been identified as contributing to the pathogenesis of scleroderma include excessive collagen deposition, microvascular injury, and changes in humoral and cellular immunity.

Excessive Collagen Deposition

Excessive deposition of collagen in the skin and viscera is a characteristic feature of scleroderma. The mechanism that causes increased production of collagen is unclear; however, it is known that the excessive synthesis of collagen is caused by scleroderma fibroblasts rather than a decrease in degranulation. Although an abnormal amount of collagen is synthesized, it is otherwise qualitatively normal. Collagen types I and III are the predominant types deposited in the affected tissues.

Vascular Injury

Although the mechanisms of microvascular damage are not completely understood, vascular injury is another major feature of systemic scleroderma. Close pathologic examination will reveal a characteristic vascular lesion of scleroderma. This lesion typically affects small arteries, demonstrating intimal proliferation and fibrosis without disrupting the internal elastic lamina; the result is a narrowing of the vascular lumen. Because of this, it has been suggested that the endothelial lining of the blood vessels is a major target in systemic scleroderma.

Endothelial damage and cell death result in platelet activation and amplification of the perivascular inflammatory response. Once activated, platelets release a number of potent substances, leading to vasoconstriction, increased capillary permeability, and recruitment of fibroblasts and inflammatory cells to the target area. Ischemia develops as a result of fibrin deposition in the vessel and changes in the function and morphology of the microvasculature tissue.

Clinical evidence of vascular alteration and injury in scleroderma is demonstrated by Raynaud's phenomenon, telangiectasia, and nail fold capillary abnormalities.

Humoral Immunity

Humoral immunity to collagen has been observed. It consists primarily of antibodies to type I and type IV collagen. These antibodies may be significant, particularly antibodies to type IV collagen (basement membrane), in that they may promote immunogenicity and perpetuate endothelial cell injury.

Another factor in the relationship between humoral immunity and systemic scleroderma is that a significant number of patients develop hypergammaglobulinemia, with the largest elevation in IgG. In addition, immune complexes have often been detected in the serum of patients with systemic scleroderma, especially those with pulmonary or renal involvement. A few patients test positive for rheumatoid factor, and autoantibodies are

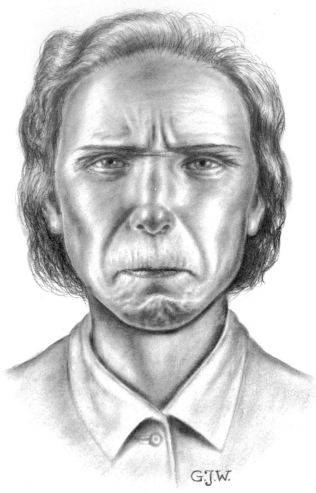

FIGURE 6-3
Characteristic facial changes of scleroderma: a nonexpressive and masklike appearance; tight, thick, and rigid skin; thin constricted lips, beaklike nose; smooth and immobile forehead; telangiectasia; and hair loss.

found in approximately 95% of patients. In addition, Raynaud's syndrome often coexists with scleroderma.

Cell-Mediated Immunity

In systemic scleroderma, circulating T lymphocytes may be normal or slightly decreased. Skin biopsies show that most cells in affected areas are T lymphocytes, with macrophages and plasma cells present in smaller numbers. It has been suggested that accumulation of T lymphocytes in the tissue is responsible for the decrease in circulating T lymphocytes. Also, the degree of skin thickening has been correlated with the degree of lymphocytic infiltration.[148] It has also been postulated that cytokines produced by T lymphocytes and macrophages may contribute to the altered regulation of fibrotic deposition seen in scleroderma.

Skin changes similar to those in scleroderma have been described in graft-versus-host disease. These skin changes are thought to be due to a reaction of donor T lymphocytes against host antigens, resulting in clinical features similar to those of scleroderma. The host antigen responsible for the immune response in graft-versus-host disease, and possibly scleroderma, is not known.

Changes in the endothelial lining of the small vessels in scleroderma may contribute to the persistent immune response and release of inflammatory mediators capable of modulating connective tissue metabolism.

CLASSIFICATION

Scleroderma is divided into two categories, **localized** and **generalized. The latter is also called systemic sclerosis.**

Localized scleroderma is the least severe form of the disease and affects primarily the skin. It may involve the muscles and bone but does not affect the internal organs. The two types of localized scleroderma are **morphea scleroderma** and **linear scleroderma.** Morphea is the development of skin lesions that are hard, oval, whitish patches with a purple ring around them. They typically appear on the face, arms, and legs but can appear anywhere on the body. Morphea often improves over time.

Linear scleroderma usually occurs in childhood. It is also a skin lesion and appears as a thickened line of skin. It generally develops on the arms, legs, or forehead, but like morphea scleroderma can occur anywhere on the body. This lesion frequently extends deep into the skin, involving the bones and muscles and affecting motion and growth in the affected area.

> **En coup de sabre means strike of a sword. It is the development of a thickened line of skin that forms a crease, often on the head or neck in linear scleroderma.**

Generalized scleroderma, or progressive systemic scleroderma, involves the skin and many internal organs such as the lungs, kidneys, joints, muscles, cardiovascular system, and digestive tract. The severity of the

---

CLASSIFICATION OF SCLERODERMA

Localized type	Generalized scleroderma (PSS)
Morphea scleroderma	Limited cutaneous scleroderma (CREST syndrome)
Linear scleroderma	Diffuse cutaneous scleroderma

disease depends on the organs affected and the extent of involvement. Basically there are two types of generalized scleroderma, **limited subcutaneous scleroderma,** also called **CREST syndrome,** and **diffuse subcutaneous scleroderma.**

Limited subcutaneous scleroderma generally has a slow onset, with the initial symptoms appearing 10 to 20 years before the complete disease develops. It also tends to have a more protracted course and better prognosis than the diffuse type. However, as the disease progresses, the internal organs may become affected.

CREST syndrome
  C = Calcinosis
  R = Raynaud's phenomenon
  E = Esophageal motility
  S = Sclerodactyly
  T = Telangiectasia

Patients with limited scleroderma typically have skin changes that are confined to the hands, fingers, and face. They generally have one or more of the features that make up CREST syndrome. CREST syndrome is a combination of symptoms that develop with limited subcutaneous scleroderma, including calcinosis, Raynaud's phenomenon, esophageal dysfunction, sclerodactyly, and telangiectasia (see Table 6-3).

Diffuse subcutaneous scleroderma is a systemic disorder that involves the entire body. It generally affects the skin, blood vessels, heart, lungs, gastrointestinal tract, joints, muscles, and kidneys. The area affected and the severity of involvement determine the nature and manifestations of the disease. This type of scleroderma often causes hypertension, muscle weakness, dysphagia, and dyspnea.

CLINICAL MANIFESTATIONS

Scleroderma is a systemic disease in which 90% of patients demonstrate Raynaud's syndrome. Systemic scleroderma affects primarily the skin, joints, muscles, lungs, heart, kidneys, and gastrointestinal tract. The onset often is nonspecific and mild. It frequently starts with skin changes. However, in approximately one third of patients, the initiating symptoms are polyarthralgias and polyarthritis.

Raynaud's phenomenon is a vascular disorder caused by an episodic and reversible spasm of arteries and arterioles. Although many attacks occur spontaneously, it is triggered primarily by cold or emotional stress. Although Raynaud's phenomenon typically affects the hands and feet, other parts of the body may also be affected, such as the ears, tip of the nose, and nipples. Raynaud's syndrome has three phases: pallor, cyanosis, and hyperemia. The syndrome is manifested initially by pallor caused by arterial constriction, which leads to a decrease in cutaneous blood flow. Cyanosis

Table 6-3

CREST SYNDROME IN SCLERODERMA

Symptom	Pathophysiology	Clinical feature
Calcinosis	Development of small, white calcium lumps under the skin	Hard white lumps under the skin; often distributed on the hands, fingers, and forearms; lumps may break and drain a chalky, gritty, white liquid
Raynaud's phenomenon	Episodic digital ischemia triggered by cold or emotional stress	Fingers, hands, and forearms become numb, tingle, and appear pale, followed by cyanosis and hyperemia; may result in fingertip ulcerations that heal with pitted scars or gangrene
Esophageal dysmotility	Weakened esophagus resulting from excessive accumulation of scar tissue, fibrosis, and muscle atrophy, causing inflammation, erosion, ulcerations, and stricture of the esophageal mucosa	Difficulty swallowing, heartburn, bloating, anorexia, nausea, vomiting, and weight loss
Sclerodactyly	Localized scleroderma of the digits, both fingers and toes	Skin on the fingers and toes becomes hard, leatherlike, and shiny; movement of these joints is difficult, and contractures may develop
Telangiectasia	Permanent dilation of small blood vessels (capillaries, arterioles, and venules)	Small, focal red lesions, typically on the fingers, palms, face, lips, and tongue

follows as a result of deoxygenated hemoglobin in the capillary vessels, where blood flow is significantly reduced. Finally, the hyperemic phase occurs when the vessels dilate and fill rapidly with arterial blood, causing redness. Prolonged or severe episodes can lead to ischemic necrosis and ulceration of the fingers. These ulcerated areas often heal with pitted scars. Occasionally gangrene develops in the distal phalanges.

Raynaud's phenomenon is generally diagnosed based on history rather than examination. However, in severe cases, on physical examination the distinct, triphasic color change, pallor, cyanosis, and hyperemia, can be seen. The fingers often are cool, with possible nail dystrophy, ulcerations, or small, pitting scars. The Allen test generally is positive in the ulnar artery in patients with even mild disease.

It is important to note that Raynaud's phenomenon can occur as an isolated event or secondary to a number of disorders besides scleroderma.

Skin changes are common in scleroderma. There are three primary stages of cutaneous involvement, edematous (inflammatory), fibrotic (sclerotic), and atrophic. The edematous stage is characterized by nonpitting edema that affects primarily the hands. It can extend to the forearms, arms, upper anterior chest, abdomen, back, and face. Patients frequently complain of puffy fingers and hands and morning stiffness.

The fibrotic stage is demonstrated by skin that is thick, smooth, taut, and shiny and that appears tightly connected to the underlying tissue. Hardening and thickening of the skin occur, particularly on the hands, arms, neck, upper chest, and face. Skin changes may stabilize for long periods of time, soften, and return to normal or progress to the atrophic stage.

After many years the skin thins, and atrophy of the epidermis develops. During the atrophic stage the skin appears hidebound and leathery. Flexion contractures of the fingers and other joints can develop. The hands often are shiny and red, and approximately half the patients have healing ulcerations. The fingers may become tapered and flexed, with depressed scars and loss of fingertips from poor arterial circulation and atrophy. Nails frequently atrophy and shed. The facial appearance is nonexpressive and masklike, lips become thin, and the mouth may not open completely. The nose may appear beaklike, and the forehead becomes smooth and immobile. Wrinkles and skin folds frequently disappear. Affected skin shows areas of hypopigmentation (especially in blacks) and hair loss. Telangiectases may be present on the fingers, palms, and face and tend to occur in greater number in patients with limited disease.

Subcutaneous calcium deposits (calcinosis circumscripta) that vary in size typically affect the fingertips and friction points over bony prominences throughout the body. These calcium deposits may lead to ulceration of the overlying skin, with the extrusion of a gritty substance consisting mainly of calcium hydroxyapatite. This process can lead to secondary infections in the affected area.

Musculoskeletal symptoms develop as the disease begins to affect the microcirculation to the muscles, bones, synovial membranes, and joints. Changes that develop include lymphocytic infiltration into the perivascular and interstitial tissues, deterioration of muscle fibers, and fibrosis. The number of capillaries is reduced, and arteriolar walls thicken. Synovial fluid generally is noninflammatory or may show mild mononuclear infiltrates. In addition, there is extensive fibrin deposition on the surface of the synovium.

Bone involvement consists of reabsorption of the tufts of the terminal phalanges, often in the second or third decade of disease. This often is accompanied by atrophy of adjacent soft tissue and subcutaneous calcinosis.

Articular complaints are a prominent feature, particularly early in the disease when arthralgias, edema, and stiffness often occur. As the disease progresses, range of joint motion becomes limited and contractures develop, mainly in the fingers. Severe flexion contractures are not uncommon.

Muscle involvement is characterized by easy fatigability, muscle weakness, and pain in the proximal muscles of both the upper and lower extremities. Later in the course of the disease, muscle atrophy develops. Muscle biopsies reveal increased collagen deposition and accumulation of lymphocytes and plasma cells.

Pulmonary manifestations are very common in scleroderma and are one of the leading causes of death. There are three primary types of pulmonary involvement: diffuse interstitial fibrosis, pleuritis, and pulmonary hypertension. Dyspnea on exertion is the most common symptom reported. It may be associated with a dry, nonproductive cough, orthopnea, chest pain, and

---

SCLERODERMA RENAL CRISIS

This is a medical emergency characterized by the following:
  Malignant hypertension
  Encephalopathy
  Pulmonary edema
  Retinopathy
  Microangiopathic hemolytic anemia
  Azotemia

hoarseness. Physical examination shows inspiratory crackles that are more prominent at the bases. Chest x-rays may be normal but frequently reveal basilar fibrosis or diffuse infiltrates. Pulmonary function tests show a restrictive pattern with a decrease in lung volume, manifested by decreases in forced vital capacity, total lung capacity, and functional residual capacity. Histologic findings often are similar to those for idiopathic pulmonary fibrosis with interstitial and alveolar fibrosis.

Cardiac involvement is unusual; it includes fibrosis of the myocardium, conduction system, small coronary arteries, and pericardium. Cor pulmonale may occur as the result of pulmonary fibrosis in systemic scleroderma. Myocardial fibrosis can cause arrhythmias and conduction disturbances, manifested as palpitations and syncope. In severe cases it can lead to left-sided heart failure that is resistant to digitalis. The characteristic pathologic cardiac feature in scleroderma is a contraction-band necrosis that develops in the myocardium when it has been reperfused after a transient interruption in blood flow.

Renal manifestations of scleroderma vary from mild, asymptomatic proteinuria to malignant hypertension. The prevalence of renal involvement varies, depending on the diagnostic criteria employed. Nonetheless, mild proteinuria is observed in approximately 35% of patients with scleroderma and mild hypertension in 25%.

Histologic examination shows intimal thickening of the renal interlobular arteries, fibrosis, and deposition of immunoglobulin and complement in small renal arteries. Diminished cortical perfusion is present, often with maintenance of normal glomerular filtration.

The renin-angiotensin system plays a pivotal role in the development of renal ischemia and hypertension in patients with scleroderma. Cortical ischemia is thought to result in the activation of the juxtaglomerular apparatus to secrete renin. As renin levels increase, specific enzymes assist with the generation of the potent vasoconstrictor angiotensin II, resulting in a decrease in renal blood flow. Increased levels of angiotensin II cause further vasospasm in the renal cortex, with ensuing renal ischemia. Plasma renin activity is often significantly higher in patients with scleroderma. Other causes of decreased renal blood flow may be due to sodium or volume depletion that further stimulates the renin-angiotensin system.

Lower urinary tract involvement has included microscopic hematuria with or without urgency. Biopsy of the urinary bladder often reveals interstitial fibrosis.

Gastrointestinal disorders are the most common visceral manifestation of systemic scleroderma. Esophageal involvement occurs most frequently, affecting approximately 80% of patients with systemic scleroderma. Characteristic symptoms include dysphagia, particularly for solid foods, and heartburn that is exacerbated by a recumbent position, which promotes a more active esophageal reflux. As a result of gastric reflux, inflammation, erosion, or ulceration of the mucosa may occur. Stricture of the esophagus may develop after a prolonged course of peptic esophagitis.

Special studies demonstrate aperistalsis of the distal portion of the esophagus, dilation or strictures, and free gastroesophageal reflux. Microvascular alterations seen in scleroderma may contribute to the pathogenesis of esophageal dysmotility by decreasing the blood supply to this area. Smooth muscle atrophy and fibrosis are other contributing factors.

Gastric involvement is the result of delayed gastric emptying and reduced gastric contractions. Symptoms

---

OVERVIEW OF THE CLINICAL FEATURES OF PROGRESSIVE SYSTEMIC SCLERODERMA

Vascular: generalized small vessel pathologic condition, Raynaud's phenomenon, telangiectasia, nail fold capillary abnormalities

Skin: tight, leathery, hard skin; masklike facial expression, beaked nose, small mouth opening and thin lips, loss of distal epidermal phalanges, flattened distal phalanges, hypopigmentation or hyperpigmentation, subcutaneous calcinosis

Musculoskeletal: arthralgias, muscle weakness and pain, joint stiffness, flexion contractures, soft tissue reabsorption of fingertips

Pulmonary: dyspnea, nonproductive cough, orthopnea, chest pain, hoarseness, crackles on auscultation

Cardiac: arrhythmias, chest pain, signs of congestive heart failure

Renal: hypertension, azotemia with progressive renal insufficiency

Gastrointestinal: dysphagia, bloating and cramping, heartburn and reflux, diarrhea, constipation, nausea and vomiting, anorexia with weight loss

of gastric and small bowel involvement include nausea, vomiting, bloating, distention, and anorexia; weight loss may result from intestinal atony. The onset of acute abdominal pain may be due to pseudoobstruction secondary to segmental bowel atony. Hypomotility may result in bacterial overgrowth, leading to malabsorption.

The colon frequently is involved and demonstrates changes similar to those seen in the esophagus and small intestine. Symptoms tend to be less common and include chronic constipation and bloating. Pseudoobstruction and perforation are rare complications of colonic involvement but are considered life threatening when they occur.

COMPLICATIONS

Nephrosclerosis and renal failure
Bowel obstruction or perforation (or both)
Aspiration pneumonia
Malignant hypertension
Pulmonary hypertension
Congestive heart failure
Cor pulmonale
Respiratory failure (due to fibrotic lung disease)
Cardiomyopathy
Death

DIAGNOSTIC STUDIES AND FINDINGS

Diagnostic test	Findings
Baseline data*	
Hematocrit and hemoglobin	Normochromic, normocytic anemia
Erythrocyte sedimentation rate (ESR)	Mild to moderate elevation
Blood T lymphocytes	Normal or slightly decreased
Blood immunoglobulins	Polyclonal hypergammaglobulinemia is common; presence of antibodies to collagen types I and IV
Immune complexes	Present in 20%-50% of patients, particularly those with pulmonary or renal involvement
Antinuclear antibody	Positive speckled or nucleolar pattern present in approximately 90% of patients
Rheumatoid factor	May be present
Complement	Normal or slightly elevated
Muscle enzymes (e.g., CPK, aldolase)	Elevations indicate inflammatory myositis, and muscle biopsy is recommended
Blood urea nitrogen (BUN) and creatinine	Slightly elevated; varies, depending on renal involvement
Creatinine clearance	May be decreased or normal, depending on renal involvement
Urinalysis	Mild proteinuria (<1 g/24 h)
X-rays	
Bone x-ray	Thickening of periarticular tissues; osteoporosis; digital cuff reabsorption; flexion contractures; subcutaneous calcinosis
Chest x-ray	May be normal; may show basilar fibrosis or diffuse infiltrates, or disseminated pulmonary calcifications in advanced cases
Upper gastrointestinal study	Often demonstrates decreased or absent esophageal peristaltic activity; dilation of lower 70% of esophagus; ulcers or strictures of lower esophagus are common
Barium enema	Wide-necked diverticula on antimesenteric border of transverse and descending colon
Miscellaneous studies	
Electrocardiogram (ECG)	May show arrhythmias characteristic of pericarditis or myocardial disease

*Baseline data are obtained according to the patient's specific needs and to assist with classification of the type of scleroderma.

DIAGNOSTIC STUDIES AND FINDINGS—cont'd

Diagnostic test	Findings
Miscellaneous studies—cont'd	
Pulmonary function tests	Restrictive pattern; decreases in lung volume, forced expired vital capacity (FEVC), total lung capacity (TLC), and functional residual capacity (FRC)
Nail fold capillaroscopy (to detect microvascular changes)	Two patterns have been identified: *Active:* correlates with diffuse sclerodema, characterized by capillary enlargement, distortion, and dropout *Slow:* correlates with cutaneous scleroderma, characterized by capillary enlargement without capillary loss
Muscle biopsy	Increased collagen deposition and focal accumulation of lymphocytes and plasma cells

MEDICAL MANAGEMENT

There is no specific treatment or cure for scleroderma. Proper classification is the key to management of patients with systemic scleroderma. Patients at highest risk for developing internal organ involvement are those with early diffuse disease and rapidly progressive skin thickening. These patients should be considered for aggressive disease-modifying therapy.

GENERAL MANAGEMENT

Psychosocial: Anticipate depression, withdrawal, and anger; obtain psychiatric consultation to assist patient and family with ongoing adjustment process.

Physical therapy: Develop a routine exercise program to preserve joint function and prevent contractures.

Smoking: Should be avoided; if patient smokes, provide access to a stop smoking program to minimize the effects of Raynaud's phenomenon.

Nutrition: Encourage patient to eat small, frequent meals to minimize esophageal reflux; encourage a well-balanced diet high in fiber to prevent constipation and diarrhea; implement parenteral alimentation or hyperalimentation when indicated.

Instruct patient to avoid exposure to cold and stressful situations and to wear gloves and extra clothing during cold weather: To prevent arterial spasms and decreased blood flow to hands and fingers.

Oxygen therapy: Used as a supportive measure in advanced pulmonary fibrosis.

ECG monitoring: Instituted to detect cardiac arrhythmias.

Blood pressure monitoring: Instituted to detect hypertension.

Skin lubricants: Used for dry skin.

Renal monitoring: Instituted for early detection of proteinuria and renal insufficiency (elevated BUN, creatinine, decreased creatinine clearance).

DRUG THERAPY

Vasodilators: To relieve pain in patients with severe Raynaud's phenomenon: calcium channel blockers (e.g., nifedipine, diltiazem); direct vasodilators (e.g., hydralazine, topical nitrates [Ketanserin]); sympatholytic agents (e.g., prazosin [Minipress], methyldopa [Aldomet]).

Antihypertensive agents: To control blood pressure; particularly successful are the angiotensin-converting enzyme inhibitors (e.g., enalapril [Vasotec], captopril [Capoten]).

MEDICAL MANAGEMENT—cont'd

Antiinflammatory agents: May be used to treat joint pain and swelling: acetylsalicylic acid (aspirin); nonsteroidal antiinflammatory drugs; ibuprofen (Motrin, Advil), and indomethacin (Indocin) should not be used in patients with renal involvement.

Corticosteroids: Reserved for treating inflammatory myopathy and pericarditis and for patients who fail to respond to nonsteroidal antiinflammatory drugs.

Penicillamine: Slow acting NSAID may be effective in slowing visceral disease and treating cutaneous slceroderma.

Antacids (e.g., Mylanta or Amphogel) or H$_2$-receptor blockers (e.g., ranitidine [Zantec]): To relieve heartburn and to protect the esophageal mucosa from acid damage.

Gastrointestinal stimulants (e.g., metoclopramide [Reglan]): To increase upper GI tract emptying; to treat esophageal reflux and gastric stasis.

Antibiotics: To decrease bacterial overgrowth that can lead to malabsorption and to treat episodes of pneumonia or other types of infection (e.g., infected skin ulcers).

Analgesics: To minimize pain; they may be given PO or topically.

Vitamin supplements: For nutritional support.

Immunosuppressive agents (controversial): Chlorambucil, cyclophosphamide (Cytoxan), azathioprine (Imuran).

Experimental drugs: Colchicine, cyclosporine, ketanserin, recombinant gamma-interferon, antilymphocyte globulin.

ADJUNCTIVE THERAPY

Esophageal dilation, plasmapheresis, plasma exchange, dialysis for renal support.

SURGERY

Sympathectomy provides transient relief of vascular symptoms; intestinal resection for obstruction or repair of perforation; ulcer debridement and care; reconstructive surgery; bowel resection for bowel obstruction or perforation; pericardiocentesis or pericardiectomy for tamponade.

1 ASSESS

ASSESSMENT	OBSERVATIONS
General appearance	Withdrawn; masklike face; tight, smooth facial skin; drawn, wrinkled mouth with small opening; beaklike nose
Skin	Dry, tough, hardened skin with thinning and atrophy in some areas, hair loss over affected areas, and hypopigmentation; usual skin creases absent; telangiectasias on fingers and palms, subcutaneous calcinosis, and small ulcerated areas on fingers; digits become pale and cyanotic when exposed to cold
Gastrointestinal	Dysphagic with esophageal reflux; anorexia and demonstrated weight loss; alternating constipation and diarrhea

ASSESSMENT	OBSERVATIONS
Musculoskeletal	Finger contractures; joint stiffness; decreased ROJM; increased fatigue with minimal exertion; weakness; diffuse muscle atrophy; tenderness and pain in proximal muscles of upper and lower extremities
Pulmonary	Dyspnea; orthopnea; hoarseness; dry, nonproductive cough; dependent, dry crackles
Renal	Hypertension; proteinuria <1 g/24 h; slightly elevated BUN and creatinine
Cardiac	Clinical features of pericarditis (dyspnea, dependent edema); fever; chest pain; possible intermittent pericardial friction rub

2 DIAGNOSE

NURSING DIAGNOSIS	SUBJECTIVE FINDINGS	OBJECTIVE FINDINGS
Impaired skin integrity related to altered peripheral perfusion and changes in skin turgor	Reports pain, numbness, and tingling in hands and fingers; complains that skin feels tight and leathery over entire body	Triphasic color changes in hands and fingers; fingers are cool to touch and have several small ulcerations; skin generally has hidebound appearance, with loss of normal wrinkles and folds
Potential for aspiration related to difficulty swallowing and esophageal disease	Reports difficulty swallowing and heartburn	Coughing follows swallowing; barium studies show aperistalsis of distal portion of esophagus and gastroesophageal reflux; delayed gastric emptying
Altered nutrition: less than body requirements related to esophageal reflux, difficulty swallowing, reduced mouth opening, and malabsorption	Complains of difficulty swallowing, midsternal discomfort when eating, loss of appetite, and intermittent diarrhea and constipation	Weight loss, inadequate food and fluid intake, dysphagia, muscle atrophy, and wasting; steatorrhea, with bacterial overgrowth in the stool; x-rays show dilation of duodenum and possibly jejunum
Activity intolerance related to joint contractures and weakness	Complains of being unable to complete ADLs because of joint discomfort, stiffness, swelling, and weakness	Joint tenderness and limited ROJM, particularly in hands, wrists, elbows, feet, knees, and hips; flexion contractions; muscle weakness and atrophy
Ineffective breathing pattern related to decreased lung expansion due to pulmonary fibrosis	Complains of being short of breath	Dyspnea and fatigue with minimal exertion, tachypnea, nonproductive cough, crackles in lower lung fields; decreased FEVC, TLC, and FRC
Altered renal tissue perfusion related to decreased renal blood flow	Reports a slight decrease in urinary output; complains of intermittent headaches	Proteinuria <1 g/day; elevated BP, decreased urine output rising BUN and creatinine

→ › ›

NURSING DIAGNOSIS	SUBJECTIVE FINDINGS	OBJECTIVE FINDINGS
Body image disturbance related to inability to integrate body changes and appearance	Complains of feeling ugly and not looking the same	Masklike face; tight, hard skin; thin lips; drawn, wrinkled mouth; smooth, immobile forehead; wasted musculature; hands contracted

Other related nursing diagnoses: **Social isolation** related to alterations in physical appearance; **Altered sexuality patterns** related to body image disturbances; **Impaired gas exchange** related to altered blood flow and pulmonary fibrosis; **Constipation** related to chronic colonic diverticular lesions; **Diarrhea** related to malabsorption; **Hopelessness** related to progressive deterioration in physiologic condition; **Pain** related to skin ulcerations and joint contractures; **Altered family processes** related to deteriorating physical condition; **Potential decreased cardiac output** related to reduced ventricular filling resulting from pericarditis.

3 PLAN

Patient goals

1. The patient will demonstrate progressive healing of skin ulcerations and regain skin integrity.
2. The patient will have improved arterial blood flow to fingers and hands.
3. The patient will not aspirate.
4. The patient will have an increased nutritional intake adequate for body demands and healing.
5. The patient will have increased tolerance for daily activities.
6. The patient will have an effective breathing pattern without dyspnea or fatigue.
7. The patient will have adequate renal perfusion.
8. The patient will have a positive body image.

4 IMPLEMENT

NURSING DIAGNOSIS	NURSING INTERVENTIONS	RATIONALE
Impaired skin integrity related to altered peripheral perfusion and changes in skin turgor	Assess and monitor extremities, particularly hands and fingers, for adequacy of peripheral arterial blood flow (e.g., skin color, pulses, capillary refill, sensation, temperature).	Severity of symptoms reflects degree of decreased arterial blood flow and guides therapy.
	Instruct patient not to smoke or to use other nicotine products (e.g., chewing tobacco, nicotine patch).	Nicotine causes vasoconstriction, damaging intimal cells of both large and small blood vessels.
	Instruct patient to avoid exposure to cold (e.g., outdoors, refrigerator).	To prevent vasoconstriction and decreased tissue perfusion.
	Instruct patient to wear suitable clothing (e.g., extra insulation on body) and to protect hands with gloves when in a cold environment.	To maintain blood flow and vasodilation.
	Instruct patient to avoid synthetic fabric and to wear wool or cotton.	Cotton next to skin moves perspiration away from body and prevents sweat from cooling the body; wool is warmer than synthetic fabric.

NURSING DIAGNOSIS	NURSING INTERVENTIONS	RATIONALE
	Maintain a warm environment.	To promote vasodilation and tissue perfusion.
	Monitor for complaints of tingling, numbness, or burning.	These indicate lack of oxygenation, leading to ischemia.
	Administer topical vasodilators (nitroglycerin paste, procaine jelly) or oral vasodilators as ordered, and monitor response.	To improve arterial blood flow to affected areas and maintain tissue perfusion and cellular oxygenation.
	Protect affected areas (fingers and hands) from trauma; keep fingernails short to prevent scratching.	To promote healing; trauma may cause vasoconstriction and eventual ulceration.
	Encourage intake of adequate diet; consult nutritionist.	Adequate nutritional intake promotes healing; consulting expert team member promotes individualized care.
	Instruct patient in importance of routine skin care (i.e., using tepid water, mild soap, and patting completely dry).	To promote healing and maintain skin integrity.
	Apply lanolin-based lotions to skin.	To decrease dryness and improve skin turgor.
	Ambulate frequently; if patient is unable, change position at least q 2 h.	To maintain circulation to skin.
	Use aseptic wound care in ulcerative areas; cover impaired skin as ordered with dressings, ointments, etc. Monitor changes.	To regain skin integrity and prevent bacterial invasion.
	Teach patient relaxation strategies (e.g., self-hypnosis, visualization).	Emotional stress contributes to peripheral vasoconstriction in Raynaud's syndrome; decreasing stress diminishes vasoconstriction.
Potential for aspiration related to difficulty swallowing and esophageal disease	Elevate head of bed to 90-degree angle during meals and for 30 min after meals; avoid recumbent position after meals.	To provide proper position for adequate swallowing and to prevent esophageal reflux.
	Provide small, frequent meals.	To help manage esophageal hypomotility and reflux.
	Cut food into small pieces, and remind patient to take small bites and to chew food well before swallowing.	Lack of chewing may cause aspiration of large pieces of food.
	Tell patient to think, "Remember to swallow."	Conscious thought may enhance swallow reflex.

→ › ›

NURSING DIAGNOSIS	NURSING INTERVENTIONS	RATIONALE
	Monitor for signs of coughing, gagging, nasal regurgitation, holding food in mouth, decreased breath sounds, or signs of air hunger.	These are signs of possible aspiration.
	Administer metoclopramide (Reglan) as ordered, and monitor response.	To promote gastric motility, and to increase lower esophageal sphincter pressure and upper GI contractions.
	Administer antacids or H_2-receptor blockers as ordered, and monitor response.	Antacids protect esophageal mucosa from acid damage; H_2-receptor blockers reduce gastric acid secretion.
	Keep suction equipment at bedside.	For emergency use if patient chokes on food or fluids.
	Teach family members the Heimlich maneuver.	To use in emergencies if patient chokes.
Altered nutrition: less than body requirements related to esophageal reflux, difficulty swallowing, reduced mouth opening, and malabsorption	Assess dietary habits and needs; calculate for additional calories and nutrients if infection is present.	To guide therapeutic interventions and individualize diet.
	Document weight upon admission, and monitor daily.	To establish baseline and to monitor changes in weight.
	Monitor daily food and fluid intake; assist with feedings.	To determine need for supplemental or parenteral feedings.
	Help provide routine oral hygiene, particularly before meals.	To improve appetite and moisten skin that is tightly contracted around mouth.
	Provide small, frequent meals.	Esophageal hypomotility prevents intake of large amounts of food at one time; offering small, frequent meals promotes intake and absorption of nutrients.
	Encourage fluids and foods high in fiber (e.g., fruits, cereals, grains).	To minimize constipation.
	Administer antibiotics as ordered, and monitor response.	To treat steatorrhea caused by bacterial overgrowth in GI tract secondary to hypomotility.
	Administer metoclopramide (Reglan) as ordered, and monitor response.	To facilitate gastric motility.
	Begin tube feedings or hyperalimentation (or both) with intralipids as ordered.	To improve and maintain nutritional status.
Activity intolerance related to joint contractures and weakness	Assess and monitor range of motion of all joints; assess mobility and joint deformities.	To guide therapeutic interventions.

NURSING DIAGNOSIS	NURSING INTERVENTIONS	RATIONALE
	Consult exercise physiologist and occupational and physical therapists to develop routine exercise regimen consisting of ROJM, strengthening, and endurance exercises.	Professional expertise can provide a vital service in developing an individualized exercise regimen; routine exercise may minimize further contractures, increase strength, improve circulation, maintain independence, and promote psychologic well-being.
	Provide rest periods between activities.	To minimize weakness.
	Provide progressive increase in activity as tolerated.	As endurance improves, independence is facilitated.
	Provide patient and family with information about assistive devices (e.g., long-handled reachers, lightweight cooking equipment).	To promote independence and ability to perform routine activities.
	Encourage patient to take warm morning showers.	To diminish stiffness and joint discomfort.
	Administer antiinflammatory drugs or corticosteroids as ordered, and monitor response.	To reduce inflammation, swelling, and stiffness and to control symptoms.
Ineffective breathing pattern related to decreased lung expansion due to pulmonary fibrosis	Observe breathing pattern for shortness of breath, nasal flaring, pursed-lip breathing, use of accessory muscles, and intercostal retraction.	To identify increased work of breathing.
	Inspect thorax for symmetry of respiratory movement.	To determine adequacy of breathing.
	Auscultate breath sounds.	To determine adequacy of air exchange.
	Encourage use of incentive spirometry as ordered.	To maintain adequate ventilation.
	Measure tidal volume (V_T) and vital capacity (VC).	These indicate volume of air moving in and out.
	Encourage patient to use adaptive breathing techniques.	To decrease work of breathing.
	Administer oxygen as ordered, and monitor response.	To maintain adequate ventilation and decrease work of breathing.
	Assist patient to upright high Fowler's position.	To facilitate work of breathing and optimize diaphragmatic contraction.
Altered renal tissue perfusion related to decreased renal blood flow	Monitor BP q 2-4 h.	Hypertension may develop secondary to decrease in renal perfusion and activation of renin-angiotensin system.

→ › ›

NURSING DIAGNOSIS	NURSING INTERVENTIONS	RATIONALE
	Administer antihypertensive medications as ordered, and monitor response.	To decrease BP; frequently angiotensin-converting enzyme inhibitors (e.g., enalapril, captopril) are ordered to prevent generation of angiotensin II, a potent vasoconstrictor.
	Monitor serum potassium, BUN, creatinine, and creatinine clearance.	These are indicators of renal function; an elevation in potassium, creatinine, and BUN and a decrease in creatinine clearance may suggest impaired renal perfusion and function.
	Monitor urinary protein.	Increases in urinary protein (>500 mg/24 h) indicate renal impairment, suggesting alteration in the glomerular basement membrane.
	Monitor intake and output, daily weight, central venous pressure (CVP), breath sounds, and degree of peripheral edema.	As indicators of fluid status; increase in daily weight, CVP, intake over output, and rales, or diminished or absent breath sounds suggests increasing fluid volume; peripheral edema may increase; secondary to low albumin.
	Assess and monitor mental status.	Changes in mental status may indicate increasing azotemia or severe hypertension.
	If renal insufficiency requires dialysis or hemofiltration, work with nephrology nurse to provide patient and family with information about resources for these treatment modalities.	To increase patient's and family's knowledge about treatments for acute renal failure, and to minimize fear and provide support.
Body image disturbance related to inability to integrate body changes and appearance	Assess patient's concerns about body image.	To obtain an understanding of patient's specific concerns and to guide therapeutic intervention.
	Encourage patient to express feelings about joint deformities, skin abnormalities, and facial changes; offer support and understanding of patient's feelings and concerns.	Ventilation helps patient resolve grief over physical changes and clarify feelings and concerns; support and understanding may help with process of regaining a positive body image.
	Consult medical cosmetologist, and teach patient strategies for improving body image (e.g., how to dress, apply makeup or wigs, improve hygiene).	Expert team members can help provide individualized care and promote a positive body image.
	Help significant others understand impact of disease limitation on patient, and elicit their help in identifying methods to promote patient's efforts toward a positive body image.	Significant others can play a pivotal role in helping patient regain a positive body image.

NURSING DIAGNOSIS	NURSING INTERVENTIONS	RATIONALE
	Refer patient to community resources and self-help groups.	To provide access to individuals who may have effective alternative strategies and to provide ongoing support.

5 EVALUATE

PATIENT OUTCOME	DATA INDICATING THAT OUTCOME IS REACHED
Patient has regained and maintains skin integrity.	Skin is intact, warm, dry, and of natural color; patient has no pain; capillary refill is normal (2-4 sec), fingers and toes natural color without tingling, nails blanch within 2-4 sec and there is no evidence of skin breakdown.
Patient does not aspirate.	There is no evidence of aspiration; breath sounds are clear to all lobes; patient has no air hunger and appears well oxygenated.
Patient has improved and maintains her nutritional status.	Weight has increased and remains stable; albumin is normal; patient eats an adequate and nutritionally sound diet.
Patient performs daily activities.	Patient performs all self-care activities and maintains routine household maintenance expectations with decreased joint discomfort and stiffness; she reports that strength has improved.
Patient has an effective breathing pattern.	Patient's VC measurements are optimum for her status, including FEVC, TLC, FRC; patient has no dyspnea with activity; respiratory rate is normal; and breath sounds are clear to auscultation.
Renal perfusion is adequate.	Patient is normotensive; BUN, creatinine, potassium, and creatinine clearance are normal or optimum for patient; urinary protein is <500 mg/24 h.
Patient has achieved a positive body image.	Patient verbalizes acceptance of limitations and demonstrates resolution of grief; she shows an effort to improve her appearance and participates in a self-help support group.

PATIENT TEACHING

1. Teach the patient and family the Heimlich maneuver, to be performed in emergencies when the patient has aspirated.
2. Teach the patient and family about the disease trajectory of progressive systemic scleroderma, management strategies, and medications.
3. Teach the patient and family the purpose, administration, and side effects of all medications.
4. Teach the patient strategies for avoiding trauma and protecting her joints (see Patient Guide).
5. In collaboration with the exercise physiologist, teach the patient range of joint motion exercises to be performed at home.
6. Teach the patient how to monitor her blood pressure at home.
7. Teach the patient routine skin care to prevent breakdown and ulceration.
8. Teach the patient cold protection strategies (e.g., wear gloves in cold weather and when going into the refrigerator or freezer; keep torso well insulated in cold weather; wear hat and scarf to cover nose and ears; avoid synthetic fabric; keep heater on in the home and in the car when driving).
9. Teach the patient ways to minimize diarrhea and constipation (e.g., maintain activity, eat high-fiber foods [grains, bran, fresh fruits, and vegetables]).

10. Teach the patient methods of stress management (e.g., breathing exercises, visualization, self-hypnosis, listening to music, providing diversional activities).

11. Teach the patient to cut food into small pieces, to chew thoroughly, to drink water to soften food, and to eat slowly.

12. Teach the patient to avoid foods that cause gas (e.g., cauliflower, broccoli) or heartburn (e.g., spicy foods).

13. Teach the patient to sit up during meals and for at least 30 minutes afterward.

14. Refer the patient and family to organizational resources.

Sjögren's Syndrome

Sjögren's syndrome is a chronic autoimmune disorder. It is characterized by a combination of ocular (xerophthalmia) and oral (xerostomia) membrane dryness, called the sicca complex (see the box below). Generally it is of no systemic consequence; however, it is often seen in association with other immunologic disorders.

EPIDEMIOLOGY

Although controversial, Sjögren's syndrome may appear as a primary entity; however, it may also be associated with systemic lupus erythematosus (SLE), progressive systemic sclerosis (scleroderma), rheumatoid arthritis, or other immunologic disorders. For example, Raynaud's syndrome is clinically present in 20% of patients with Sjögren's syndrome, and extraglandular infiltrates are present in 10% of patients with the disorder. Extraglandular infiltrates may be found in the lungs, kidneys, lymph nodes, and muscles.

Sjögren's syndrome is also like other autoimmune disorders associated with HLA antigens DR3 and B8, indicating that the syndrome may be regulated by the genes governing the immune response.[28]

Although 90% of those with Sjögren's syndrome are middle-aged women (mean age is 50 years), the disorder has also been detected in children. In addition, there is evidence that sex hormones play an etiologic role in the disease, and the ratio of female to male patients is 9:1.[158]

PATHOPHYSIOLOGY

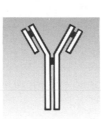

Some researchers think that the pathogenesis of Sjögren's syndrome is related to an abnormal immunologic response to one or more unidentified antigens that are probably viral in nature. However, the exact etiology remains unclear.[116,169]

Sjögren's syndrome is characterized by an excessive increase in B-cell and plasma cell activity, producing large amounts of IgG and IgM and decreasing the number of suppressor T cells. The increase in lymphocyte activity is manifested by polyclonal hypergammaglobulinemia, the production of rheumatoid factor, antinuclear factor, cryoglobulins, and anti–salivary duct antibodies. The excessive B-cell activity may be due to a primary B-cell defect or to the inability of the T cells to regulate appropriately. This abnormal immune response is demonstrated by cellular lymphoid infiltration into the exocrine glands, a reduction in endogenous and interferon-induced natural killer (NK) cell activity in the blood, an absence of NK cells in the salivary glands, diminished production of interferon, autoantibodies, and benign and malignant lymphomas.[169]

Biopsy specimens from glandular lesions have shown replacement of secretory acinar tissue with infiltrating B lymphocytes, plasma cells, and macrophages. Immunofluorescence studies show both B-cell and T-cell infiltrates in involved tissues.

SICCA COMPLEX

The hallmark of Sjögren's syndrome is a nonspecific lymphocytic infiltration of exocrine glands, primarily the lacrimal and salivary glands, which results in a decrease in lacrimal and salivary secretions. The cellular infiltration insidiously destroys glandular tissue, producing the combination of ocular and oral membrane dryness. Persistent dryness is caused by insufficient secretion from the lacrimal, salivary, and mucous glands.

In most patients with Sjögren's syndrome, the lymphoproliferation is localized to the salivary, lacrimal, and mucosal tissue. It usually results in a benign, chronic course of xerostomia and keratoconjunctivitis. Persistent dryness in keratoconjunctivitis sicca generally results when all the mucous glands of the conjunctival sac are involved, rather than just the lacrimal glands. Approximately 5% of patients with Sjögren's syndrome have enlarged lacrimal glands, and the enlargement usually is bilateral.[28]

The course and prognosis for patients with Sjögren's syndrome who also have rheumatoid arthritis or one of the connective tissue disorders almost always are determined by the underlying disease. The symptoms of the sicca complex in this group usually are mild; more severe symptoms develop in patients who have the sicca syndrome alone or primary Sjögren's syndrome.

The most severe long-term prognosis is subsequent total destruction of tissues as a result of decreased secretion by involved glands. Although unusual, this would be characterized by keratoconjunctivitis sicca, with complete loss of the integrity of the corneal epithelium due to desiccation, and extensive xerostomia, with both conditions leading to severe complications. Generally, keratoconjunctivitis is effectively treated with artificial tears.

Lymphoproliferative disease in Sjögren's syndrome ranges from benign to malignant; however, patients rarely develop extraglandular lymphoid infiltration or neoplasms. Benign lesions generally are a glandular infiltration (progressing to ductal proliferation) of plasma cells and lymphocytes into major and minor salivary and lacrimal glands. This process will result in myoepithelial islands, doing minor damage to the duct but preserving the architecture.

These benign lesions may develop into a pseudolymphoma, which is identified by an extraglandular lymphoproliferation that does not meet the histologic requirements for a malignancy. Polyclonal B cells usually are the predominant cell type in this associated condition. Clinically cellular infiltrates and lymphadenopathy affect the involved organs, primarily the salivary glands, lungs, and kidneys. Clinical features that increase the risk of malignancy in patients with Sjögren's syndrome are chronic parotid swelling, systemic lymphadenopathy, splenomegaly, and a progressive decrease in previously elevated immunoglobulin and/or rheumatoid factor.

CLINICAL MANIFESTATIONS

Sjögren's syndrome manifests clinically with dryness of the eyes and mouth. Dryness of the nose, trachea, bronchi, vagina, and skin can occur. Scaly skin and decreased sweating may also be present.

Ocular Symptoms

Ocular manifestations of Sjögren's syndrome often are mild and nonspecific. The primary clinical feature affecting the eyes is keratoconjunctivitis sicca. Symptoms include hyperemia of the conjunctivae, lacrimal deficiency (decreased tearing and dryness), thickening of the corneal epithelium with or without ulceration of the cornea, ropy (an accumulation of a thick, mucoid material at the inner canthus of the eye, particularly in the early morning), itching and burning of the eyes, photosensitivity, pain, a "sandy" or "gritty" feeling in the eyes, the sensation of having a foreign body in the eyes, and a reduction in visual acuity (although this is uncommon). By far the most common complaints are itchy, dry eyes that feel gritty, which occurs in more than 50% of patients with the disorder.

Although rare, severe or untreated keratoconjunctivitis sicca may lead to the development of erosions, ulcerations, and sloughing of the corneal epithelium (filamentary keratitis), as demonstrated by rose bengal staining and slitlamp examination. If the condition is not treated, visual acuity may be impaired.

Oral Symptoms

Xerostomia is one of the most distressing symptoms of Sjögren's syndrome and is observed in 90% of these patients. It often interferes with mastication and the swallowing of dry food. Swallowing a bolus of food or food fragments may be so difficult that the food adheres to the gums and palate, requiring the patient to remove it manually.

Patients typically are intensely thirsty as a result of the persistent dryness and discomfort. In an attempt to relieve the dryness, they often increase their fluid intake between meals; this in turn usually results in polyuria and nocturia.

Xerostomia frequently is associated with burning in the mouth and has been shown to progress to oral ulcerations and fissures at the corners of the mouth, in the buccal mucosa, and on the tongue. In advanced cases of tongue and buccal mucosa ulcers, the mucous membrane lining in the mouth can be peeled off. These factors frequently contribute to changes in taste and smell.

Salivary Glands

Parotid swelling and firmness with rapid fluctuation in the size of the gland are observed in 50% of patients with Sjögren's syndrome, and submaxillary swelling is observed in 20% of these patients. Glandular swelling may be associated with fever, pain or tenderness, and local heat and redness. Salivary glands that are erythematous and very tender may indicate an infection, often caused by *Staphylococcus aureus*.

Enlargement of the parotid gland usually is unilateral and episodic. On palpation the gland is smooth and irregular, not nodular as in the case of a neoplasm. Histologically, salivary glands in Sjögren's syndrome show acinar atrophy and polylymphoid infiltration consisting primarily of mature lymphocytes and plasma cells. Immunofluorescence studies have shown production of rheumatoid factor by plasma cells in these infiltrates.[28]

Enlargement of the submaxillary gland is less common and can be unilateral or bilateral; metaplastic and proliferative changes are more common in this gland.

About 60% to 70% of patients with Sjögren's syndrome also develop focal sialadenitis, a chronic inflammatory disease of the major salivary glands characterized by intermittent edema that progresses to fibrotic degeneration.

Other Symptoms

Other clinical findings might include dryness of the nose, posterior oropharynx, larynx, nasal mucosa, and respiratory tract. Prolonged, persistent drying of these mucous membranes may result in a chronic nonproductive cough, epistaxis, dysphonia, recurrent otitis media (hearing impairments may ensue), and tracheobronchitis or pneumonia. The vaginal mucosa is also dry, and dyspareunia may be problematic.

It has also been reported that patients with Sjögren's syndrome have an increased susceptibility to drug reactions, specifically penicillin.[28] Arthralgias and myopathies are not infrequent, and peripheral vasculitis is seen, particularly in patients with antibody to the Sjögren's syndrome A (SS-A) antigen.

CONDITIONS ASSOCIATED WITH SJÖGREN'S SYNDROME

Systemic lupus erythematosus (SLE)
Rheumatoid arthritis
Raynaud's syndrome
Primary biliary cirrhosis
Chronic active hepatitis
Autoimmune diseases of the liver
Hyperglobulinemic purpura
Myasthenia gravis
Graft-versus-host disease
Polyarteritis
Hashimoto's thyroiditis
Pemphigus
Systemic sclerosis (scleroderma)
Polymyositis
Cryoglobulinemia
Pancreatitis
Waldenström's macroglobulinemia
Myeloma

From Buchanan and Kean[28]; Kammer.[86]

COMPLICATIONS

Ocular:
Corneal ulceration
Ocular vascularization with opacification
Ocular or corneal perforation with subsequent loss of the eye
Ocular infection (secondary to lack of bactericidal action of lysozyme
Symblepharon (lids adhere to globe with contracture of conjunctivae)

Oral:
Oral infections (particularly candidal type)
Oral ulcerations
Dental complications (gingivitis and dental caries; teeth may crumble and fillings may fall out because of reduction in saliva, which has antibacterial factors)

Pulmonary/respiratory:
Painful hard, dry crusting of nasal mucosa with subsequent epistaxis and atrophy of nasal mucosa
Hoarseness (secondary to dryness or presence of thick, tenacious mucus on vocal cords)
Dysphagia (secondary to pharyngeal dryness or abnormal esophageal motility)
Conduction-type deafness or otitis media caused by dry crusts obstructing the nasopharyngeal opening of the eustachian tubes (relieved by removing the crusts)
Lower respiratory complications (less common)

Gastrointestinal:
Splenomegaly
Decreased output of gastric acid
Constipation
Pancreatic and hepatic insufficiency

Renal:
Renal tubular acidosis, aminoaciduria, glycosuria (pathogenesis is unknown; may be related to autoimmunity or hyperviscosity secondary to hyperglobulinemia)
Renal tubular acidosis (RTA) from infiltrative interstitial nephropathy (patients with RTA have antibody-producing lymphocytes in medulla of kidneys)
Increased fluid intake (secondary to xerostomia; may result in diabetes insipidus, provoking lack of response to antidiuretic hormone [ADH] by renal tubules)
Hypergammaglobulinemic purpura with renal tubular acidosis

Other:
   Rare extraglandular lymphoid infiltration or neoplasm (lymphoma often is a monoclonal B-cell neoplasm with intracellular IgM)
   Leukopenia
   Vasculitis with leg ulcers
   Chronic autoimmune thyroiditis (5%)
   Lymphoproliferative disease

DIAGNOSIS

The varied nature of Sjögren's syndrome may obscure the diagnosis; however, it generally can be made on the basis of two of the three classic manifestations. The criteria for diagnosis include keratoconjunctivitis sicca, a minor salivary gland biopsy taken from the lower lip, demonstrating a lymphocytic infiltrate, and an associated connective tissue or lymphoproliferative disorder.[172]

Any patient with systemic lupus erythematosus, rheumatoid arthritis, or scleroderma should be assessed and monitored for Sjögren's syndrome. In addition, any patient with Sjögren's syndrome should be completely examined for other immunologic disorders.

DIAGNOSTIC STUDIES AND FINDINGS

Diagnostic test	Findings
Slitlamp examination (an examination of the cornea for punctate keratitis or filamentary keratitis; the most reliable test for diagnosing keratoconjunctivitis in Sjögren's syndrome)	Indicates more advanced keratoconjunctivitis sicca; demonstrated by abnormalities of tear film stability and decreased volume of tear film meniscus in the lower lid; in severe cases, damaged corneal and conjunctival cells with rose bengal; may progress to ulceration
Rose bengal (1%) stain (staining of the cornea and conjunctivae to identify corneal erosions)	Interpretations vary; may not be conclusive; may cause pain in severe cases and should not be used
Schirmer test	Decreased tear production (<15 mm of wet filter paper after 5 min; however, if environment is hot and dry and ammonia is not used, test may not be conclusive for keratoconjunctivitis)
Biopsy (biopsy from the minor salivary glands [lower lip] is the most significant and diagnostic test for Sjögren's syndrome)	*Specific:* lymphocytic infiltration of acinar glands and progressive destruction of glandular tissue. The extent of inflammation can be scored using a "focus score"; for example, each aggregate of 50 or more lymphocytes is considered a focus. The number of foci in 4 mm² of tissue is the focus score. In Sjögren's syndrome, a focus score greater than 1 is considered a criterion for diagnosis
	General: there may also be lymphocytic, B-cell, and macrophage infiltration involving exocrine glands of the respiratory, gastrointestinal, and vaginal tracts and the glands of the ocular and oral mucosa
Salivary scintigraphy (measured by parotid salivary flow [normal is 5 ml/10 min/gland]; the uptake, concentration, and excretion of technetium pertechnetate by the major salivary glands are recorded)	Decreased uptake, concentration, and excretion of intravenous 99mTc pertechnetate by major salivary glands; measured by a sequential scintigraphic technique that shows a decrease in parotid secretory function
Secretory sialography (uses radiopaque dye to measure secretory flow)	Glandular disorganization, dilations, and other changes such as atrophy in intrasalivary duct system; demonstrates abnormalities of ducts and atrophy of gland
Complete blood count	Mild anemia (50% of cases), leukopenia
Erythrocyte sedimentation rate (ESR)	Elevated
Immunologic tests	
Rheumatoid factor	Elevated in 90% of patients; titer ≤1:80; this is the most common autoantibody in Sjögren's syndrome

Continued.

DIAGNOSTIC STUDIES AND FINDINGS—cont'd

Diagnostic test	Findings
Immunologic tests—cont'd	
Antinuclear antibody (ANA)	Elevated titers in 68% of patients; antibody against antigen SS-B is relatively specific for Sjögren's syndrome; antibody against antigen SS-A is seen in Sjögren's syndrome with SLE
Immunoglobulins	Diffuse elevation in all classes of immunoglobulins, with major elevation in IgG fraction and slight elevation in IgA and IgM; high levels of gamma globulin are seen in patients who also demonstrate hyperglobulinemic purpura; β_2 microglobulin may be elevated in urine, serum, and saliva; this is a useful predictor of salivary gland involvement
Serum protein electrophoresis	Hypergammaglobulinemia is seen in about 50% of patients
T-lymphocyte mitogenic stimulation	About 30% of patients have decreased response; some patients show a decline in circulating T cells

MEDICAL MANAGEMENT

Management of Sjögren's syndrome is directed primarily at alleviating the symptoms and complications of xerophthalmia and xerostomia. These conditions generally are well controlled with palliative treatment.

GENERAL MANAGEMENT

Mouth care: Mouth rinses with 1% methylcellulose qid and prn; oral hygiene with frequent brushing, flossing, and fluoride rinses; mouth sprays; regular dental examinations; glycerin or gelatin lozenges to alleviate dryness; mild electrical stimulation to produce saliva in severe cases; regular dental visits.

Eye care: Routine conjunctival cultures to detect ocular infections. Quarterly evaluation by an ophthalmologist.

Diet: Fluids are encouraged to stimulate salivary secretion; regular diet if tolerated, otherwise soft diet with nutritional supplements; hard sweet or sour candies or sweetened drinks to combat xerostomia should be avoided, unless they are sugarless, because they contribute to dental caries.

Medical therapy for refractory ocular complications: Mucolytic agents (5%-10% acetylcysteine); punctal occlusion (to increase accumulation of residual tears); soft contact lenses; partial tarsorrhaphy (suturing together a portion of or the entire upper and lower eyelids).

MEDICAL MANAGEMENT—cont'd

DRUG THERAPY

Artificial tears (0.5% carboxymethylcellulose eye drops): prn.

Nystatin (Mycostatin): To treat oral candidal infections.

Antibiotics: To treat the development of: parotiditis (surgical drainage is avoided), staphylococcal blepharitis, and bronchopulmonary infections.

Acetylcysteine in a 5%-10% solution (mucolytic agent): To treat patients with large amounts of inspissated mucus.

Nonsteroidal antiinflammatory agents: To manage and treat nonerosive arthritis.

Corticosteroids or immunosuppressive agents (corticosteroids do not prevent progression of the syndrome): Dosage titrated for relief of severe symptoms; generally administered only late in the course of the disease when symptoms are not relieved by supportive approaches; frequently confined to only the more severe cases involving the kidneys or bronchopulmonary tract and systemic vasculitis.

Antineoplastic agents: Cyclophosphamide has been reported to improve lacrimal and salivary secretion.[28]

---

1 ASSESS

ASSESSMENT	OBSERVATIONS
Eyes	Keratoconjunctivitis; sensation of foreign body; "gritty" or sandy feeling in the eyes; burning; accumulation of thick ropy strands at inner canthus, particularly in the morning; decreased tearing (ask, do your eyes tear when you peel an onion?); redness; photosensitivity; eye fatigue; pruritus; filmy sensation that interferes with vision; *late:* corneal erosion or ulceration, vascularization, and opacification, decreased visual acuity
Salivary glands	Episodic unilateral parotiditis with rapid fluctuation in gland size, often associated with fever, tenderness or pain, and erythema; on palpation the gland is smooth and irregular, not nodular
Skin	Dryness of skin and scalp; vasculitic lesions
Respiratory tract	Dry nasal mucosa, epistaxis, nonproductive cough, dysphonia, recurrent and persistent otitis media secondary to frequent blockage of eustachian tubes, bronchitis, pneumonia
Gynecologic	Dry vaginal mucosa; dyspareunia
Renal	Polyuria secondary to increased fluid intake (this may progress to diabetes insipidus due to tubules' inability to respond to ADH); renal tubular acidosis; aminoaciduria; glycosuria
Gastrointestinal	Choking on food, changes in gag reflex; dry oral mucous membranes; halitosis; a small percentage of patients demonstrate clinical symptoms associated with pancreatitis, hepatosplenomegaly, chronic active hepatitis, primary biliary cirrhosis, and autoimmune liver disease

Nursing care plan is directed at those patients with severe Sjögren's syndrome.

→ 〉〉

2 DIAGNOSE

NURSING DIAGNOSIS	SUBJECTIVE FINDINGS	OBJECTIVE FINDINGS
Sensory/perceptual alteration (visual) related to keratoconjunctivitis	Complains of decreased visual acuity; burning, itchy eyes; increased sensitivity to sun; filmy feeling in eyes, especially in the morning; feeling of sand in eyes	Red, irritated eyes with ropy strands at inner canthus; positive slitlamp examination; decreased tear production on Schirmer test
Altered oral mucous membrane related to xerostomia	Complains of dry mouth, difficulty swallowing and chewing, increased fluid intake, inability to tolerate dry foods, and burning in mouth	Finger passed over buccal mucosa may adhere to it; diminished flow on salivary flow studies; hoarseness; oral candidiasis; red, irritated buccal mucosa; mouth with milk curds that may adhere to buccal mucosa and may be mistaken for monilial infection; *late:* fissures and ulcerations at corners of mouth and on buccal mucosa, tongue, and lips
Impaired swallowing secondary to xerostomia	Complains of difficulty swallowing dry foods; reports that food often adheres to buccal mucosa and must be removed manually	Stasis of food in mouth, coughing, and choking
Pain related to parotiditis, conjunctivitis, xerostomia, and otitis media	Complains of chronic gland, eye, and ear pain, discomfort, or tenderness and difficulty hearing	On a scale of 1-10, pain is rated at 6; glandular pain on palpation; conjunctivae red and irritated; erythema and decreased motility of the tympanic membrane; purulent ear drainage, altered hearing, reddened oral cavity with fissures or ulcerations
Ineffective breathing related to dry nasal mucosa and bronchitis	Complains of difficulty breathing, cough, and dry nose	Dyspnea at rest; mouth breathing; persistent, productive or nonproductive cough; positive sputum culture; dry, crusting nasal airways; sputum may be clear, thin or thick; tenacious or purulent; epistaxis; diffuse chest crackles and rhonchi throughout
Potential for impaired skin integrity related to skin dryness	Complains of itchy skin, dandruff, cracks around mouth, and epistaxis; women report "problems" with intercourse	Dry, scaly, inelastic skin that is red and irritated from scratching; poor skin turgor; vaginal examination shows dry mucous membranes; crusting in nasal mucosa
Potential for altered nutrition: less than body requirements secondary to dysphagia and xerostomia	Reports altered taste sensation, difficulty swallowing food, increased fluid intake, difficulty with mastication, and inadequate food intake	Weight loss; food particles adhere to oral mucosa; choking, coughing
Potential for fluid volume deficit due to compromised regulatory mechanisms	Complains of frequent urination and profound thirst	Output exceeds intake; specific gravity is low, indicating dilute urine; dry mucous membranes; poor skin turgor

3 PLAN

Patient goals

1. The patient will have no changes in visual acuity.
2. The patient will demonstrate an intact oral mucous membrane, as evidenced by moist, pink, smooth mucosal surfaces and no oral caries; she will maintain a comfortable, functional oral cavity.
3. The patient will be able to swallow certain foods and fluids without choking or coughing.
4. The patient's pain will be eliminated or controlled.

5. The patient's breathing pattern will improve. Dyspnea and dry nasal passages will resolve.
6. The patient's skin will remain intact with adequate circulation.
7. The patient will maintain an adequate nutritional balance.
8. The patient will maintain an adequate fluid and electrolyte balance.
9. The patient will show she understands self-care requirements.

4 IMPLEMENT

NURSING DIAGNOSIS	NURSING INTERVENTIONS	RATIONALE
Sensory/perceptual alteration (visual) related to keratoconjunctivitis	Assess degree of visual deficit.	To determine baseline visual acuity for monitoring changes.
	Administer 0.5% methylcellulose eye drops as needed and monitor patient response.	To maintain moisture at conjunctival surface and to protect against ocular complications.
	Obtain regular cultures of the eyes.	To monitor for infection.
	In collaboration with physician, administer antimicrobial ointment and monitor patient response.	To treat or prevent ocular infections.
	Administer hot or cold therapy to eyes as needed and monitor patient response.	To control pain.
	Encourage use of sunglasses as needed, particularly when in the sun or wind.	To prevent photophobia and to protect against drying effects of wind.
	Assess eyes every shift.	To evaluate for signs of erosion or ulceration.
	In collaboration with physician, administer acetylcysteine 5%-10% and monitor patient response.	To break up mucus in patients with large volumes of inspissated mucus.
	Encourage semiannual ophthalmic examinations.	To prevent complications secondary to keratoconjunctivitis.
Altered oral mucous membrane related to xerostomia	Assess oral skin and buccal mucosa for ulcerations, fissures, and candidiasis; check for caries, gingivitis, and tooth erosion; monitor changes.	To determine extent of oral injury and identify need for medical treatment (antibiotics).

NURSING DIAGNOSIS	NURSING INTERVENTIONS	RATIONALE
	Provide or encourage patient to perform frequent (tid) oral hygiene (brushing with a soft toothbrush, flossing, and using fluoride rinses).	To prevent further breakdown of buccal membrane and prevent infection of ulcerated or eroded areas.
	Force fluids and use of aerosolized preparations of artificial saliva.	To keep oral membranes moist, to prevent burning and pain in oral membrane, and to prevent further damage to buccal mucosa.
	Urge patient to use sugarless gum or candy and to avoid sour or sweetened liquids and candies.	To stimulate salivary secretion, which can sometimes relieve xerostomia; hard candies and sweet drinks increase risk of dental caries and cause burning of buccal mucosa.
	Advise patient not to drink large amounts of water.	To prevent hyponatremia and maintain fluid and electrolyte balance.
	Have patient use a bedroom humidifier.	To decrease nocturnal xerostomia.
	Advise patient to avoid spicy foods and hot fluids, since buccal mucosa may be sensitive.	Hot fluids and spicy foods may disrupt buccal mucosa, causing erosions and pain.
	Encourage semiannual dental checkups.	To prevent dental complications secondary to xerostomia.
Impaired swallowing secondary to xerostomia	Assess gag, swallowing (have patient swallow saliva), and cough reflexes before feeding.	To prevent aspiration.
	Auscultate breath sounds.	To monitor for previous aspiration.
	Provide periods of rest before and between meals.	Fatigue can impair swallowing; also, to prevent aspiration.
	Identify patient's food preferences.	To obtain patient's cooperation.
	Encourage patient to wear properly fitting dentures.	To promote adequate chewing before swallowing and thus prevent choking.
	Help patient assume a 90-degree sitting position during meals and for 30 minutes afterward.	To prevent aspiration and allow gravity to assist in peristaltic motion.
	Have suction ready at the bedside.	In case patient chokes or aspirates food particles.
	Assist with oral hygiene before and after eating.	To stimulate salivation before eating and to keep oral cavity clean and prevent infection or breakdown after eating.

NURSING DIAGNOSIS	NURSING INTERVENTIONS	RATIONALE
	Have patient progress slowly from swallowing saliva, to thick juice or nectar, semisolids, pureed diet, soft diet, and regular diet.	To prevent aspiration and to boost patient's confidence that food will be swallowed.
	Massage over patient's throat prn as she swallows; teach her how to perform this maneuver.	May be necessary to stimulate laryngopharyngeal muscles; may offer patient a sense of control to ensure swallowing and prevent choking.
	Accurately measure intake and output.	To monitor and ensure appropriate hydration.
	Provide an environment free of distractions such as television, radio, or visitors.	Patient may need to concentrate on swallowing until mechanism becomes routine.
	Have patient tilt head forward 45 degrees while swallowing.	To help keep esophagus patent and thus aid swallowing.
	Inspect patient's mouth frequently if she cannot do so.	To ensure that food is being swallowed and not collected in the mouth.
Pain related to parotiditis, conjunctivitis, xerostomia, and otitis	Assess pain: location, onset, duration, impact on quality of life, and provocative and palliative factors; have patient rate intensity on scale of 0-10.	To determine quality of pain and guide therapeutic intervention.
	In collaboration with physician, administer appropriate analgesics; if pain is due to inflammatory or infectious episode, also administer antibiotics and antiinflammatory agents as ordered and monitor patient response.	To alleviate pain and resolve infection.
	Assess effectiveness of pain medication and note side effects; identify and explore strategies that helped to eliminate or control pain in the past.	To determine whether pain relief regimen should be changed.
	Parotiditis: Ensure prompt antibiotic treatment.	To avoid surgical drainage.
	Conjunctivitis: Apply cool to warm, moist packs to eyes, apply eye drops frequently, and use antibiotic ointments.	To provide moisture, eliminate or control pain, and prevent or treat infection.
	Xerostomia: Provide oral lubricants and frequent sips of water or mouth sprays to keep mouth moist.	To provide moisture and prevent erosion, breakdown, and infection of mucous membrane.
	Otitis media: Ensure prompt antibiotic treatment of otitis, instruct patient in relaxation techniques and imagery, and use counterstimulation (massage, vibration, heat or cold).	To prevent further infection and possible hearing loss, to promote distraction from pain and provide a mechanism for pain control, and to eliminate or control pain.

→ > >

NURSING DIAGNOSIS	NURSING INTERVENTIONS	RATIONALE
Impaired breathing pattern related to dry nasal mucosa and bronchitis	Assess degree of respiratory impairment; monitor rate, rhythm, and quality of respirations; assess degree of dyspnea and cough.	Increased respiratory rate and rhythm reflect the body's attempt to compensate for respiratory compromise and work of breathing.
	Auscultate breath sounds for rhonchi and rales.	Determines adequacy of gas exchange and degree of airway obstruction due to secretions.
	Monitor for hemoptysis and epistaxis.	To detect bronchial erosion and nasal dryness, crusting, and erosion.
	In collaboration with physician, administer appropriate antibiotics and other respiratory medications for bronchitis or pneumonia; monitor effectiveness of medications, and note side effects.	To treat the infection and promote effective gas exchange.
	Obtain sputum specimens for culture and monitor results.	To detect specific pathologic condition and effectiveness of antibiotics.
	Administer nasal saline soaks and lubricant.	To prevent dryness of nasal mucosa and provide comfort.
	Monitor ABGs and Hgb, and administer humidified oxygen as ordered.	To ensure adequate ventilation and maintain moist airways.
	Monitor vital signs.	Rise in temperature may indicate an inflammatory process, tachycardia, and elevated B/P, which often accompany hypoxemia.
	Monitor chest x-ray results.	X-rays show the severity of pulmonary compromise.
	Promote pulmonary hygiene by increasing mobility as tolerated and encouraging use of incentive spirometry, coughing, and deep breathing.	To assist in clearing airways and preventing further complications.
	Provide rest periods; plan activities accordingly.	To prevent patient from becoming dyspneic and to promote recovery.
	Provide comfort measures (back rub, position changes).	To help patient relax, to promote recovery, and to allow effective ventilation.
Potential for impaired skin integrity related to skin dryness	Inspect skin (color, moisture, lesions, vascularity); provide and encourage use of lotions, creams, or ointments.	Dryness of skin causes changes in color, with subsequent cracking and skin breakdown; lotions, creams, and ointments prevent potential skin dryness and breakdown.

NURSING DIAGNOSIS	NURSING INTERVENTIONS	RATIONALE
	When itching is a problem, encourage patient not to scratch; pressing on the area or applying ice decreases sensation; cool environment is less irritating than a warm one; other soothing measures include lubricating skin with oil or lotion, oatmeal powder baths, corn starch baths at 32°-38° C (98.6°-100.4° F); loose clothing; antihistamines as ordered by physician.	Scratching can cause skin to break down, resulting in infection.
	Keep skin completely clean and dry after bathing; maintain moisture in skin by encouraging sufficient fluids and by keeping skin lubricated.	To remove bacteria and prevent maceration from excessive moisture; moisture prevents skin breakdown.
Potential for altered nutrition: less than body requirements secondary to dysphagia and xerostomia	Monitor daily calorie count to ensure adequate nutritional intake; consult nutritionist to determine patient's requirements.	To prevent weight loss; calculate amount of calories based on patient's basal metabolic rate to prevent weight loss.
	Provide supplemental feedings high in calories and protein.	To ensure adequate caloric intake.
	Assess and monitor patient's ability to swallow and oral discomfort; provide liquids, and progress to regular diet as tolerated.	Prevents aspiration; regular food may exacerbate dysphagia and oral cavity dryness.
	Encourage large amounts of liquids with meals.	To decrease dryness and facilitate swallowing.
	Offer small, frequent feedings and encourage patient to chew food completely before swallowing.	Large meals and food particles may be too difficult to swallow and may aggravate xerostomia.
	Ensure patient's comfort during meals, and encourage patient to select foods.	To stimulate appetite and tolerance.
Potential for fluid volume deficit due to compromised regulatory mechanisms	Measure intake and output and daily weight.	When output exceeds intake, there may be a fluid volume loss and potential dehydration.
	Monitor vital signs.	Hypovolemia is marked by tachycardia (as the heart attempts to circulate adequate volume), decreased BP (because of the shift of fluid out of the vascular space), elevated temperature, and increased metabolic rate.
	Measure urine specific gravity.	With normal renal function, patient will have an increase in specific gravity as he or she becomes more dehydrated.
	Assess skin turgor and oral mucous membranes.	Dry mucous membranes indicate a fluid deficit; loss of skin turgor occurs as fluid moves into interstitial spaces.

→ > > >

5 EVALUATE

PATIENT OUTCOME	DATA INDICATING THAT OUTCOME IS REACHED
Visual acuity is stabilized.	Visual acuity is at patient baseline as documented by the Snellen chart; no complaints of eye burning, itching, gritty feeling, or sun sensitivity; demonstrates ability to use eye drops.
Oral mucous remains intact.	Demonstrates activities to minimize dry and burning mouth; able to swallow without difficulty; mucous membrane pink, moist, with no evidence of infection or dental caries.
Patient is able to maintain an adequate diet without choking, coughing or aspiration during a meal.	The patient is able to swallow adequate fluids and food particles without them adhering to the buccal mucosa or aspiration; weight and hydration are maintained.
Patient is able to identify strategies that eliminate or control pain.	The patient has no complaints of gland, eye, or ear pain; no glandular discomfort with palpation; conductive clear; tympanic membrane pearly gray; hearing deficit is resolved.
Breathing pattern is improved.	Nasal passages are moist and intact; breathing is regular without consistent mouth breathing; no complaints of dyspnea; breath sounds are clear.
Skin integrity is maintained.	Skin remains moist; patient demonstrates strategies to cope with itching and dry skin; nasal mucosa is moist; female patients report no discomfort with intercourse.
Nutritional status has improved.	Recommended body weight is maintained; adequate fluid and nutritional intake is maintained; dysphagia is resolved; no evidence of choking, coughing or difficulty swallowing.
Fluid status is maintained.	Adequate intake is maintained; fluid status remains balanced; mucous membranes remain moist; urine output is adequate; specific gravity is normal.

PATIENT TEACHING

1. Provide information about Sjögren's syndrome and the purpose of the treatment.
2. Encourage the patient to have semiannual ophthalmic and dental examinations, and stress the importance of seeing the dentist at the first signs of gum disease.
3. Teach family members the Heimlich maneuver for use in an emergency if the patient is choking.
4. Teach the patient how to instill and use artificial tears.
5. Explain the importance of fastidious oral hygiene: frequent brushing of the teeth with a soft toothbrush and fluoride toothpaste and use of dental floss and mouth rinses.
6. Encourage the patient to increase fluid intake to control xerostomia; advise her to avoid sour or sweetened drinks, candies, or gum and to use only artificially sweetened products.
7. Teach the patient how to check her mouth for signs of developing lesions, fissures, and ulcerations.
8. Emphasize the importance of regular follow-up care to detect underlying autoimmune or neoplastic disease.
9. Explain that the use of unnecessary antibiotics should be avoided because of the increased incidence of drug allergy, especially to penicillin.
10. Explain that regular application of saline soaks may help nasal dryness.
11. Explain that skin dryness often responds to a variety of lotions, creams, and emollients; vaginal dryness leading to dyspareunia generally responds to lubricants such as K-Y Jelly (oil-based lubricants should not be used vaginally).
12. Explain to the patient that she should avoid scratching, and teach her ways to prevent or treat itching.

CHAPTER 7

Hemopoietic Disorders

Autoimmune Hemolytic Anemia

Autoimmune hemolytic anemia is a disorder of the immune system in which normal erythrocytes are attacked and destroyed by antibodies.

PATHOPHYSIOLOGY

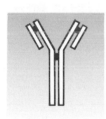

Autoimmune hemolytic anemia (AIHA) is divided into two classifications: (1) warm autoimmune hemolytic anemia, which is characterized by IgG- mediated lysis or by IgG- and complement-mediated lysis and (2) cold autoimmune hemolytic anemia, which is characterized by IgM- and complement-mediated lysis. These two types of AIHA show important differences in their etiology, response to therapy, mechanisms of red blood cell (RBC) lysis, and clinical and laboratory characteristics[4] (see Table 7-1). Autoimmune hemolytic anemia is a relatively uncommon disorder, afflicting approximately 1 in 80,000 individuals every year. It is associated with idiopathic thrombocytopenic purpura in a childhood disease known as Evans' syndrome and recently has also been associated with graft-versus-host disease and AIDS.[2]

Warm autoimmune hemolytic anemia (WAHA) occurs when an IgG autoantibody interacts with red blood cells at the body's own temperature (37° C [98.6° F]). Complement usually is bound to the red blood cells as well, which can lead to a more pronounced hemolysis. A direct antiglobulin test (DAT) will be positive, and if all sites on the red blood cell are covered with IgG, an indirect antiglobulin test will also detect antibody in the plasma. Warm autoimmune hemolytic anemia most often occurs with other diseases such as malignancy, systemic lupus erythematosus, immunodeficiency, or leukemia.[3,4] It also occurs idiopathically or may be drug induced.

Red blood cells coated with IgG are phagocytized by the reticuloendothelial cells, located in the spleen. If a portion of the red blood cell membrane is torn but the reticuloendothelial cells fail to destroy it, the red blood cell forms a microspherocyte (a small, rigid, spherical red blood cell), which is then trapped and destroyed in the spleen. Red blood cells may also be destroyed in the liver if they are coated with large quantities of IgG or complement.[3]

Intravascular lysis usually is not caused by the IgG antibody. However, it can occur in certain instances when complement component C1 binds to the red blood cell. The entire complement cascade must be activated before intravascular lysis results, and this is an uncommon physiologic occurrence due to the instability of the terminal attack sequence of the complement cascade.[2,4]

Cold autoimmune hemolytic anemia (CAHA) is the result of an IgM autoantibody reacting with the body's red blood cells at below body temperature. Each person with CAHA has his or her own specific group of antibodies that react at a specific temperature range, called thermal amplitude.[9] The thermal amplitude for a patient's antibodies may be very narrow, with only a few degrees' range, or quite broad, extending to just

TABLE 7-1 _____

COMPARISON OF WARM AND COLD AUTOIMMUNE HEMOLYTIC ANEMIAS

Clinical features	WAHA	CAHA
Autoantibody	IgG + complement	IgM + complement
Associated factors	Lymphoma, systemic lupus erythematosus, chronic lymphocytic leukemia, non-Hodgkin's lymphoma, AIDS and AIDS-related illnesses, graft-versus-host disease, certain medications, pregnancy[2]	*Mycoplasma pneumoniae*, Epstein-Barr virus, infectious mononucleosis, Legionnaires' disease, lymphatic cancer, cytomegalovirus, anemia that is associated with cold weather[6]; complication of syphilis, certain viral illness such as mumps and measles[7]; precipitated by cold operating rooms[9]
Clinical manifestations	Hemolysis, splenomegaly, thrombocytopenia, hemoglobinuria, shock, hemoglobinemia, anemia[4,6]	Hemolysis, hemoglobinuria, acrocyanosis, jaundice, chills, fever, pain, purpura, Raynaud's phenomenon, pallor, gangrene, immune complex nephritis[6,9]
Incidence*	~49%-70%[11,12]	~24%-30%[11,12]
First-line treatment	Steroids	Keep patient warm
Antibody's critical temperature	37° C	Usually <20° C
Major site of hemolysis	Spleen	Part of body exposed to cold

*~15% mixed IgG warm and IgM cold autoantibodies; ~10% unclassifiable.[11]

below body temperature. The maximum temperature above which the antibodies cease functioning is called the critical temperature, which usually is less than 20° C (68° F). The severity of hemolysis is affected by these previously mentioned factors and by the environmental temperature, duration of exposure to cold, and the cold agglutinin titer (the titer of the cold-reacting IgM autoantibody).[9]

All normal, healthy people produce antibodies called cold agglutinins, but the titer is very low (less than 1:64), and only an extremely cold temperature (4° C [39.2° F]) will activate them.[3] A clinically significant titer is 1:1,000.[6] It is thought that the critical temperature increases as the cold agglutinin titer increases, thus producing agglutination and even hemolysis at close to body temperatures, especially if the individual becomes chilled.[3]

Cold autoimmune hemolytic anemia can occur acutely or chronically. In the chronic form, more than 95% of the IgM antibodies react with the I antigen, an antigen present on red blood cells after 18 months of age as the adult expression of the I-i blood system. However, these antibodies can also react with the i antigen (the fetal expression of the I-i system found on red blood cells into infancy) in other acute diseases, such as infectious mononucleosis.[10] Certain other infections have been reported in the etiology of acute CAHA, including *Mycoplasma pneumoniae*, Legion-

naires' disease, Epstein-Barr virus, and cytomegalovirus.[4,6] Idiopathic acute CAHA has also been reported.[2] The chronic form of the disease occurs most frequently in men and women over 60 years of age and can occur with malignancies.[6]

CLINICAL MANIFESTATIONS

Anemia
Fatigue/weakness
Pallor/jaundice
Bleeding tendencies/easy bruising
Pruritus
Dyspnea
Hypotension
Chills
Fever

COMPLICATIONS

Hemodynamic and cardiovascular instability
Gallstones
Renal insufficiency
Raynaud's disease (CAHA)
Tissue necrosis (CAHA)

NURSING CARE

See pages 218-233.

DIAGNOSTIC STUDIES AND FINDINGS

Diagnostic Test	Findings
Red blood cell smear	Spherocytes (WAHA)
Bilirubin	Elevated
Bone marrow biopsy	Usually hyperplasia
Platelet count	Decreased
Reticulocyte count	Elevated
Red blood cell count	Decreased
Hemoglobin/hematocrit	Decreased
Direct antiglobulin test (DAT or direct Coombs' test)	Positive if IgG or complement or both are detected; IgM usually is not demonstrated with DAT
Indirect antiglobulin test (antibody screen)	Detects IgM or IgG: IgG at body temperature (37° C [98.6° F]) and IgM at cooler temperatures[4]
Cold agglutinin titers (CAHA)	Elevated
Urinalysis	High specific gravity, hemoglobinuria[7]

MEDICAL MANAGEMENT

GENERAL MANAGEMENT

CAHA: keep patient warm to reduce hemolysis; treat underlying precipitating cause; keep patient well hydrated; and maintain optimum urine output (most important during acute, intravascular hemolytic complement-mediated crises[2,4]).

WAHA: treat underlying cause.

DRUG THERAPY

CAHA: high-dose corticosteroids to improve RBC survival by decreasing their phagocytosis and by decreasing autoantibody and IgM production, although with inconsistent results. Immunosuppressive drugs may be effective, although the intravascular hemolysis in CAHA may be refractory to cytotoxic medications.[4]

WAHA: therapeutic level of corticosteroids to inhibit autoantibody formation; may also decrease the autoantibody's adherence to the erythrocyte.[3]

Immunosuppressants (e.g., oral cyclophosphamide, azathioprine, cyclosporine): to suppress autoantibody production.

Sodium bicarbonate or sodium lactate: IV infusions to alkalinize urine in cases of severe hemolysis.[5]

ADJUNCTIVE THERAPY

Plasma exchange: to reduce the amount of autoantibodies, although benefit may be transient.[1]

Plasmapheresis.

Transfuse with carefully cross-matched packed red cells or washed red cells to further eliminate possible complement transfusion; however, transfused RBCs may be destroyed as rapidly as the patient's own.

Platelet transfusion should be given if indicated.

Red cell exchange.

SURGERY

Splenectomy: performed if RBC destruction is not halted by steroid therapy, since the spleen is a prominent site of red cell sequestration and destruction in WAHA. Splenectomy is not a therapeutic option in CAHA, since the spleen is not a prominent factor in the extravascular hemolysis usually seen with that disorder.[4]

Idiopathic Thrombocytopenic Purpura

Idiopathic thrombocytopenic purpura is a primary immune disorder manifested by persistent thrombocytopenia, normal to elevated levels of megakaryocytes in the bone marrow, and increased platelet destruction by the mononuclear phagocyte system.[2,3]

EPIDEMIOLOGY

The transient nature of idiopathic thrombocytopenic purpura (ITP) makes it difficult to estimate its incidence or prevalence. Many patients show spontaneous remission, especially children. A true patient population is also difficult to determine because some individuals have subclinical cases of ITP, in which platelet counts are below normal but not so dangerously low as to cause purpura or bleeding or both. These individuals are very susceptible to clinical ITP with any stress to platelet longevity. An estimated 1 in 10,000 people will develop clinical ITP each year in the United States.[1,5]

Idiopathic thrombocytopenic purpura can be categorized into three types: the acute form, which occurs mainly in children after either a viral illness or a vaccination; the intermittent form, which may develop in children and adults; and the chronic form, which appears primarily in adults. The chronic form of ITP has a female-to-male ratio of 2-4:1, with women of childbearing age afflicted most often. The most severe complication of ITP is central nervous system hemorrhage, which is seen most frequently in patients over 50 years of age.[1,4]

The acute form of ITP usually persists for 1 to 2 months and has a better prognosis than the chronic form. Chronic ITP may last years, with no improvement in clinical or laboratory abnormalities except for occasional transient remission of purpura. Intermittent ITP may occur approximately every 3 months, but the intervals between bouts of the disease are characterized by normal platelet counts and normal platelet life span. Disease periods generally persist for less than 6 months.[1]

PATHOPHYSIOLOGY

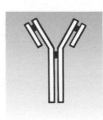

The destruction and phagocytosis of antibody-coated platelets by the mononuclear phagocytic system (mainly in the spleen and liver), rather than a decrease in platelet production, seem to account for the thrombocytopenia noted in ITP. The pathogenesis is unclear, but one theory postulates that platelet-associated IgG (PAIgG) may result in platelet destruction in the adult chronic form of ITP.[3] A circulating platelet-reactive immune complex that causes a platelet-antibody reaction has been implicated in the acute ITP seen in children and also when ITP is associated with HIV in adults.[3,6] The role of complement in the development of ITP is also unclear and merits further investigation.

Idiopathic thrombocytopenic purpura can also occur secondary to an underlying disease. The diseases most often associated with ITP include systemic lupus erythematosus, chronic lymphocytic leukemia, Evans' syndrome, a viral illness such as HIV disease, hemolytic uremic syndrome, aplastic anemia, hypogammaglobulinemia, Hodgkin's disease, other malignancies, and lymphoproliferative disorders.[5,7] Heredity has also been reported as a factor.[5] Classic examples of drugs that can produce thrombocytopenia are quinidine, quinine, sulfonamides, and methyldopa.[4] Transient ITP after a transfusion has been reported, as has ITP with iron-deficiency anemia.[7]

CLINICAL MANIFESTATIONS

Purpura, ecchymosis, petechiae
Hemorrhagic oral blisters
Epistaxis
Hematemesis, melena, hematuria
Irritability, seizures
Hypotension
Dyspnea
Fatigue

COMPLICATIONS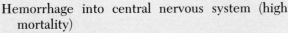

Hemorrhage into central nervous system (high mortality)
Iron-deficiency anemia (chronic ITP, leading to blood loss into the gastrointestinal tract)
Infection leading to overwhelming sepsis after splenectomy (especially in children)

NURSING CARE

See pages 218-233.

DIAGNOSTIC STUDIES AND FINDINGS

Diagnostic Test	Findings
Platelet count	Thrombocytopenia at dangerously low levels (<50,000/mm^3)
Bleeding time	Prolonged
Red blood cell count	Decreased; anemia
Bone marrow aspirate	Increased young megakaryocytes[1]
Coulter counter	RBC and platelet fragmentation with severe thrombocytopenia[1]
White blood cell count	Normal or slightly increased

MEDICAL MANAGEMENT

GENERAL MANAGEMENT

Routine monitoring of CBC and platelet counts, fluid status, and neurologic status; consult physical and/or occupational therapy to begin a progressive program of rehabilitation when indicated; RBC transfusions to correct anemia; platelet transfusion in life-threatening situations to replace clotting factors.[6]

DRUG THERAPY

Corticosteroids: to prevent further sequestering of destroyed or damaged platelets by the spleen.[1]

Immunosuppressive drugs (oral cyclophosphamide, azathioprine, vinca alkaloids, cyclosporine, and antiviral agent zidovudine [AZT]): may benefit a small number of patients refractory to corticosteroids, although their side effects and/or effects from long-term use limit their therapeutic potential.[4,6]

IV immune globulin: may diminish the destruction of antibody-coated platelets[3]; administered primarily to children (and some adults) who do not respond to steroid therapy before splenectomy; may be a less expensive alternative to splenectomy, especially in preschool age children.[5]

Analgesics for pain management: no aspirin-containing products are administered, because they interfere with platelet function; nonsteroidal antiinflammatory medications are also avoided.

EXPERIMENTAL DRUG THERAPY

IV anti-D (RhoGAM, anti-Rhesus globulin): an experimental therapy administered to pediatric Rh-positive patients before splenectomy; IV anti-D apparently blocks a mononuclear phagocyte receptor, thereby interfering with platelet destruction.[5]

Staph protein A pheresis: removes protein A antibodies, thereby reducing the number of antiplatelet antibodies; an expensive, controversial therapy that has been used in a limited number of patients.[5]

3G8: a monoclonal antibody, specific for a monocyte-macrophage receptor, that has raised platelet counts in a small number of patients; currently considered experimental.[5,6]

ADJUNCTIVE THERAPY

Plasmapheresis.

SURGERY

Splenectomy: removes the site of platelet sequestration and destruction. If the patient relapses after some time, an accessory spleen may be located and also removed.[6]

Idiopathic Neutropenia

Idiopathic neutropenia is a decrease in the absolute neutrophil count to less than 1,000/mm^3 for an unknown or obscure reason.[1,2]

EPIDEMIOLOGY

Idiopathic neutropenia has been noted predominantly in women. Interestingly, the incidence of infections is relatively low, considering the patients' neutropenic state. This phenomenon has been attributed to humoral mechanisms (B lymphocytes) and the stress-induced mobilization of bone marrow neutrophil reserves.[10]

PATHOPHYSIOLOGY

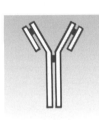 Neutropenia is the result of several pathogenetic mechanisms. A number of bone marrow disorders can cause decreased production of neutrophils, as can malignancies, exposure to toxic drugs or chemicals, some bacterial or viral infections, and malnutrition. However, idiopathic neutropenia (IN) occurs without a primary cause or underlying illness. Insufficient or ineffective neutrophil production and/or release from the bone marrow, an abnormally short life span for neutrophils, an increased number of neutrophils that shift from the circulating to the marginal blood pools (neutrophils that adhere to blood vessel walls), or a combination of these processes can precipitate IN.[1,8] Antineutrophil antibodies (neutrophil binding), as well as antibodies to specific neutrophil precursors, have been implicated in certain cases of IN, and immune complexes have been discovered in patients' blood that can also be linked to the disorder. These immune complexes can generate certain complement components, such as C5a, that aggregate neutrophils.[8] IgG and/or IgM antineutrophil antibodies have been detected in about one third of all adult patients with IN.[10] The neutropenia may be acute, cyclic, or chronic.

CLINICAL MANIFESTATIONS

Recurrent infections
Rash, cellulitis
Oral ulcerations
Anorexia and weight loss
Fatigue/lethargy
Weakness
Dyspnea

COMPLICATIONS
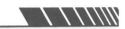

Severe, life-threatening infections that may progress to overwhelming sepsis
Pneumonia or recurrent upper respiratory infections
Lung or liver abscesses
Acute leukemia or aplastic anemia (rare)[1]
Furunculosis[9]
Otitis media, especially in children[9]

NURSING CARE

See pages 218 to 233.

DIAGNOSTIC STUDIES AND FINDINGS

Diagnostic Test	Findings
White blood cell count	Absolute neutrophil count (ANC) <1,000/mm^3
Bone marrow aspiration	Increased ratio of immature to mature neutrophils; defective development of neutrophils (hypoplasia) or normal cellular appearance (a shift to the left)
Blood neutrophil kinetic studies	May note antineutrophil antibodies[1]

MEDICAL MANAGEMENT

GENERAL MANAGEMENT

Initiation of treatment for underlying cause of neutropenia, if applicable.

Bed rest while severely neutropenic for safety; activity increases as neutrophil count rises and patient's strength increases.

Close monitoring of vital signs, especially temperature.

Routine monitoring of laboratory values, especially WBC with differential, and ABGs if patient has respiratory difficulty or is intubated.

Dietary consult to instruct and assist patient in selecting nutritious and microbe-free food.

Physical and/or occupational therapy consult to protect patient from complications of immobility during neutropenic episodes and to assist in providing appropriate exercise regimen and diversional activities.

Protective isolation until ANC is over 1,000/mm^3 for a consecutive number of days, according to protocols.

Portable chest x-rays to monitor pulmonary status if fever is present.

Cultures of blood, urine, stool, sputum, throat, all invasive lines, and all lesions if fever is present.

DRUG THERAPY

Antibiotics for empiric therapy for infection.

Glucocorticoids have been beneficial for some patients.[1]

IV immune globulin has increased ANC in some patients, especially those refractory to steroids.[3]

Antipyretics and analgesics as appropriate. Fever patterns may be diagnostic if cause is unknown, so antipyretics are not always administered routinely[2]; however, a fever over 39.4° C [102.9° F]) constitutes a medical emergency in a neutropenic patient and must be treated immediately.[4]

Recombinant human granulocyte–stimulating factor (rhG-CSF): administered IV or SQ, it increases the ANC in some patients.[5,6]

Stool softeners to prevent patient from straining and to protect tissues.

ADJUNCTIVE THERAPY

Granulocyte transfusions may be administered for short-term management during Gram sepsis.

Plasmapheresis.

Pernicious Anemia

Pernicious anemia is a disease characterized by (1) anemia with the production of large, irregular, red blood cells known as megaloblasts; (2) an atrophic gastric wall that does not produce an enzyme known as intrinsic factor, which is necessary for the absorption of vitamin B_{12}; and (3) a vitamin B_{12} deficiency.

EPIDEMIOLOGY

Pernicious anemia (PA) is a disease primarily of people over 40 years of age, with a preponderance in women. It occurs in almost 1% of people over 60 years of age, and its frequency increases with age.[4] Certain groups are more commonly affected, particularly Scandinavians, other northern Europeans, and American blacks. Other racial groups and nationalities are affected, especially individuals with prematurely gray hair and blue eyes, but the disease occurs infrequently among Orientals.[1,6] Pernicious anemia is responsible for 85% of all vitamin B_{12} deficiency disease.[5]

Pernicious anemia is also associated with certain human leukocyte antigen (HLA) types, placing it with other autoimmune diseases that appear to be inherited.[1] Other diseases that increase the incidence of PA have also been identified as autoimmune. Some of the more frequently mentioned diseases are disorders of the thyroid, insulin-dependent diabetes mellitus, hypoparathyroidism, Addison's disease, ulcerative colitis, agammaglobulinemia, and vitiligo.[1,6] Infertility problems in men and in women under 40 years of age have also been associated with PA.[1]

A small number of patients develop pernicious anemia secondary to poor dietary intake of protein or years of strict vegetarianism. Dietary causes are uncommon, however, because vitamin B_{12} stores take years to deplete.[7,8]

PATHOPHYSIOLOGY

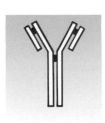

Pernicious anemia may manifest itself with a multitude of clinical symptoms. The variety of symptoms is due to atrophy of the gastric wall, which drastically reduces the amount of intrinsic factor secreted; this leads to decreased absorption of vitamin B_{12} (cobalamin), which is necessary for the maturation of red blood cells. The production of large, irregular red blood cells with abnormal maturation of the nucleus is known as **megalo-**

blastosis. These megaloblasts are classic signs of pernicious anemia.[1,4]

Neuropathy or psychiatric changes may be some of the first symptoms of PA, before anemia or other hematologic changes occur. Any unexplained psychiatric symptoms merit an evaluation of vitamin B_{12} levels. The more recent the onset of neurologic symptoms and the earlier treatment is begun, the more likely it is that the symptoms will fully resolve. Treatment begun 3 to 6 months after the onset of symptoms may produce only partial recovery. Intensive physical therapy, in addition to cobalamin therapy, is necessary for normal function to return. Notable changes in mental status that may occur include memory lapses, motor and sensory deficits, abnormal muscle tone, impairment of proprioception in the extremities, abnormal deep tendon reflexes, and neurogenic bowel or bladder. Demyelination of the spinal cord with degeneration of the central and peripheral nervous systems, stemming from a malfunction of both DNA synthesis and fatty acid metabolism, is responsible for the neurologic manifestations of PA.[5] Spinal cord involvement usually occurs in the thoracic segment but may also involve patchy areas throughout the cord.[8]

Achlorhydria, an absence of free hydrochloric acid in the stomach, is another classic symptom of PA. It may precede the development of other symptoms by years. A gastric pH over 3.5 without a significant decrease after stimulation with histamine constitutes achlorhydria.[1] Because both hydrochloric acid and intrinsic factor are secreted by the parietal cells in the gastric wall, atrophy commonly produces both deficiencies in patients.

A firm diagnosis of pernicious anemia depends on the findings of the Schilling test. For this test a fasting patient is given a standard dose of radioactive vitamin B_{12} orally, then an intramuscular injection of nonradioactive vitamin B_{12} 2 hours later. If the radioactive oral vitamin has been absorbed (i.e., there is no intrinsic factor deficiency), the "flushing" dose of intramuscular vitamin B_{12} saturates the normal plasma binding sites, and the radioactive vitamin B_{12} is excreted by the kidneys into the urine. Radioactivity is measured in a 24-hour urine specimen, and if only small amounts (less than 9%) are recorded, this implies lack of absorption as a result of intrinsic factor deficiency. This is verified by repeating the test with the addition of exogenous intrinsic factor administered with the oral vitamin B_{12}. If the 24-hour urine collection then reveals more radioactive vitamin B_{12} excretion, PA is confirmed. One major drawback to the Schilling test is the logistics of a complete 24-hour urine collection.[7]

Current studies suggest that pernicious anemia may be of autoimmune origin, but this theory cannot be applied to all patients. As many as 90% of patients with PA demonstrate multiple antigastric antibodies, particularly against the parietal cells of the gastric wall. Two antibodies to intrinsic factor have also been reported: type I antibody, also called the blocking antibody, impedes intrinsic factor from combining with vitamin B_{12}; type II antibody, or binding antibody, prevents the vitamin B_{12}–intrinsic factor complex from reacting with receptor sites in the ileum. Also, a greater number of T lymphocytes are present in the gastric mucosa with PA, which may contribute to mucosal destruction.[1,6]

CLINICAL MANIFESTATIONS

Anemia/pallor
Oral infections
Constipation/diarrhea/nausea/vomiting
Anorexia/weight loss
Urinary incontinence
Palpitations
Dyspnea
Fatigue

COMPLICATIONS

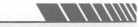

Congestive heart failure
Dehydration (due to anorexia, diarrhea, and vomiting)
Psychiatric disturbances (secondary to cerebral dysfunction and neurologic damage)
Chronic gastric ulcers

NURSING CARE

See pages 218-233.

DIAGNOSTIC STUDIES AND FINDINGS

Diagnostic Test	Findings
Red blood cell count	Decreased; anemia with large, irregular RBCs
Fasting plasma gastrin levels	Elevated in most patients[1]
Gastric analysis	Diminished volume; achlorhydria
Schilling test	Decreased vitamin B_{12} absorption
Red cell folate level	Decreased
Serum vitamin B_{12} level	Decreased
Bone marrow aspiration	Megaloblastosis[4]
Mean corpuscular volume (MCV)	Increased[4]
Serum intrinsic-factor autoantibody	Positive for antibody to intrinsic factor in half of patients with PA[8]
Segmented neutrophils	More than five lobes (abnormal[8])

MEDICAL MANAGEMENT

GENERAL MANAGEMENT

Packed red blood cell transfusion to correct anemia.

Bed rest, with gradual increase in activity, to conserve energy while anemic.

Close monitoring of neurologic status.

Routine monitoring of laboratory values.

MEDICAL MANAGEMENT—cont'd

Dietary consult to instruct and assist patient in planning nutritious meals.

Physical therapy consult to protect patient from complications of immobility during anemic episodes, to correct any neurologic motor deficits, and to assist in providing an appropriate exercise regimen.

DRUG THERAPY

Vitamin B_{12} IM injections daily or several times a week initially to correct acute deficiency (protocols may vary), then monthly IM injections to provide maintenance therapy.

Oral cobalamin (vitamin B_{12}) in very high doses to ensure absorption of sufficient amount of medication; this currently is not accepted treatment in the United States but has found favor in Sweden.[2]

Folic acid PO, since a folate deficiency often occurs simultaneously with cobalamin deficiency.[8]

Ferrous sulfate PO to improve anemia.

Hydrochloride if achlorhydria persists, to enhance digestion, absorption, and metabolism of food.

Analgesics for pain management.

Steroids to correct atrophy of the gastric mucosa, to enhance cobalamin absorption, and to increase the secretion of intrinsic factor by the gastric mucosa.[1,6]

1 ASSESS

	OBSERVATIONS			
ASSESSMENT	AUTOIMMUNE HEMOLYTIC ANEMIA	IDIOPATHIC THROMBOCYTOPENIC PURPURA	IDIOPATHIC NEUTROPENIA	PERNICIOUS ANEMIA
History	Personal or family history of any immunologic disorders and/or hospitalizations; current or recent medications, especially penicillins, quinidine, phenacetin, cephalosporins, or methyldopa; any known underlying illness	Personal or family history of bleeding or bruising tendencies and/or hospitalizations with or without transfusions; current or recent medications, especially quinidine, quinine, sulfonamides, methyldopa[4]; any alcohol or illegal drug problems; any known underlying illness or recent viral infection; note any risk factors for HIV	Personal or family history of underlying illness, especially malignancy, bacterial or viral infection, chronic gingivitis or periodontitis, SLE; current medications to rule out drug-induced neutropenia (e.g., glucocorticoids, cancer chemotherapy, chloramphenicol, phenothiazines, and antithyroid medications[1]);	Personal or family history of any known illness, especially stomach problems such as ulcers; any hospitalizations; any psychiatric disturbances or evaluations; any current medications (to rule out medication reactions); alcohol consumption (to rule out alcoholism as a possible cause for an increased MCV)

ASSESSMENT	AUTOIMMUNE HEMOLYTIC ANEMIA	IDIOPATHIC THROMBOCYTOPENIC PURPURA	IDIOPATHIC NEUTROPENIA	PERNICIOUS ANEMIA
			tricyclic antide-pressants, anti-convulsants, and antimicrobials have been linked to neutropenia[4]; patients taking several drugs of any kind are also at risk for neutro-penia due to drug reactions[1]; daily alcohol consumption	
Skin	Appears dry, jaun-diced; with CAHA may be cyanotic or pale; bruising, pruritus	Purpura, ecchy-moses, petechiae; If thrombocytope-nia is severe, hemorrhagic blis-ters may be noted on lips and oral mucosa; epistaxis[5]	Local erythema with infection; may have rash, cellulitis, axillary and/or groin ulcer-ations	Pallor due to ane-mia; areas of hy-perpigmentation may also be not-ed[3]
Gastrointestinal	Splenomegaly or hepatomegaly; accumulation of bilirubin may cause formation of gallstones; hemolytic crisis may cause nau-sea	Hematemesis; me-lena	Sore throat and mouth ulcerations; anorexia leading to weight loss; at risk for perirectal fissures	Oral sores and glossitis (smooth, red tongue); dis-turbance of bowel function, constipa-tion or diarrhea; anorexia leading to weight loss; nausea and/or vomiting; indigestion
Neurologic	Normal	Signs and symp-toms of intracra-nial bleeding and increased ICP: irritability, listless-ness, pupillary changes, abnor-mal reflexes, al-tered levels of consciousness, seizures, postur-ing, coma; symp-toms of nerve damage may be noted (paresthe-sia, paralysis)	May manifest gen-eral malaise, but as neutropenia progresses, fa-tigue increases to lethargy and stu-por	Cerebral dysfunc-tion (e.g., confu-sion, hallucinations, irritability, depres-sion, memory lapses, paranoia, impaired judg-ment)
Genitourinary	Normal	Hematuria; women may have heavy menstrual bleed-ing, bleeding from vaginal mucosa	Normal	Neurogenic blad-der

	OBSERVATIONS			
ASSESSMENT	AUTOIMMUNE HEMOLYTIC ANEMIA	IDIOPATHIC THROMBOCYTOPENIC PURPURA	IDIOPATHIC NEUTROPENIA	PERNICIOUS ANEMIA
Cardiovascular	Phlebitis in extremities, particularly deep vein thrombosis; intravascular hemolysis producing fever, chills, and back and extremity pain; hypotension; fatigue due to anemia	Tachycardia, hypotension (with copious blood loss)	May be tachycardic with weak pulses	Palpitations and/or angina pectoris on exertion; tachycardia; congestive heart failure may occur
Respiratory	Dyspnea on exertion or at rest if in crisis; decreased O_2 saturation by pulse oximeter or decreased Pa_{O_2} by ABG analysis during hemolytic crises or on moderate exertion	Tachypnea (with copious blood loss); may note decreased O_2 saturation by pulse oximetry or decreased Pa_{O_2} by ABG analysis	Weak respiratory effort producing shallow breaths with extreme fatigue; may exhibit normal air exchange or may note decreased O_2 saturation by pulse oximetry or decreased Pa_{O_2} by ABG analysis	Dyspnea on exertion; may note decreased O_2 saturation by pulse oximetry or decreased Pa_{O_2} by ABG analysis
Psychosocial	Depression due to extreme fatigue	Feelings of depression, loss of control, isolation	Feelings of depression and isolation, especially if patient requires strict or protective isolation during neutropenic crisis	Depression and paranoia as part of cerebral dysfunction that may occur

2 DIAGNOSE

NURSING DIAGNOSIS	SUBJECTIVE FINDINGS	OBJECTIVE FINDINGS
Activity intolerance related to generalized weakness, an imbalance between oxygen supply and demand, and immobility; related to possible depression if in protective isolation	Complains of fatigue during ADLs; complains of heart "racing" during exertion; with AHA, may complain of pain associated with exertion; with PA, may complain of numbness and tingling in hands and feet and difficulty walking "normally"; may express frustration at lack of physical mobility	Dyspnea, tachypnea, tachycardia on exertion; generalized muscle weakness; poor range of motion; pain on movement, causing patient to remain stationary when possible; lack of social outlets may lead to depression **PA:** Palpitations may occur with exertion, along with paresthesia in bilateral extremities; gait disturbances may be evident due to neuromuscular impairment

NURSING DIAGNOSIS	SUBJECTIVE FINDINGS	OBJECTIVE FINDINGS
Fluid volume deficit related to failure of regulatory mechanisms; with ITP, possible fluid losses due to bleeding	Complains of dry, itchy skin; reports occasional lightheadedness; states that urinary output is decreased and that urine looks darker **ITP:** Women may complain of heavy menstrual bleeding	Tachycardia, hypotension, decreased capillary fill time with poor skin turgor; dry skin and mucous membranes, weight loss; high specific gravity with low output **AHA:** Elevated bilirubin **ITP:** Large number of sanitary pads used during menstruation
Fatigue related to anemia and neurologic changes (PA)	**PA:** Complains of inability to concentrate; reports irritability	**PA:** Mental impairment, listlessness; emotionally labile with alternating tears, anger, and laughter
Altered nutrition: less than body requirements related to inflamed buccal mucosa (PA and N) and decreased vitamin B_{12} levels (PA)	**PA:** Reports no interest in eating due to abdominal discomfort, nausea; reports vomiting and diarrhea **IN** and **PA:** Sore mouth and tongue	Weight loss, evidence of muscle wasting; laboratory findings consistent with poor nutrition (e.g., hypoalbuminemia, hypoglycemia) **PA** and **IN:** Oral cavity sores **PA:** Glossitis (smooth, red, painful tongue) and decreased vitamin B_{12} levels
Altered oral mucous membrane related to gastrointestinal changes (PA); bleeding (ITP); infection and ineffective oral hygiene due to pain (IN)	Complains of sore mouth and tongue **ITP:** Complains of oral bleeding	**ITP:** Oral hemorrhagic lesions **PA** and **IN:** Painful oral lesions **PA:** Glossitis
Impaired skin integrity related to altered nutritional state, altered circulation, and immunologic disorder (AHA; potential in ITP and IN)	**AHA:** Complains of intense itching with dry, flaky skin	**AHA:** Evidence of scratching on various parts of body; poor skin turgor, dehydration; jaundice **ITP:** Risk because of decreased tissue perfusion secondary to poor platelet function **IN:** Risk because of possible development of furunculosis, a skin condition manifesting in lesions such as boils
Impaired home maintenance management related to inadequate knowledge about home safety regarding CAHA; related to impaired cognitive and emotional functioning with (PA)	**CAHA:** Complains of drafty rooms that contribute to chills; fingertips get cold when reaching into refrigerator **PA:** Family members complain of high stress of taking care of patient at home due to impaired mental status	**CAHA:** Fingertips sensitive to cold; elevated cold agglutinin titers **PA:** Exhausted, anxious, stressed family members

➙ ❯ ❯

NURSING DIAGNOSIS	SUBJECTIVE FINDINGS	OBJECTIVE FINDINGS
Potential for injury related to thrombocytopenia (ITP); related to abnormal blood profile (neutropenia), possibility of broken skin with hospital procedures, nosocomial agents, environment (IN)	**ITP:** Complains of easy bruising; reports using aspirin **IN:** Complains of weakness, generalized discomfort	**ITP:** Ecchymoses, purpura **IN:** Inability to mount a defense against pathogens in environment, or with hospital procedures, thus is vulnerable to injury
Potential for infection related to suppressed inflammatory response due to neutropenia (IN)	**IN:** Complains of weakness; unable to perform ADLs	**IN:** If ANC >1,000/mm^3, reverse isolation usually is not practiced, but strict isolation with meticulous handwashing is necessary; oral ulcers are noted; skin is otherwise intact but merits close observation for breakdown
Altered tissue perfusion and potential altered cerebral tissue perfusion related to circulatory and capillary blood supply changes (ITP)	**ITP:** Complains of slow healing of lesions, listlessness and lethargy	**ITP:** Ecchymoses, purpura; unable to focus, short attention span; responds only to yes/no questions; withdrawn
Altered bowel elimination related to neuromuscular impairment and malabsorption by the bowel (PA)	**PA:** Complains of inability to have a bowel movement, then of having diarrhea; reports occasional bowel incontinence	**PA:** Intermittent bouts with constipation and diarrhea; infrequent bowel incontinence
Sensory/perceptual alterations (kinesthetic and tactile) related to neurologic impairment (PA)	**PA:** Complains of tingling in hands and feet and inability to feel normal sensations when touching objects	**PA:** Paresthesia in bilateral upper and lower extremities; disturbances in tactile perceptions; inability to maintain straight, erect posture while sitting or standing unsupported
Social isolation related to altered mental status and unacceptable social behavior (PA); patients are potentially at risk for this diagnosis if they must be isolated for lengthy periods (IN)	**PA:** Expresses indifference regarding family and friends **IN:** Expresses feelings of frustration and loneliness when strict isolation is required	**PA:** Flat affect, uncommunicative; labile emotional behavior hinders social acceptance **IN:** Misses social contact when isolated
Altered patterns of urinary elimination related to neuromuscular impairment (PA)	**PA:** Complains of occasional urinary incontinence and inability to void at will	**PA:** Neurogenic bladder, frequent episodes of incontinence

3 PLAN

Patient Goals

1. The patient will demonstrate improved activity tolerance and optimum energy level.
2. The patient will demonstrate optimum fluid balance.
3. The patient will demonstrate that emotional and mental fatigue have diminished.
4. The patient will demonstrate an improved nutritional state.
5. The patient will demonstrate improved oral mucous membranes and improved oral hygiene and be pain free (PA and IN); the patient will have no bleeding from oral mucous membranes (ITP).
6. The patient will demonstrate improved skin integrity (AIHA, CAHA, PA, IN).
7. The patient will demonstrate increased knowledge about home safety (CAHA) and improved home maintenance management (PA).
8. The patient will remain free of injuries (ITP and IN) and infection (IN).
9. The patient will demonstrate optimum tissue perfusion and will maintain optimum cerebral perfusion (ITP).
10. The patient will demonstrate normal bowel and urinary function (PA).
11. The patient will demonstrate optimum sensory/perceptual status (PA).
12. The patient will demonstrate improved social behavior (PA).

4 IMPLEMENT

NURSING DIAGNOSIS	NURSING INTERVENTIONS	RATIONALE
Activity Intolerance related to generalized weakness, an imbalance between oxygen supply and demand, and immobility (related to bleeding tendencies in ITP; related to possible depression if in protective isolation with IN)	Assess patient's activity level.	To use as a baseline for activity tolerance and to guide therapeutic interventions.
	Assist patient with movement when necessary and with grouping of ADLs.	Grouping activities allows for longer periods of uninterrupted rest.
	Encourage patient to ask spouse or family for assistance when necessary.	To promote spouse's and family's understanding of patient's course and capabilities.
	Provide walker, cane, or wheelchair as needed.	To help keep patient as mobile and independent as possible.
	Working with physical therapists, teach passive range of motion (PROM) and active range of motion (AROM), and pace the exercise-rest regimen to maximize patient's ability.	To provide consistency through a team approach and to maintain full range of motion (ROM) in extremities, yet help patient avoid overworking easily fatigued muscles.
	In cooperation with physical therapists, help patient establish an exercise routine consistent with her ability.	As fatigue decreases, a fitness regimen retrains muscles and helps patient's self-esteem.
	Limit number and length of stay of visitors.	To allow patient longer periods of uninterrupted rest and to decrease O_2 demand.
	Give pain medication as ordered, especially before physical exertion or painful procedure. **ITP:** Avoid aspirin-containing products, nonsteroidal antiinflammatory drugs (NSAIDs), and alcohol.	To relieve discomfort and maximize mobility. To avoid deleterious effect on platelets.[6]

→ › ›

NURSING DIAGNOSIS	NURSING INTERVENTIONS	RATIONALE
	Instruct patient in relaxation techniques, assist with comfortable positioning, and use massage therapy if appropriate.	As an adjunct to medication for pain relief and comfort measures.
	Teach patient's spouse or family techniques for safely assisting patient as appropriate.	To help patient's spouse or family better understand how disease limits movement and to provide emotional support.
	Encourage patient to express her feelings about the course of her illness, symptoms, and recovery.	To allow patient to vent any anger, anxiety, and feelings of depression or isolation and to help her find constructive methods of dealing with these feelings.
Fluid volume deficit related to failure of regulatory mechanisms; with ITP, possible fluid losses due to bleeding	Assess patient's fluid status.	To establish a baseline fluid status and to guide therapeutic interventions.
	Monitor intake and output; follow daily weights and urine specific gravity; examine skin turgor daily.	Assessment of intake and output gives a rapid evaluation of fluid balance discrepancy; daily weights, specific gravity, and skin turgor are other measures of fluid balance that assist in detecting dehydration or overhydration; elevated specific gravity may indicate sodium and water retention secondary to hypovolemia. **AHA:** Renal problems caused by severe hemolysis will occur if urine does not remain alkaline.
	Administer IV fluids and crystalloid and colloid replacement as ordered, using a small-gauge needle; encourage PO fluids as appropriate. **CAHA:** Use blood warmer for colloid.	To restore circulating volume and depleted blood counts, yet minimize local tissue trauma from injections. **CAHA:** To avoid increasing cold agglutinin titers.
	Monitor for signs of fluid deficit or circulatory overload (e.g., elevated CVP reading, shortness of breath, copious amounts of dilute urine).	To guard against patient's becoming dehydrated or overhydrated.
	CAHA: Administer sodium bicarbonate as ordered and monitor patient response.	**CAHA:** To maintain urine alkalinity as necessary.
	CAHA: Assess pulses, core and skin surface temperature, and color daily.	**CAHA:** To monitor for circulatory complications.
	WAHA: Check for Homans' sign if deep vein thrombosis is suspected (i.e., dorsiflex foot, assess for pain in calf); if present, elevate patient's leg and apply warm compresses; notify physician.	**WAHA:** Deep vein thrombosis can be a dangerous complication that may lead to pulmonary embolism.[7]

NURSING DIAGNOSIS	NURSING INTERVENTIONS	RATIONALE
	ITP: Monitor for signs of overt and covert bleeding, including laboratory values; test all drainage (NG, urinary catheter, stool) for occult blood; avoid IM injections; apply pressure and/or cool compresses as appropriate; report findings to physician.	**ITP:** To prevent unnecessary blood loss or to control losses already occurring; therapeutic regimen may require changing as ordered.
Fatigue related to anemia and neurologic changes (PA)	Assess patient's fatigue and energy levels and patterns.	To establish a baseline for measuring patient's fatigue and to guide therapeutic interventions.
	Monitor for orthostatic hypotension during patient's first attempts at physical exertion.	To help maintain adequate blood pressure during patient's physical therapy program.
	PA: Reassure patient that cardiac symptoms (tachycardia, palpitations) will resolve over time with vitamin B_{12} therapy.	**PA:** To support patient in her efforts to comply with prescribed medication regimen and to persist with physical therapy.
	Help patient establish a daily pattern of activity, rest, and sleep.	To ensure that patient is getting sufficient, reasonable quantities of exercise, rest, and uninterrupted sleep.
Altered nutrition: less than body requirements related to inflamed buccal mucosa (PA and IN) and decreased vitamin B_{12} levels (PA)	Assess patient's nutritional status.	To establish a baseline and to guide therapeutic interventions.
	Encourage small, frequent meals.	To prevent distention and nausea, yet allow for maximum nutritive intake.
	Administer antiemetic medications as ordered	To allow patient to consume orally as much food and fluids as possible without nausea and vomiting
	Monitor laboratory values.	To monitor fluid balance, albumin, glucose, and nitrogen balance. **AHA:** To monitor erythropoiesis and liver function as well. **PA:** To monitor RBC count, red cell folate level, vitamin B_{12} level, MCV, and megaloblastosis; report discrepancies, and make necessary adjustments in therapy.
	AHA: Encourage an iron-rich, high-protein, high-vitamin diet and discourage fatty foods.[5]	**AHA:** To promote erythropoiesis, yet avoid satiety and abdominal discomfort from high-fat intake.
	AHA: Palpate abdomen as part of daily assessment.	**AHA:** To monitor for liver and/or spleen enlargement.
	IN: Collaborate with registered dietitian in providing a low-microbial diet.	**IN:** To prevent introduction of pathogens in patient's diet and provide individualized care.
	IN: Encourage patient to choose soft, bland foods while oral lesions are present.	**IN:** To avoid traumatizing sensitive and painful oral tissues.

NURSING DIAGNOSIS	NURSING INTERVENTIONS	RATIONALE
	IN: Administer antiseptic, antimicrobial, anesthetic oral rinses and medications as ordered and monitor patient response.	**IN:** To prevent further infection, empirically treat current infections, and provide comfort measures so patient can consume foods orally.
	IN: In collaboration with the physician, assess the need for and administer total parenteral nutrition (TPN) via a central line.	**IN:** To ensure that the patient receives adequate nutrition, protein, and fluids despite inability to ingest them orally.
Altered oral mucous membrane related to gastrointestinal changes (PA); bleeding (ITP); infection and ineffective oral hygiene due to pain (IN)	Assess oral mucous membranes daily, more frequently if necessary.	To establish a baseline and to guide therapeutic interventions.
	Help patient establish a mouth care routine.	To provide an opportunity for patient to assess her own mouth and to prevent further inflammation and infection.
	Perform meticulous oral care for patient as required.	To ensure optimum cleansing and promote comfort.
	Instruct patient to use a soft toothbrush or toothette.	To clean and refresh the mouth without aggravating oral tissue trauma and pain.
	Instruct patient to remove dentures when mouth is sore.	To maximize comfort and minimize oral tissue trauma.
	Instruct patient to avoid extreme temperatures in foods and fluids; encourage soft foods and room-temperature fluids.	To avoid trauma and bleeding in oral cavity.
	Encourage routine dental check-ups as part of discharge planning.	To encourage patient to continue good dental maintenance at home. **IN:** Stomatitis and periodontitis occur frequently with neutropenia, and regular dental check-ups provide expert examination of oral tissues.
	Administer analgesics as appropriate.	To maximize comfort.
	ITP: Monitor for any oral bleeding.	**ITP:** To detect and prevent further blood loss.
	Suction mouth and trachea as infrequently as possible; when necessary, use low suction and gentle technique.	To minimize oral tissue trauma while removing excess secretions that may inhibit respiratory effort and gas exchange.
Impaired skin integrity related to altered nutritional state, altered circulation, and immunologic disorder (AHA; potential in ITP and IN)	Assess patient's skin condition daily.	To establish baseline and assess therapeutic regimens.
	Promote optimum environmental temperature.	To provide maximum comfort.
	Discourage patient from scratching irritated skin; provide lotions and teach appropriate use, or teach other coping mechanisms for avoiding scratching.	To prevent further skin irritation, to avoid a possible route of infection, and to help restore optimum skin integrity.

NURSING DIAGNOSIS	NURSING INTERVENTIONS	RATIONALE
	Instruct patient in positioning, and assist with position changes as appropriate.	To prevent further irritation at pressure points on sensitive, dry skin and to avoid positions that may impair circulation.
	Teach proper skin care to patient and spouse or family.	To promote knowledge of appropriate skin care.
	Instruct patient to stop smoking and assist in instituting a stop-smoking regimen.	To minimize vasoconstriction caused by cigarette smoking.
	Instruct patient in the use of egg-crate mattress, sheepskin, or whatever method provides the most therapeutic benefits.	To prevent any risk of impaired circulation and pressure sores with skin that is already tissue hypoxic.
Impaired home maintenance management related to inadequate knowledge about home safety regarding CAHA; related to impaired cognitive and emotional functioning with PA	Assess home maintenance management techniques of patient and spouse or family.	To establish a baseline and to guide therapeutic interventions.
	CAHA: Teach patient to avoid exposure to cold (e.g., bathe in warm water, minimize drafts, use warm blankets when appropriate, and dress warmly [e.g., wear mittens when reaching into freezer]); instruct patient to use electric razors and to avoid all constrictive clothing, jewelry, eyeglasses, and shoes.	**CAHA:** To minimize altered circulation related to cold agglutinins and to avoid elevated cold agglutinin titers and subsequent hemolysis; fingertips are especially vulnerable, so they should be protected; cuts, scrapes, and bruises should also be avoided due to increased bleeding tendencies and possible decreased O_2-carrying capacities; anything that may impair circulation should be avoided.
	Instruct patient to keep a hall or bathroom light on at night and to remove throw rugs.	To avoid bumping or bruising legs and feet and to prevent slips and falls.
	Instruct patient to call 911 if injured at home and to wear a medical alert bracelet.	To ensure that appropriate medical assistance is only minutes away, even when patient is at home.
	PA: Provide emotional support to patient and to spouse or family; if appropriate, refer for counseling.	**PA:** To provide a forum for patient and spouse or family to express anxieties and frustrations about patient's illness.
	PA: Reassure patient and spouse or family that patient's emotionally labile state is related to illness and most likely will improve with medication.	**PA:** To assist patient and spouse or family in understanding the disease and to help ensure rigid adherence to medical therapies.
	Begin discharge planning. Contact local organizations to facilitate home management.	To help focus patient and family on discharge planning and to begin home health care referrals if necessary.

NURSING DIAGNOSIS	NURSING INTERVENTIONS	RATIONALE
Potential for injury related to thrombocytopenia (ITP); related to abnormal blood profile (neutropenia), possibility of broken skin with hospital procedures, nosocomial agents, environment (IN)	Instruct patient in proper body alignment and position changes; assist when appropriate.	To prevent patient from inadvertently injuring herself during position changes.
	IN: Avoid any unnecessary invasive procedure (e.g., no rectal temperatures); avoid indwelling urinary catheters if possible; minimize blood drawing.	**IN:** To protect skin and tissues from trauma and to preserve a line of defense against pathogens.
	IN: Avoid using suppositories and enemas if possible; administer stool softeners as ordered; assist patient with proper personal hygiene.	**IN:** Perirectal tears and abscesses can be life threatening to neutropenic patients; area must be kept as clean and dry as possible to prevent breakdown and infection.
	IN: Instruct women to use sanitary pads rather than tampons during menstruation.	**IN:** To prevent trauma to tissues and avoid introducing an avenue for infection.
	IN: If urinary catheterization is necessary, use generous amounts of lubricant on insertion, and use as small a catheter as possible.	**IN:** To avoid tissue trauma.
	Instruct patient and family on techniques to make home environment safer.	To prevent injury. **ITP:** To minimize risk of covert bleeding.
	ITP: Monitor for bleeding from any orifice.	**ITP:** To detect bleeding early and prevent further blood loss.
Potential for infection related to suppressed inflammatory response due to neutropenia (IN)	**ITP** and **IN:** Instruct patient to avoid crowds and people with colds or other infectious diseases.	**ITP** and **IN:** To minimize risk of viral infection.
	IN: Monitor ANC, and institute appropriate isolation measures according to results.	**IN:** ANC dictates susceptibility to infection and should be used as a reference for isolation protocols.
	Perform head-to-toe assessment q 8-12 h, more frequently if fever develops.	To meticulously inspect all skin areas for breakdown or local infection.
	IN: Monitor vital signs, especially temperature, at least q 2 h around the clock; notify physician if temperature reaches 38.3° C (100.9° F).[7]	**IN:** To establish baselines and to guide therapeutic interventions; prompt intervention for fever is vital for neutropenic patients, since fever may indicate a life-threatening illness.
	IN: Auscultate patient's lungs with vital sign checks.	**IN:** To evaluate for symptoms of pneumonia (decreased breath sounds, rales, rhonchi), since pulmonary infiltrates may not be present on chest x-ray due to neutropenia.
	IN: Enforce protective isolation, including meticulous handwashing, before nursing and medical care.	**IN:** To protect patient from pathogens and to prevent nosocomial infection.

NURSING DIAGNOSIS	NURSING INTERVENTIONS	RATIONALE
	IN: Assist patient with skin care as required; meticulous skin observation and care, especially with any fever; daily baths with mild antimicrobial soap and light oil or lubricant; report and culture any suspicious lesion; if fever is present, culture throat, sputum, urine, blood, stool, all IV lines, and catheters.	**IN:** To promote optimum skin function and integrity; close inspection of skin is essential to prevent infection (especially vulnerable are the axillae, groin, any indwelling IV or catheter site, biopsy sites, and skin folds). Patient may not be capable of a typical local response to infection; exudate and swelling may be absent due to neutropenia, but fever, pain, and erythema may still occur. Daily bathing helps promote optimum personal hygiene and offers an opportunity for assessment.
	IN: Assess patient's response to tape and transparent dressing covers, and use what is least irritating.	**IN:** Dressings require frequent changing for asepsis and site observation; nonallergenic tape makes the process less painful.
	IN: Use strict aseptic technique when performing dressing changes, manipulating IV tubing or catheters, or drawing blood from indwelling IV lines; do not allow blood to stand in stopcock caps after blood sampling.	**IN:** To protect patient from pathogens and nosocomial infections; blood is an excellent medium for pathogens.
	IN: Avoid fresh flowers, any standing water, or potted plants in patient's room.	**IN:** For patient's protection against pathogens, especially *Pseudomonas aeruginosa* and *Serratia marcescens.*[7]
	IN: Collaborate with registered dietitian to provide a low-microbial, nutritious, and appealing diet; instruct patient to drink only sterile water.	**IN:** To avoid introducing pathogens in patient's diet, yet provide food that entices consumption; all foods must be cooked—no fresh fruit or vegetables.
	IN: Inspect patient's mouth daily, and report any white patches or other lesions; administer antibacterial and antifungal oral rinses as ordered.	**IN:** To evaluate any changes in oral mucosa and to ensure immediate treatment if infection develops.
	IN: Instruct patient to wipe from front to back after bowel movements, and assist with meticulous hygiene if required; instruct patient to take sitz baths twice a day, especially after bowel movements.[4]	**IN:** Perirectal abscesses and rectal fissures are frequent occurrences with neutropenia if strict hygiene is not maintained; infections from *Escherichia coli* are minimized with scrupulous personal hygiene.
	IN: Monitor for vaginal discharges.	**IN:** To evaluate any discharge, culture if necessary and notify physician to begin treatment if required.
	IN: Instruct patient to wear a mask if she must leave her room while neutropenic.	**IN:** To prevent respiratory transmission of pathogens.
	IN: Prevent staff and visitors from entering patient's room if they have been exposed to or currently have a cold or infection.	**IN:** To protect patient from exogenous pathogens while she is neutropenic and vulnerable to infections.

→ > >

NURSING DIAGNOSIS	NURSING INTERVENTIONS	RATIONALE
	IN: Assist and instruct patient in proper oral hygiene.	**IN:** To promote meticulous mouth care and avoid infection.
	IN: Collaborate with respiratory therapist and housekeeping personnel to ensure that patient's equipment and room are as sterile as possible.	**IN:** To protect patient from infection.
Altered tissue perfusion and potential altered cerebral tissue perfusion related to circulatory and capillary blood supply changes (ITP)	Assess patient's tissue perfusion, and closely monitor levels of consciousness to assess cerebral perfusion.	To establish a baseline and to use as a tool to guide therapeutic interventions.
	ITP: Administer stool softeners and instruct patient to avoid Valsalva maneuver.	**ITP:** To minimize potential risk of increased intracranial pressure and possible bleeding.
	ITP: Heme-test urine, and instruct patient in use of heme-test equipment.	**ITP:** To detect any renal bleeding and intervene immediately.
Altered bowel elimination related to neuromuscular impairment and malabsorption by the bowel (PA)	**PA:** Assess patient's bowel function.	**PA:** To establish a baseline and to guide therapeutic interventions.
	PA: Collaborate with other health team members in teaching patient pelvic floor strengthening exercises, and instruct in practice sessions.	**PA:** Team approach provides essential consistency with reestablishing a bowel routine.
	PA: Help patient establish a toilet routine, and provide privacy during these times.	**PA:** Daily private routine helps patient learn a bowel regimen to prevent incontinence.
	PA: Maintain a sensitive attitude during patient's bowel retraining.	**PA:** To help maintain patient's dignity.
Sensory/perceptual alterations (kinesthetic and tactile) related to neurologic impairment (PA)	**PA:** Assess patient's kinesthetic and tactile perceptual status.	**PA:** To establish a neurologic baseline and to guide therapeutic interventions.
	PA: Reassure patient that neuropathies often are associated with pernicious anemia and will improve with medical therapy.	**PA:** To help restore patient's self-esteem and to assure her that neurologic symptoms are amenable to treatment.
	PA: Encourage patient to share any neurologic event she experiences; avoid suggesting that it is a real event.	**PA:** To help patient focus on reality, not on hallucinations, in order to begin separating fantasy from reality.
	PA: Orient patient to person, place, and time when necessary.	**PA:** To keep patient in touch with her real environment.

NURSING DIAGNOSIS	NURSING INTERVENTIONS	RATIONALE
Social isolation related to altered mental status and unacceptable social behavior (PA); patients with IN are potentially at risk for this diagnosis if they must be isolated for lengthy periods	Evaluate social history.	To establish a baseline and to guide therapeutic interventions.
	PA: Reassure patient that unacceptable social behavior is based on her disease and will improve with medical therapy.	**PA:** To provide emotional support and encouragement.
	PA: Reinforce all social progress.	**PA:** To provide incentives for further improvement.
	PA: Involve spouse or family in patient's increasingly social behavior.	**PA:** To allow spouse or family a better understanding of patient's neurologic involvement and to encourage improvement.
	IN: Use a team approach with other services (physical and occupational therapy), nursing personnel, family, and friends to provide diversional activities while patient is isolated.	**IN:** Early and consistent involvement of all available personnel decreases feelings of social isolation.
Altered patterns of urinary elimination related to neuromuscular impairment (PA)	**PA:** Assess patient's bladder function.	**PA:** To establish a baseline and to guide therapeutic interventions.
	PA: Assist patient in establishing a pattern of regular voiding.	**PA:** To begin a bladder retraining program.
	PA: Instruct patient in Kegel's exercise.	**PA:** To strengthen pelvic muscles.
	PA: Instruct patient in use of absorbent undergarments if necessary.	**PA:** To prevent stained clothing while patient is relearning urinary elimination.
	PA: Provide any necessary written guidelines for patient and family to use during bladder retraining.	**PA:** To provide a readily available resource to patient and to involve spouse or family in retraining efforts.
	PA: Maintain a sensitive attitude when assisting patient in bladder regimen.	**PA:** To preserve patient's dignity.

5 EVALUATE

PATIENT OUTCOME	DATA INDICATING THAT OUTCOME IS REACHED
Activity level has increased.	Patient reports decreased periods of fatigue and can complete ADLs without tiring; patient is participating in a light exercise program that contributes to increased cardiovascular fitness, better muscle tone, and increased self-esteem. **PA:** No tachypnea or palpitations are reported; patient exhibits a normal gait, and paresthesias from upper and lower extremities have resolved; patient is participating in physical therapy. **ITP** and **AHA:** Medication is required less often before exercise, and pain-free periods have increased; patient freely communicates feelings to spouse and family, who assist when appropriate; oxygen therapy is not required. **AHA:** In CAHA, cold antibody titers are down significantly.

PATIENT OUTCOME	DATA INDICATING THAT OUTCOME IS REACHED
Fluid volumes are normal.	Weight has stabilized; oral fluids are consumed without distention or discomfort; skin has good turgor with no flaking noted or itchiness reported; capillary refill time is 1-2 seconds; urine specific gravity, alkalinity, and bilirubin levels are within normal limits. **ITP:** Laboratory blood tests are normal, including a normalizing platelet count.
Emotional and mental fatigue have diminished significantly.	Emotional status is stable, mental alertness is normal, and ability to concentrate has improved.
Nutritional status has improved.	Patient reports increased appetite; weight has stabilized; patient has no nausea or vomiting; laboratory results are normal (e.g., albumin >3.5 mg/dl, BUN 10-20 mg/dl, glucose 60-105 mg/dl).
Oral mucous membranes have improved.	Patient reports no oral bleeding, and no oral pain with food or fluids; patient's mouth and tongue are clean and free of sores or white patches. **PA:** Glossitis has resolved.
Skin integrity has improved.	Patient reports no pruritus; no scratching is evident; patient has no jaundice, and skin turgor is good; there is no evidence of vasoconstriction. **ITP:** No bleeding is reported or noted.
Home maintenance management is optimal.	**AHA:** Patient, spouse, and family can describe a proper environment and appropriate action in case of an emergency. **PA:** Patient and family members report no frustrations or anxieties attributed to patient's course; home care is going well.
Patient remains free of injuries and infection.	Patient no longer smokes. **ITP:** Patient reports no new bruising and reports using appropriate safety precautions. **IN:** No tissue trauma or tears are noted; ANC is within normal limits ($2,500/mm^3$-$9,000/mm^3$).[4] Patient remains afebrile with stable vital signs; lungs are clear to auscultation bilaterally; no skin breakdown, local pain, or erythema is noted; routine blood cultures are negative for microbial growth.
Tissue perfusion is improved, and optimum cerebral tissue perfusion is maintained.	**ITP:** There is no evidence of intracranial bleeding or increased pressure; patient reports normal mental capabilities and is alert and oriented.
Bowel and urinary elimination patterns are normal.	**PA:** Patient reports a normal bowel and urinary routine, with no incontinence; no perianal tissue breakdown.
Sensory/perceptual reception has improved.	**PA:** Patient is oriented to person, place, and time and reports no hallucinatory events; paresthesia has resolved, so tactile perceptions are normal.
Social interactions have improved.	**PA:** Patient reports an increasing social life with spouse and family members and exhibits socially correct behavior. **IN:** Patient received sufficient social stimulation to combat loneliness during protective isolation.

PATIENT OUTCOME	DATA INDICATING THAT OUTCOME IS REACHED
Patient is knowledgeable about her disease, rationale for hospitalization, need for medical follow-up, and discharge instructions. **IN: Patient understands rationale for isolation.** **PA: Patient understands need for lifelong medical therapy for pernicious anemia.**	Patient describes course of disease, precipitating factors, and appropriate action regarding diet, activity, and environmental precautions. Patient states name, dosage, time and route of administration of medications, possible side effects, and when to notify a health care practitioner.

PATIENT TEACHING

1. Teach the patient about the course of the disease, the prognosis, medication requirements, and the need for medical follow-up.
2. Review signs and symptoms of an infection, necessary precautions, and proper course of action if an infection is noted (IN).
3. Review proper mouth care techniques and stress the importance of thorough self-examinations and regular dental examinations to prevent the occurrence of stomatitis and periodontitis (IN).
4. Instruct the patient to utilize the 911 emergency system if he requires immediate assistance from a health care professional.
5. Review proper nutrition and assist the patient in establishing a healthy diet high in protein, vitamins, and calories, with appropriate fluid intake.
6. Instruct the patient to avoid crowds and people with colds and other infectious diseases (IN).
7. Review purpose dosages, routes of administration, schedule, and any side effects of all medications. Emphasize the importance of avoiding self-medication without consulting a health care professional because of possible hypersensitivity reactions.
8. Explain signs and symptoms of worsening course and when to notify the patient's physician.
9. Instruct the patient in proper skin care.
10. Teach relaxation techniques, imagining, and appropriate comfort measures as an adjunct to medication.
11. Instruct the patient and family on the correct method of intramuscular injections for vitamin B_{12} therapy (PA).
12. Instruct the patient on appropriate activity level and encourage participation in a fitness program.
13. Instruct the patient to avoid extreme heat and cold (compresses or heating pads) until all paresthesias have fully resolved (PA).

CHAPTER 8

Vasculitis

Vasculitis is a rare disorder characterized by inflammation and progressive necrosis of blood vessels. Vasculitis is described as necrotizing when the vessel is obliterated as a result of thrombosis or hemorrhage and when the mediators of inflammation cause infarction. No single cause accounts for all the vascular disorders, but the most likely mechanism is an immune complex–mediated response. Further, immunofluorescent studies of biopsied tissue have confirmed the presence of immunoglobulins and complement in the vessel walls.

Vasculitis can affect any blood vessel, causing a variety of symptoms depending on the location of the insult. It may arise as a primary disorder or as a component of another systemic disorder. Vascular diseases are divided into two main groups, small vessel vasculitis and systemic necrotizing vasculitis.

Small Vessel Vasculitis

Small vessel vasculitis is primarily an immune complex–mediated disease that causes inflammation of small vessels, including the arterioles, capillaries, and venules. The disease is characterized by a group of syndromes that may or may not appear simultaneously. These syndromes frequently accompany other systemic disorders (e.g., systemic lupus erythematosus, rheumatoid arthritis, infections, and Goodpasture's syndrome).

The proposed etiologies for small vessel vasculitis include exposure to chemicals (e.g., insecticides), infection, foreign proteins (e.g., animal dander, monoclonal antibodies), drugs (e.g., antiinflammatory agents, NSAIDs, and antirheumatic medications), and certain foods (e.g., milk, fish, and eggs). The involved vessels typically demonstrate both acute and chronic inflammation simultaneously. Clinical manifestations often affect the skin, reflected as palpable purpuric lesions, nonblanching petechiae, erythema, ulcerative lesions, and edema. Lesions occur most often on the lower extremities and are accompanied by pain and burning. The diagnosis is based on the patient's history, a physical examination, skin biopsy, and the following supportive laboratory tests: erythrocyte sedimentation rate (elevated); immune complexes (present); rheumatoid factor (may be present); and serum complement levels (elevated). Treatment focuses on identifying and eliminating the causative agent or treating the underlying disease. Other management tactics have included short-term corticosteroid therapy, analgesics for pain relief, and rest.

Table 8-1

ASSOCIATED SMALL VESSEL SYNDROMES

Syndrome	Specific clinical features	Probable mediator
Behçet's disease	Venulitis appearing as recurrent eye lesions, genital and oral ulcers, thrombophlebitis, and various cutaneous lesions	Antibody or T cell mediated
Henoch-Schönlein purpura	Systemic venulitis, skin lesions, nonthrombocytopenic purpura, fever, renal impairment, abdominal pain with possible bleeding, arthralgias	IgA mediated with complement activation
Hypocomplementemic urticarial vasculitis	Persistent urticaria, skin erythematosus, angioedema, joint pain, abdominal discomfort, glomerulonephritis, neurologic impairments	Complement mediated, selective depression of Clq
Essential mixed cryoglobulinemia	Arthralgia, purpura, weakness, recurrent palpable purpura of the lower extremities, hepatosplenomegaly, polyarthralgia, glomerulonephritis	Antibody mediated

Systemic Necrotizing Vasculitis

Systemic necrotizing vasculitis comprises a group of disorders that manifest a multisystem, necrotizing vasculitis of both small and medium muscular arteries. These disorders are polyarteritis nodosa, Wegener's granulomatosis, Churg-Strauss syndrome (allergic granulomatosis and angiitis), temporal arteritis (giant cell arteritis), and polyangiitis overlap syndrome (characteristics of both polyarteritis nodosa and Churg-Strauss syndrome). The diagnosis is based on clinical presentation, a complete history, and one or more of the following tests: biopsy, complete blood count, platelets, erythrocyte sedimentation rate, presence of immune complexes, rheumatoid factor, and complement levels. Treatment generally consists of treating the specific organ system and the underlying disorder, rest, analgesia for pain, and corticosteroids or cyclophosphamide, or both.

POLYARTERITIS NODOSA

Polyarteritis nodosa (PAN) is an immune complex–mediated necrotizing vasculitis that affects small and medium-sized muscular arteries.

Polyarteritis nodosa is an uncommon disease that can affect either sex at any age. It primarily targets men (at a ratio of 2.5:1) between 40 and 45 years of age. As yet no human leukocyte antigen (HLA) association has been identified.

The etiology of PAN is not completely clear. It has been associated with a number of infections, particularly hepatitis B but also tuberculosis and streptococcal infections. Following exposure to an infectious agent, immune complexes are thought to develop and be deposited in selected tissues, primarily the kidneys, skin,

Table 8-2

SYSTEMIC NECROTIZING VASCULITIS

Disorder	Probable mediator	Primary organ systems affected
Polyarteritis nodosa	Immune complex	Kidneys, heart, and gastrointestinal and nervous systems
Wegener's granulomatosis	Cell mediated Hypersensitivity Immune complex	Upper and lower respiratory tract, renal system
Churg-Strauss syndrome (allergic granulomatosis and angiitis)	Allergic Elevated IgE Hypereosinophilia	Upper and lower respiratory tract
Temporal arteritis (giant cell arteritis)	Immune complex Antibody mediated Cell mediated	Systemic panarteritis of large and medium-sized arteries
Polyangiitis overlap syndrome (polyarteritis nodosa and Churg-Strauss syndrome)	Immune complex Allergic Elevated IgE	Kidneys, respiratory tract, and gastrointestinal and nervous systems

heart, abdominal organs, and nervous system. Evidence that an external antigen may be the triggering agent is demonstrated in patients who develop polyarteritis nodosa in association with the hepatitis B virus. Early in the course of the viral infection, the vascular lesions of these patients demonstrate hepatitis B antigen, IgM antibody, and complement components.

PATHOPHYSIOLOGY

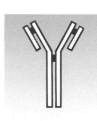

The triggering event that ultimately leads to vascular inflammation is unknown. The inflammatory response that follows is a characteristic infiltration of polymorphonuclear leukocytes, followed by the invasion of monocytes, lymphocytes, and plasma cells. These cells typically accumulate within the small and medium muscular arteries. Generally the arterioles, venules, and veins are not affected, and granuloma formation is unusual. As the disorder progresses, the media and internal elastic lamina are destroyed, and aneurysms form. New lesions continue to develop, often surrounded by older lesions. PAN is considered a chronic inflammatory condition, because lesions at varying stages of evolution are involved. The chronic inflammation within the vessel wall subsequently leads to endothelial proliferation, degeneration of the vessel wall, ischemia, necrosis, infarction, and possibly hemorrhage of the affected organ or tissue.

CLINICAL MANIFESTATIONS

Patients generally complain of headaches, weakness, fever, anorexia, weight loss, and fatigue. Clinically this process affects primarily the kidneys (glomerulitis, glomerulosclerosis, progressive renal failure), heart (coronary arteritis, myocardial ischemia or infarction, pericarditis, congestive heart failure), abdominal organs (appendicitis, cholecystitis, hepatitis), skin, and nervous system. Patients may also have myalgias, arthralgia, and retinopathy. The primary clinical characteristics are listed in Table 8-3.

The prognosis of polyarteritis nodosa depends on the extent of vascular damage and renal involvement. Renal symptoms typically indicate a rapid downward trajectory in the illness. Death usually results from myocardial infarction, heart failure, infection, or gastrointestinal bleeding.

COMPLICATIONS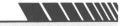

Severe hypertension
Necrotizing vasculitis
Spontaneous hemorrhage
Renal failure
Intestinal obstruction, perforation, rupture of mesenteric aneurysms
Myocardial infarction
Pericarditis
Ischemic strokes

Table 8-3

POLYARTERITIS NODOSA: CLINICAL MANIFESTATIONS AND INCIDENCE OF ORGAN INVOLVEMENT

Renal (85%)	Cardiac (75%)	Gastrointestinal (50%)	Neurologic: peripheral (27%); central (20%)	Skin (20%)
Hematuria, proteinuria, hypertension, glomerulitis, glomerulosclerosis, progressive renal failure	Angina pectoris, chest pain, hypertension, myocardial ischemia, congestive heart failure	Nausea, vomiting, abdominal pain, anorexia, weight loss, malabsorption, steatorrhea, appendicitis, cholecystitis, hepatitis	Neuropathies, paresthesias, pain, weakness, sensory loss, mononeuritis multiplex, encephalopathy, severe hypertension, seizures	Maculopapular rash, purpuric, urticarial exanthema, subcutaneous hemorrhage, ulcerations, livedo reticularis, and/or small painful subcutaneous nodules along the arteries of the extremities, ischemic changes in distal digits

From Samter et al.[148]

DIAGNOSTIC STUDIES AND FINDINGS*

Diagnostic test	Findings
Erythrocyte sedimentation rate (ESR)	Elevated during acute phase
Complete blood count (CBC)	Elevated WBC due to neutrophilia; decreased hematocrit; anemia
Platelets	Elevated
Urinalysis	Cellular casts; proteinuria >500 mg/24 h with glomerular disease; hematuria
Angiography	To detect characteristic aneurysms (circular vascular dilations), typically at bifurcation points; to determine changes in vessel caliber (asymmetric narrowing pattern); this test establishes a diagnosis in approximately 80% of cases
Histologic tissue studies (biopsies from symptomatic sites such as skeletal muscle and nerves have a greater yield)	Necrotizing vasculitis of small and medium arteries; invasion of tissue by polymorphonuclear leukocytes and monocytes
Rheumatoid factor	May be present
Complement components	May be reduced
Immune complexes	May be present

*There is no one specific laboratory test for polyarteritis nodosa; the features observed are associated with the organs or tissues affected.

DIFFERENTIAL DIAGNOSIS

Systemic lupus erythematosus (SLE)
Trichinosis
Heart failure
Infection

NURSING CARE

See pages 241-247.

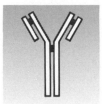

WEGENER'S GRANULOMATOSIS

Wegener's granulomatosis is a multisystem necrotizing vasculitis that involves primarily the small and medium muscular arteries. It is characterized by a granulomatous vasculitis of the upper and lower respiratory tract, a necrotizing glomerulonephritis, and varying degrees of small vessel vasculitis.

Wegener's granulomatosis occurs equally in men and women. Although it may develop at any age, the peak incidence is in the fourth and fifth decades.

PATHOPHYSIOLOGY

The exact cause of Wegener's granulomatosis is not known, but it has been suggested that the triggering event is an infectious or inhaled antigen that stimulates either a hypersensitivity response or a cell-mediated reaction.

Wegener's granulomatosis is characterized histologically by a widespread, necrotizing vasculitis of the small arteries, venules, arterioles, and some capillaries, together with granuloma formation. Early neutrophilic infiltration is followed by mononuclear cells and subsequent fibrotic healing. The vasculitic lesion demonstrates all stages of inflammation.

Clinical Manifestations

Most patients (85%) have some degree of upper and lower pulmonary involvement. Approximately 95% of patients have some degree of sinus involvement that often is complicated by recurrent secondary bacterial infections. Pansinusitis may result in the erosion of adjacent bones and septal perforation. As the nasal septum is destroyed, a characteristic saddle-nose deformity may be observed.

In the lungs a diffuse bilateral nodular lesion develops that tends to cavitate and alter pulmonary function; this can result in dyspnea, pleuritic chest pain, and productive cough and can progress to hemoptysis and massive pulmonary hemorrhage.

Renal involvement, seen in approximately 80% of cases, is demonstrated by a focal segmental glomerulonephritis that may progress to a diffuse proliferative disease and renal failure.

If detected and treated early, the prognosis for Wegener's granulomatosis is good. However, extensive renal involvement indicates a poor prognosis.

COMPLICATIONS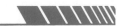

> Hemorrhage
> Renal failure
> Airway obstruction

DIFFERENTIAL DIAGNOSIS

Chronic sinusitis
Otitis media
Associated diseases (SLE, Goodpasture's syndrome, thrombotic thrombocytopenic purpura)

NURSING CARE

See pages 241-247.

Table 8-4

WEGENER'S GRANULOMATOSIS

System affected	Clinical manifestations
Upper respiratory system (85%)	Sore throat, sinusitis, nasal obstruction, nasal ulcers, rhinorrhea, otitis media, hearing loss
Lower respiratory system (35%)	May be asymptomatic; otherwise dyspnea, cough, sputum production, pleuritic chest pain, hemoptysis, and massive pulmonary hemorrhage
Renal system (80%)	May be asymptomatic; otherwise proteinuria, hematuria, progressive glomerulonephritis (on biopsy)
Skin (50%)	Subcutaneous nodular lesions with purpuric papules, petechiae, vesicles, ulceration
Joints (50%)	Joint pain
Eyes (40%)	Proptosis due to orbital inflammation (e.g., conjunctivitis, episcleritis, scleromalacia, corneal ulcers, and retinal artery thrombosis), retinal vasculitis (10%)
Heart (25%)	Pericarditis
Nervous system (25%)	Cranial neuritis, mononeuritis multiplex

DIAGNOSTIC STUDIES AND FINDINGS

Diagnostic Test	Findings
Tissue biopsy	Granuloma formation; vasculitic lesions (open lung biopsy provides greatest yield)
Chest x-ray	Most common pattern is multiple bilateral nodular cavitary infiltrates
Complete blood count (CBC)	Mild anemia (normochromic, normocytic), leukocytosis
Platelets	Elevated
Erythrocyte sedimentation rate (ESR)	Elevated during active disease
C-reactive protein	Present
Polyclonal hypergammaglobulinemia	Elevated IgG and IgA, normal levels of IgM
Antineutrophil cytoplasmic autoantibodies	Present in most cases
Renal involvement	Elevated BUN and creatinine, proteinuria, hematuria, cellular casts

CHURG-STRAUSS SYNDROME (ALLERGIC GRANULOMATOSIS AND ANGIITIS)

Churg-Strauss syndrome, also known as allergic granulomatosis and angiitis, is characterized by a systemic vasculitis of the medium and small muscular arteries, allergic rhinitis, and/or asthma and hypereosinophilia.

Churg-Strauss syndrome is a rare disorder that produces a vascular lesion very similar to the pattern found in polyarteritis nodosa. It has a slight male predominance, and onset generally occurs within the fourth decade, often appearing in three phases. The first phase is a prodromal period that may last for many years. The primary clinical findings during this period are atopic (e.g., allergic rhinitis followed by asthma). Hypereosinophilia and infiltration of eosinophils into the tissue mark the second phase, and the third phase is characterized by a systemic necrotizing vasculitis.

PATHOPHYSIOLOGY

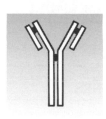

The pathophysiology of Churg-Strauss syndrome is very similar to that of polyarteritis nodosa, with the exception that asthma or some other type of pulmonary involvement often is seen in Churg-Strauss syndrome. The vascular lesions are also similar to those in polyarteritis nodosa, but the vasculitis in Churg-Strauss syndrome affects the small and medium muscular veins and capillaries as well as the arteries. Eosinophilic infiltration and granuloma formation are frequently found in the tissue of patients with Churg-Strauss syndrome.

CLINICAL MANIFESTATIONS

The clinical manifestations of Churg-Strauss syndrome are also similar to those of polyarteritis nodosa, except for the higher incidence of pulmonary involvement. Pulmonary symptoms usually precede systemic vasculitis by several years; these symptoms include dyspnea, cough, bronchospasms, and pleuritic pain. The onset of vasculitis is characterized by weight loss, intermittent fever, fatigue, and myalgias. The prognosis is similar to that for polyarteritis nodosa.

COMPLICATIONS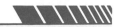

Same as for polyarteritis nodosa (page 236)

DIAGNOSTIC STUDIES AND FINDINGS

Diagnostic Test	Findings
Complete blood count (CBC) with differential	Eosinophilia in 85% of cases, anemia
Erythrocyte sedimentation rate (ESR)	Elevated during acute phase
Platelets	Elevated
Serum IgE	Elevated
Urinalysis	Cellular casts with renal involvement; proteinuria >500 mg/24 h with glomerular disease; hematuria
Chest x-ray	Pulmonary infiltrates
Histologic tissue studies (biopsies from symptomatic sites such as the lungs have a greater yield)	Necrotizing vasculitis of medium and small arteries; invasion of tissue by polymorphonuclear leukocytes and monocytes

DIFFERENTIAL DIAGNOSIS

Same as for polyarteritis nodosa (page 237)

NURSING CARE

See pages 241-247.

TEMPORAL ARTERITIS (GIANT CELL ARTERITIS)

Temporal arteritis is a systemic panarteritis that affects the large and medium arteries in elderly people.

Temporal arteritis affects both sexes, although predominantly women. It generally affects individuals older than the fifth decade, and the average age of onset is 70 years. The annual incidence increases with age; there are 1.7 cases per 100,000 in individuals over 50 years of age and 55.5 per 100,000 in those over 80 years.[170]

Although the etiology of temporal arteritis is unknown, immune complex–mediated, cell-mediated, and antibody-mediated mechanisms have been suggested. Temporal arteritis tends to affect any medium or large arteries, with symptoms resulting primarily from the vasculitis of the carotid artery.

PATHOPHYSIOLOGY

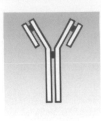

Temporal arteritis differs from other vasculitides in that it does not involve the small vessels such as the arterioles and capillaries. Histologic characteristics include a panarteritis involving mononuclear cells, multinucleated giant cells, polymorphonuclear leukocytes, eosinophils, lymphocytes, and plasma cells. The primary target site is in the interna and media adjacent to the internal elastic lamina of medium arteries. The elastic lamina is fragmented and may be absent in some areas. In the larger arteries and the aorta, the media tends to be inflamed, with fragmentation of the elastic fibers. The intima is thickened, more so than would occur with normal aging. The lesions have a segmental pattern and do not involve long stretches of arteries. Thromboses may occur at any inflammatory site.

Table 8-5

ARTERIAL MANIFESTATIONS IN TEMPORAL ARTERITIS

Artery	Manifestations
Temporal	Temporal pain, headache, marked scalp tenderness, intermittent claudication of jaw and tongue
Aorta	Aneurysm, dissection (low back pain, hypotension, diminished or absent peripheral pulses)
Internal and external carotids	Transient ischemic attacks (dizziness, nausea, loss of vision)
Ophthalmic and central retinal	Insidious or sudden vision loss
Coronary	Myocardial ischemia and infarction (radiating chest pain to neck and left arm, ECG changes, hypotension, dyspnea)
Iliac and femoral	Intermittent claudication of lower extremities
Mesenteric	Abdominal pain, gastrointestinal bleeding, bowel infarction or obstruction

CLINICAL MANIFESTATIONS

The onset of temporal arteritis may be insidious, and it often arises as a coexisting factor with polymyalgia rheumatica. The initial presenting symptoms are nonspecific systemic signs, including malaise, fatigue, anorexia, weight loss, headache, and unexplained fevers. As the disorder progresses, the symptoms commonly are associated with the location of the temporal artery radiating to the neck, jaw, face, or tongue.

Symptoms of claudication are common and occur in certain muscle groups as a result of decreased blood flow caused by the vasculitis. The most common sites of claudication are the muscles of mastication and deglutition, the tongue, and the extremities. Common symptoms of claudication are headache, jaw pain brought on by chewing or talking, visual changes (e.g., transient blurring to complete blindness), ptosis, diplopia, and scalp tenderness. Other symptoms may include hair loss, erythema, and necrosis along the temporal artery.

COMPLICATIONS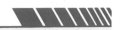

Blindness

DIAGNOSTIC STUDIES AND FINDINGS

Diagnostic Test	Findings
Temporal artery biopsy	Inflammation and characteristic panarteritis
Complete blood count (CBC)	Anemia (normochromic, normocytic), leukocytosis
Platelets	Elevated thrombocytosis
Erythrocyte sedimentation rate (ESR)	>50 mm/h
Serum IgG	Elevated
Acute-phase proteins	Elevated
Alkaline phosphatase	Mildly elevated
Hepatic transaminases	Mildly elevated

*Temporal arteritis should be suspected in any elderly individual who has a fever of unknown etiology and an elevated erythrocyte sedimentation rate.

DIFFERENTIAL DIAGNOSIS

Chronic infections
Connective tissue diseases
Abnormal thyroid function

MEDICAL MANAGEMENT: SYSTEMIC VASCULITIS

GENERAL MANAGEMENT

Follow-up clinic visits: patients should be followed routinely according to their clinical status to monitor for complications and further vascular involvement.

Monitoring of drug side effects of primarily corticosteroids and cyclophosphamide.

Renal function monitoring: blood urea nitrogen (BUN) and creatinine; creatinine clearance; urinalysis for proteinuria >500 mg/day and hematuria.

Blood pressure monitoring: frequent blood pressure checks to assess for hypertension.

Monitoring of eye involvement: regular ophthalmology exams and computed tomography (CT) scans to assess and monitor retroorbital eye involvement as indicated.

Biopsy: affected tissue.

DRUG THERAPY

Corticosteroids, 0.5-1 mg/kg/day in divided doses, tapering gradually over 2-3 mo; cyclophosphamide, 2 mg/kg qd (in severe or fulminant cases); antihypertensive agents (angiotensin-converting enzyme inhibitors [e.g., enalopril, captopril] are most effective with renal involvement); analgesics for acute pain.

1 ASSESS

| | OBSERVATIONS | | | |
ASSESSMENT	POLYARTERITIS NODOSA	WEGENER'S GRANULOMATOSIS	CHURG-STRAUSS SYNDROME	TEMPORAL ARTERITIS
History	Recent infection, especially with hepatitis B	Recent respiratory infection or exposure to environmental allergen	Asthma or other atopic disorders	Polymyalgia rheumatica
General complaints	Fever, weakness, fatigue	Malaise	Weight loss, anorexia, intermittent fever	Malaise, fatigue, anorexia, weight loss, headache, fever
Skin	Subcutaneous nodules along course of arteries on extremities (5-10 mm); purpuric, urticarial exanthema, subcutaneous hemorrhage; ulcerations, livedo reticularis, ischemic changes in distal digits	Subcutaneous nodular lesions with purpuric papules, petechiae, vesicles, and ulcerations	Subcutaneous nodules along course of arteries on extremities; purpuric, urticarial exanthema, subcutaneous hemorrhage; ulcerations, livedo reticularis, ischemic changes in distal digits	Scalp tenderness

→ › ›

ASSESSMENT	OBSERVATIONS			
	POLYARTERITIS NODOSA	WEGENER'S GRANULOMATOSIS	CHURG-STRAUSS SYNDROME	TEMPORAL ARTERITIS
Cardiovascular	Angina, hypertension	Pericarditis: chest pain relieved by sitting up or leaning forward, pericardial friction rub, tachycardia	Angina, hypertension	Claudication of lower extremities, jaw, face, and tongue; radiating chest pain from myocardial ischemia or infarction
Respiratory	Unremarkable	Paranasal sinus pain, sinusitis, purulent or bloody rhinorrhea, nasal mucosa ulceration, septal perforation, saddle-nose deformity, serous otitis media, epistaxis, dyspnea, chronic cough, hemoptysis, pleuritic pain	Asthma, inspiratory and expiratory wheezing, rhonchi; rhinitis (nasal membranes pale, bluish, edematous, and boggy); dyspnea, cough, bronchospasms, pleuritic pain	Unremarkable
Renal	Proteinuria, hematuria, signs of progressive renal failure (increased BUN and creatinine, decreased creatinine clearance)	Hematuria, proteinuria (>500 mg/24 h), progressive glomerulonephritis on biopsy	Proteinuria >500 mg/24 h	Unremarkable
Gastrointestinal	Abdominal pain, anorexia, nausea, vomiting, mucosal ulceration and hemorrhage, steatorrhea	Unremarkable	Abdominal pain, anorexia, nausea, vomiting, mucosal ulceration and hemorrhage, steatorrhea	Anorexia, weight loss, nausea, vomiting, abdominal pain, bloody stools, bloody emesis
Nervous system	Headache, paresthesia, sensory loss, seizures	Cranial neuritis, mononeuritis multiplex	Headache, paresthesia, sensory loss, seizures	Vertigo, transient ischemic attacks
Muscles/joints	Myalgia, arthralgia	Bone pain, arthralgia	Myalgia, arthralgia	Muscle pain in lower extremities, jaw, face, and tongue due to claudication
Ocular	Retinopathy	Mild conjunctivitis (bilateral conjunctival redness, edema, profuse tearing, hyperemia), proptosis, episcleritis, granulomatous sclerouveitis	Retinopathy	Transient blurring to insidious or sudden loss of vision, ptosis, diplopia

	OBSERVATIONS			
ASSESSMENT	POLYARTERITIS NODOSA	WEGENER'S GRANULOMATOSIS	CHURG-STRAUSS SYNDROME	TEMPORAL ARTERITIS
Psychosocial	Anxiety; changes in body image; feels stigmatized	Body image disturbance because of potential for nasal septal perforation and deformity	Anxiety because of difficulty in breathing	Anxiety because of changes in vision

2 DIAGNOSE

NURSING DIAGNOSIS	SUBJECTIVE FINDINGS	OBJECTIVE FINDINGS
Altered cerebral, cardiopulmonary, renal, gastrointestinal, optic, and peripheral tissue perfusion related to decreased blood flow due to vasculitis	Complains of headache, jaw, tongue, and face pain with eating or talking, chest pain, shortness of breath, nasal congestion, dizziness, mildly bloody urine, abdominal pain, nausea, anorexia, changes in visual acuity, muscle cramping, and weakness	**Cerebral:** changes in sensorium, seizures, scalp tenderness, intermittent claudication of jaw and tongue **Cardiac:** angina, pericardial friction rub, tachycardia, edema, ECG changes, hypertension **Pulmonary:** dyspnea, cough, wheezing, rhonchi, tachypnea, rhinorrhea, sinusitis, pale or bluish nasal mucosa **Renal:** proteinuria, hematuria, elevated BUN and creatinine, decreased urine output and creatinine clearance **Gastrointestinal:** abdominal tenderness with palpation, occult blood in stool, vomiting, weight loss **Optic:** retinal exudate, reddened conjunctivae, excessive tearing, decreased visual acuity, retinopathy **Peripheral:** muscle weakness, intermittent claudication of extremities, muscle atrophy
Impaired skin integrity related to impaired perfusion of cutaneous tissue from peripheral vasculitis	Complains of easy bruising, rash, and painful nodules on extremities	Ecchymosis, purpura, ulcerations, vasculitis lesions, subcutaneous nodules, maculopapular rash, subcutaneous nodules tender to palpation
Sensory/perceptual alterations (visual) related to conjunctivitis, retinopathy, or ophthalmic and retinal arteritis	Complains of altered visual acuity	Diplopia, decreased visual acuity, proptosis, corneal ulceration

→ › ›

NURSING DIAGNOSIS	SUBJECTIVE FINDINGS	OBJECTIVE FINDINGS
Impaired gas exchange related to sinusitis, pleuritic chest pain, and/or granulomatous lung disease	Complains of shortness of breath, sinus pain	Restlessness, confusion progressing to somnolence, dyspnea, tachypnea, breath sounds: decreased at bases, wheezes, rhonchi; hemoptysis, epistaxis; ABGs: Pao_2 <80 mm Hg, pH <7.35, Pco_2 >35 mm Hg
Decreased cardiac output related to myocardial ischemia	Complains of chest pain, fatigue	Skin pallor or cyanosis, diaphoresis, oliguria, arrhythmias, weak peripheral pulses

Other related nursing diagnoses: Pain related to tissue and organ ischemia resulting from vasculitis; **Impaired physical mobility** related to neuritis, paresthesia, myalgias, or muscle weakness; **Anxiety** related to actual and perceived threat to biologic integrity; **Potential for infection** related to altered tissue integrity

3 PLAN

Patient goals

1. The patient will demonstrate improved tissue perfusion and cellular oxygenation.
2. The patient will have intact skin integrity.
3. The patient will have stable or improved visual acuity.
4. The patient will demonstrate improved gas exchange.
5. The patient will demonstrate improved cardiac output.

4 IMPLEMENT

NURSING DIAGNOSIS	NURSING INTERVENTIONS	RATIONALE
Altered cerebral, cardiopulmonary, renal, gastrointestinal, optic, and peripheral tissue perfusion related to decreased blood flow due to vasculitis	Assess for signs and symptoms of altered tissue perfusion. Assess for development of headache, changes in mentation or sensorium, and seizure activity. Perform neurologic checks, observing for signs of altered sensorium.	To determine extent of involvement and to guide therapeutic interventions. To detect cerebral anoxia or cerebral edema. Altered sensorium reflects inadequate cerebral blood flow and change in systemic perfusion.
	Monitor vital signs, peripheral pulses q 1-2 h.	To monitor for hypertension and signs of vasoconstriction and tissue perfusion.
	Monitor ECG.	To detect arrhythmias.
	Auscultate and monitor heart sounds.	To assess for pericardial friction rub (best heard with patient leaning forward in third or fourth intercostal space to left of sternal border or apex).
	Auscultate and monitor breath sounds.	To assess for adequacy of air exchange, adventitious sounds, and pleuritis (dry, rubbing sound; pain with deep breathing or coughing; rapid, shallow respirations).

NURSING DIAGNOSIS	NURSING INTERVENTIONS	RATIONALE
	Monitor intake and output q 1-2 h or as indicated and daily weight; report output <30 ml/h or weight gain >2 kg/day.	To monitor renal function and volume status.
	Monitor renal laboratory results (BUN, creatinine, creatinine clearance); report any changes.	To monitor renal function (elevated BUN and creatinine and decreased creatinine clearance indicate renal insufficiency).
	Check bowel sounds and degree of abdominal pain.	To determine bowel perfusion.
	Perform Hemoccult or guaiac test on all emesis and stool.	To monitor for gastrointestinal blood loss.
	Monitor for retinopathy (changes in visual acuity, night blindness).	To gauge visual acuity and prevent complete loss of vision.
	Check eyes for orbital inflammation.	To facilitate early treatment and minimize vision loss.
	Monitor skin color, temperature, and peripheral pulses.	To determine peripheral perfusion and oxygenation.
	Instruct patient to avoid smoking.	Nicotine causes vasoconstriction and damages intimal cells of both large and small blood vessels.
	Monitor and minimize claudication of the jaw, face, tongue (e.g., assist patient in communicating by providing a writing tablet; provide small, frequent meals).	Decreasing claudication may facilitate communication and promote adequate nutrition.
	Monitor and minimize peripheral claudication by providing a balance between exercise and rest; encourage patient to stop exercising when pain develops.	To decrease claudication and peripheral pain; providing rest between activities promotes completion of ADLs.
Impaired skin integrity related to impaired perfusion of cutaneous tissue from peripheral vasculitis	Inspect skin daily, noting tissue integrity, color, temperature, and capillary refill time; observe for signs of skin breakdown or necrosis.	To detect areas of potential or actual skin breakdown and/or necrosis, allowing early intervention.
	Provide and instruct patient in daily skin care (i.e., wash with a mild soap, rinse completely and pat dry, lubricate skin with lanolin lotions).	To maintain skin integrity and reduce risk of skin breakdown.
	Do not use adhesive tape directly on skin.	To minimize stripping the epidermis when removing tape.
	Treat ulcers as they occur (bed cradle, saline soaks, topical and/or systemic antibiotics, and dressings as ordered).	To minimize or extend ulceration.

→ > ›

NURSING DIAGNOSIS	NURSING INTERVENTIONS	RATIONALE
	Use cotton or wool socks that fit properly.	Cotton and wool absorb moisture, preventing skin breakdown caused by excessive moisture.
	Instruct patient to wear properly fitting shoes and clothing and not to go barefoot when out of bed.	To avoid pressure areas that would interfere with perfusion and circulation and to prevent injury.
Sensory/perceptual alterations (visual) related to conjunctivitis, retinopathy, or ophthalmic and retinal arteritis	Assess degree of visual impairment.	To guide therapeutic intervention.
	Orient patient to bedside equipment by directing his hand over objects and controls.	To encourage independence and minimize risk of injury.
	Raise side rails, and instruct patient to use call light to get up.	To prevent injury.
	Assist patient with ADLs, meals, and ambulation.	To promote good hygiene, adequate nutrition, and exercise.
	Discuss with patient and family life-style needs and adjustments related to decreased visual acuity; refer to local center for the blind and visually impaired.	To identify patient's needs and promote adjustment to altered visual acuity.
Impaired gas exchange related to sinusitis, pleuritic chest pain, and/or granulomatous lung disease	Assess degree of impairment: auscultate lungs for decreased breath sounds, monitor ABGs, note pallor or cyanosis and respiratory distress.	To determine adequacy of gas exchange.
	Administer O_2 as indicated, and monitor patient's response.	To ensure optimum gas exchange and prevent hypoxemia.
	Position patient in optimum body alignment for breathing (semi-Fowler's or high Fowler's position).	To optimize diaphragmatic contraction and improve gas exchange.
	Teach patient abdominal breathing exercises.	To decrease work of breathing.
	Monitor chest x-rays.	To detect degree of granulomas and extent of lung disease.
	Administer pain medications as ordered and monitor patient response.	To minimize pleuritic pain and facilitate breathing and gas exchange.
	Administer antibiotics as ordered, and monitor patient's response.	To treat sinusitis and improve gas exchange.
	Observe for hemoptysis and epistaxis; report to physician.	To detect bleeding and facilitate prompt treatment of possible pulmonary hemorrhage.
Decreased cardiac output related to myocardial ischemia	Check blood pressure, apical pulse, heart rate, respirations, heart and lung sounds, and level of consciousness q 4 h.	To detect early signs and symptoms of decrease in cardiac output.

NURSING DIAGNOSIS	NURSING INTERVENTIONS	RATIONALE
	Maintain bed rest as indicated by clinical condition; elevate head of bed 30-60 degrees; administer O_2 as necessary.	To conserve energy, decrease cardiac workload by decreasing oxygen demand, and facilitate and decrease work of breathing.
	Restrict activity as indicated by condition.	To minimize fatigue, which will increase oxygen demand.
	Monitor ECG for ischemic changes.	Alteration in ST segment of ECG is possible

5 EVALUATE

PATIENT OUTCOME	DATA INDICATING THAT OUTCOME IS REACHED
Tissue perfusion and cellular oxygenation have improved.	Patient is alert and oriented and normotensive; urine output is normal ($\geq$30 ml/h); there is no evidence of GI bleeding; visual acuity has improved; skin is warm and dry and peripheral pulses are palpable.
Skin integrity is maintained.	Skin shows no signs of breakdown or ulceration; patient demonstrates appropriate daily skin care.
Visual acuity has improved.	Patient demonstrates strategies to cope with visual changes and prevent injury.
Gas exchange has improved.	Pa_{O_2} is 80-100 mm Hg, Pco_2 is 35-45 mm Hg; lungs are clear; patient is in no distress and states that breathing is easier.
Cardiac output has improved.	Patient is normotensive; cardiac output is 4-5 L/min; skin is warm and dry; patient can rest quietly without distress.

PATIENT TEACHING

1. Teach the patient about his disease and the associated symptoms and complications.
2. Teach the patient about all procedures and interventions.
3. Teach the patient the name, dosage, purpose, time of administration, and side effects of all medications; emphasize strict adherence to tapering off of steroids.
4. Teach the patient the importance of not smoking and of not promoting further vasoconstriction (e.g., going out in cold weather without warm clothing and gloves).
5. Teach the patient the importance of regular follow-up visits with his primary care provider and the need for routine eye examinations.
6. Instruct the patient to report significant changes in visual acuity, urinary patterns (hematuria, oliguria), sinuses (sinus pain, congestion), breathing and sputum (hemoptysis), or pain.
7. Teach the patient the complications to monitor that are considered emergent, and instruct him to seek immediate intervention (e.g., transient ischemic attacks, severe claudication, sudden visual loss, gastrointestinal bleeding, severe chest pain, fainting, and altered sensorium).
8. Teach the patient how to monitor his blood pressure at home.
9. Instruct the patient in skin care techniques.
10. Instruct the patient in adaptive breathing techniques as indicated.
11. Provide the patient and family with information on home management.
12. Provide the patient with information about community organizations that will assist in home management of the visually impaired.
13. Instruct the patient to carry medical identification, particularly when taking steroids.

CHAPTER 9

Renal Disorders

Goodpasture's Syndrome

Goodpasture's syndrome is an autoimmune disease characterized by three essential elements: diffuse pulmonary hemorrhage, glomerulonephritis, and circulating anti–glomerular basement membrane antibodies (anti-GBM antibodies). It is caused by anti–basement membrane antibodies that develop an affinity for the pulmonary and renal systems.

Goodpasture's syndrome was first described by Ernest Goodpasture in 1919 in the case of an 18-year-old man who died from an influenzal illness. The diagnostic findings of this illness were proliferative glomerulonephritis, hemoptysis, and alveolar hemorrhage and necrosis.

Currently Goodpasture's syndrome is characterized by pulmonary hemorrhage, glomerulonephritis, and the formation of circulating antibodies to basement membrane antigens. The presence of anti-GBM antibodies in the glomeruli and alveoli suggests that Goodpasture's syndrome is an autoimmune disorder.

The etiology of Goodpasture's syndrome is unknown. However, in 10% to 30% of patients, an upper respiratory infection precedes the onset of the disease. Environmental exposure has also been linked to Goodpasture's syndrome; such exposure may allow foreign antigens to damage alveolar walls, resulting in the release of autoantibody. Specific factors associated with Goodpasture's syndrome and the production of anti–basement membrane antibodies are exposure to mercuric chloride, inhalation of hydrocarbon solvents, and influenza A2 infections.[169]

Goodpasture's syndrome generally occurs in young men between 20 and 40 years of age, although it can occur in any age group and involve either sex. A prominent second grouping of patients comprises primarily women in the fifth decade of life. In this group glomerulonephritis without significant pulmonary involvement is seen more often.

Familial occurrences have also been reported, suggesting a genetic association with HLA-DR2. The simultaneous presence of HLA-DR2 and HLA-B8 has demonstrated a poorer prognosis, primarily because of the more severe crescent formation (see p. 249) in the kidneys.[70,135]

The anti-basement antibody response generally lasts 15 months, as measured by radioimmune assay (RIA). However, it can last from a number of weeks to 5 years. Since Goodpasture's syndrome is for the most part self-limiting, the immunologic stimulus may be transient.

Most patients have only one episode of Goodpasture's syndrome; however, it has been known to recur, even after years of remission and without anti–basement membrane antibodies. Recurrent disease has also been reported in transplanted renal allografts. It is estimated that 30% of patients with Goodpasture's syndrome involving circulating anti–basement membrane antibodies who undergo kidney transplantation will have a recurrence of the disease. Therefore renal transplantation is withheld until the circulating antibodies have disappeared.[70,198] Also, immunosuppression after transplantation has been shown to suppress the recurrence of anti–glomerular basement membrane antibodies.[192]

Goodpasture's syndrome can be a rapidly progressive, fatal disease if accompanied by severe, exsanguinating hemoptysis and acute renal failure. It must be diagnosed and treated promptly. The pulmonary disease associated with Goodpasture's syndrome may be intermittent, whereas the renal disease typically progresses rapidly to renal failure. The prognosis for renal recovery is less favorable in patients who are oliguric, who require dialytic support, or who have crescents in more than 80% of the glomeruli on renal biopsy. In addition, partial renal recovery may progress over time to end-stage renal disease. The mechanism of this progression is not well understood, but it is thought to be nonimmunologic.

PATHOPHYSIOLOGY

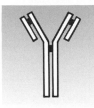

The etiology of anti–basement membrane autoantibody production remains unclear. It occasionally has been considered a type II hypersensitivity reaction, since it involves antibody-mediated cytotoxic effects directed toward normal cells.

Circulating autoantibodies (primarily IgG) are seen in more than 90% of all patients with Goodpasture's syndrome. The anti–basement membrane antibody appears to have a particular affinity for the pulmonary and renal systems, possibly because of their blood flow characteristics and filtration functions. These autoantibodies are directed against and bind mainly to the basement membranes of the renal tubules, renal glomeruli, and pulmonary alveoli.

As a result of antibody deposition in the basement membranes, the complement cascade is activated and chemotactic factors are generated to lure a number of inflammatory cells (polymorphonuclear leukocytes and monocytes) into the target area. These inflammatory cells release a variety of potent substances that eventually destroy the target tissue. In addition to anti–basement membrane antibody, it has been suggested that cytokines may play a role in the pathogenesis of Goodpasture's syndrome, specifically interleukin-1, which is released from activated monocytes and attracts fibroblasts into the area, causing further injury and scarring.[140]

Renal Effects

In the kidneys Goodpasture's syndrome is considered a form of rapidly progressive glomerulonephritis. Renal lesions are characterized by either a mild proliferative glomerulonephritis or an extensive, proliferative, necrotizing glomerulonephritis with crescent formation. **Crescents** are small masses of epithelial cells, located primarily between the glomerular capillary bed and Bowman's space, that have mixed with fibrin to form "new moon" structures. Cellular crescents consist of both proliferating urinary epithelial cells and invading tissue macrophages. Crescent formation and renal damage are aggravated by fibrin formation. The fibrin is caused by fibrinogen leaking into Bowman's space via widening gaps in the glomerular basement membrane as a result of the inflammatory process. This leakage causes the fibrinogen to be polymerized into fibrin

CHARACTERISTICS OF GOODPASTURE'S SYNDROME
Glomerulonephritis
Pulmonary hemorrhage
Anti–basement membrane antibody formation

through an enzyme associated with monocytes. Fibrin in the glomerular capillary tissue mixes with the epithelial cells, increasing deposition of crescents throughout the glomeruli and promoting progressive renal damage. The presence of crescents generally is considered an unfavorable finding with regard to renal function.

Pulmonary Effects

The exact cause of lung injury remains unclear. It may occur in the same manner as in the kidneys by nonantibody factors or as a result of anti–basement antibody-antigen immune complexes. Lung biopsy specimens have revealed pulmonary capillaritis with extensive intraalveolar hemorrhage and injury to the alveolar wall manifested by the presence of hyaline membranes, disruption of the alveolar septa, and widening of the alveolar walls by edematous connective tissue, intraalveolar hemosiderin-laden macrophages, and fibrosis of the lung parenchyma.

CLINICAL MANIFESTATIONS

Goodpasture's syndrome is clinically characterized by a triad of symptoms: pulmonary hemorrhage, glomerulonephritis, and formation of circulating anti–basement membrane antibodies. The broad spectrum of system involvement ranges from severe, massive pulmonary hemorrhage with minimal evidence of glomerular disease to fulminant crescentic glomerulonephritis with absent or mild evidence of pulmonary bleeding.

Pulmonary Manifestations

Pulmonary manifestations precede or are found simultaneously with the renal lesion in about 70% of cases. These symptoms include hemoptysis, dyspnea, cough, and bibasilar rales. Hemoptysis can vary from a few flecks of blood to exsanguinating intraalveolar hemorrhage. Bouts of severe hemoptysis that are potentially life threatening are not uncommon. The average time between the first episode of hemoptysis and the onset of renal involvement is approximately 3 months, with a range of a few weeks to several years. Pulmonary remission may occur despite progressive renal failure.

CLINICAL FEATURES OF GOODPASTURE'S SYNDROME

Pulmonary

Pulmonary hemorrhage with or without hemoptysis, ranging from mild to severe

Dyspnea, cough, bibasilar rales

Chest x-ray: hilar infiltrates; may vary with degree of intraalveolar hemorrhage

Bronchoscopy with lavage: hemosiderin-laden macrophages with or without erythrocytes

Renal

Gross or microscopic hematuria

Proteinuria >1 g/24 h

Elevated serum blood urea nitrogen (BUN) and creatinine

Decreased creatinine clearance

Peripheral edema

Renal Manifestations

Glomerular injury often is the result of rapid, progressive renal failure with oliguria. It generally occurs within a few weeks to months of clinical onset. Spontaneous renal recovery is rare, and it is not unusual for a patient to develop end-stage renal disease, necessitating renal replacement therapy, between 1 month and a year after the initial symptoms appear. Clinical manifestations of renal involvement include hematuria, proteinuria, decreased urine output, and varying degrees of peripheral edema. With severe renal involvement symptoms of chronic renal failure may be present (e.g., hypertension, anemia, and calcium/phosphorus imbalances; see box, p. 260). (See also Table 9-1, p. 259).

Other Manifestations

Fever and skin rashes tend to be uncommon, whereas complaints of arthritic pain seem to affect most patients with Goodpasture's syndrome. Anemia and pallor are common and tend to be more severe than the degree of hemoptysis and renal failure would indicate. More frequently a microcytic, hypochromic-type anemia develops that may be the result of extensive intrapulmonary iron sequestration.

COMPLICATIONS

Chronic renal failure
Severe pulmonary hemorrhage and death

DIFFERENTIAL DIAGNOSIS

Other diseases that may manifest pulmonary hemorrhage and renal failure include:

Wegener's granulomatosis
Systemic lupus erythematosus (SLE)
Polyarteritis nodosa
Renal vein thrombosis with pulmonary embolism
Hypersensitivity angiitis
Henoch-Schönlein purpura
Mixed IgG/IgM cryoglobulinemia
Congestive heart failure with uremia
Rheumatoid arthritis with systemic vasculitis
Mixed connective-tissue disease
Legionnaires' disease

DIAGNOSTIC STUDIES AND FINDINGS

Diagnostic Test	Findings
Pathology	
Light microscopy: renal biopsy	*Mild to moderate renal involvement:* focal and segmental glomerular hypercellularity, segmental necrosis of glomerular capillaries, small crescents; *severe renal involvement:* crescentic glomerulonephritis with tubulointerstitial edema and leukocytic infiltration; renal vasculitis is unusual
Immunofluorescence: renal biopsy	IgG antibody deposition with characteristic linear or ribbonlike pattern (rarely linear IgA or IgM; sometimes irregular IgM); in 70% to 80% this is accompanied by linear or segmental complement (C3) in the basement membrane; when this lesion is found in conjunction with crescent formation (>50% of glomeruli with crescents), diagnosis is confirmed

DIAGNOSTIC STUDIES AND FINDINGS—cont'd

Diagnostic Test	Findings
Electron microscopy: renal biopsy	Gaps in glomerular basement membrane: widening of subendothelial space of glomerular capillaries
Light microscopy: lung biopsy	Extensive intraalveolar hemorrhage, disruption of alveolar septa, intraalveolar hemosiderin-laden macrophages
Immunofluorescence: lung biopsy	Linear or segmental deposition of IgG antibody (rarely IgA) along alveolar capillary membranes; possible findings include pulmonary capillaritis with hemorrhage, alveolar wall injury manifested by hyaline membranes, and widening of alveolar walls by edematous connective tissue
Laboratory	
Radioimmunoassay (RIA) (to detect circulating serum anti–glomerular basement membrane antibodies, usually IgG)	90% of patients have circulating IgG anti–basement membrane antibodies that peak at the time of clinical presentation and then decline (less than 2% of patients show false-positive results)
Antinuclear antibodies (ANA)	Rarely seen
Complement C3 level	Normal
Complete blood count (CBC)	Low hematocrit (Hct) (microcytic, hypochromic-type anemia)
Serum iron level	May be low (<60 μg/dl) due to iron sequestration in lungs
Urinalysis	Proteinuria (>1 g/24 h), hematuria, RBC casts
Blood urea nitrogen (BUN)	Elevated
Serum creatinine	Elevated
Creatinine clearance	Decreased
Electrolytes	Depending on extent of renal failure, potassium may be elevated and bicarbonate may be decreased
Other tests	
Chest x-ray	Pulmonary bleeding (detected by fluffy hilar and basilar infiltrates), pulmonary edema
Sputum (broncholavage)	Hemosiderin-laden macrophages, nonspecific finding
Carbon monoxide (CO) uptake	CO has a high affinity for hemoglobin; uptake of inhaled CO is increased and excretion of CO is decreased with pulmonary bleeding

---

MEDICAL MANAGEMENT

The exact mechanism of autoantibody elimination is not known. However, patients who are treated aggressively early in the course of the disease with a combination of plasmapheresis, corticosteroids, and cytotoxic agents are more likely to recover. Approximately 20% of patients regain normal renal function; more than 50% have some degree of renal insufficiency. The greater the number of glomeruli affected by crescent formation, the less likely the chance of renal recovery.

GENERAL MANAGEMENT

Activity: Ensure bed rest during acute phase, with progressive increase in activity.

Nutrition: Provide adequate nutrition; consider altering protein, fluid, sodium, and potassium intake with regard to renal function; use parenteral support if necessary.

Monitor vital signs: Particularly blood pressure for hypertension secondary to progressive renal insufficiency

Pulmonary: Monitor pulmonary status.

Arterial blood gases: measure daily or as clinically indicated.

Serial chest x-rays: used to assess and monitor extent of intrapulmonary hemorrhage and pulmonary edema caused by bleeding.

Encourage patient to stop smoking cigarettes (cigarette smoking increases the risk of hemoptysis).

Continued.

MEDICAL MANAGEMENT—cont'd

Oxygen therapy and assisted ventilation are used if necessary.

Renal: Monitor renal function daily (BUN, serum creatinine, electrolytes); check creatinine clearance weekly.

Monitor Hct, Hb for anemia, and circulating anti—basement membrane autoantibody.

Renal biopsy may be performed to confirm diagnosis.

DRUG THERAPY

Corticosteroids often are administered in combination with cytotoxic agents.

Corticosteroids

Methylprednisolone: "pulse therapy": 7-15 mg/kg/day IV in divided doses for 3-5 days, followed by low-dose maintenance therapy, particularly in patients with hemoptysis.

Prednisone: 1-2 mg/kg PO, tapering over 2-3 wk to maintenance dosage.

Cytotoxic agents

Cyclophosphamide, 1-2 mg/kg/day; should not exceed 3 mo of therapy; not recommended in the elderly.

Azathioprine (Imuran), 1-2 mg/kg/day.

Erythropoietin: To stimulate red blood cell maturation (dose variable) in renal failure.

Anticoagulants: These medications are low on the list of therapeutic options and should not be administered during periods of active bleeding. Heparin or warfarin may help reduce the generation of fibrin as a component of crescent formation in the kidneys.

ADJUNCTIVE THERAPY

Plasmapheresis: To remove anti—basement membrane autoantibodies; 3-4 L plasma exchanges daily for 7-14 days.

Immunoabsorption using staphylococcal protein A to remove circulating anti—basement membrane antibodies.[149]

Renal replacement therapy

Dialysis support may be indicated in patients with progressive renal failure.

Continuous arteriovenous hemofiltration (CAVH) may be used in patients with renal failure who demonstrate severe cardiopulmonary compromise.

End-stage renal disease mandates chronic renal replacement therapy (transplantation, hemodialysis, or peritoneal dialysis).

SURGERY

Renal transplantation may be used to treat renal failure after the circulating anti—basement membrane antibodies have disappeared. Bilateral nephrectomy before transplantation is no longer indicated.

1 ASSESS

ASSESSMENT	OBSERVATIONS
History	Recent upper respiratory infection
Respiratory	Tachypnea; dyspnea; labored breathing; diffuse, bilateral crackles; cough with or without hemoptysis, may progress to nasal flaring, orthopnea, decreased vital capacity, confusion, restlessness, and exsanguinating hemoptysis
Renal	Decreased urine output, anuria (<30 ml/h in adults), oliguria (approximately 0.5 ml/kg/h), hematuria, proteinuria
Musculoskeletal	Generalized mild to moderate joint and muscular pain
Hematologic	Pallor; microcytic, hypochromic anemia
Psychosocial	Fear of suffocation, chronic renal failure, and dying; anxiety

2 DIAGNOSE

NURSING DIAGNOSIS	SUBJECTIVE FINDINGS	OBJECTIVE FINDINGS
Impaired gas exchange related to alveolar basement membrane changes	Complains of shortness of breath and restlessness; expresses need for additional oxygen; apprehension	Decreased breath sounds; bilateral crackles (rales); dyspnea; tachypnea; productive cough with bloody sputum; *ABGs:* decreased Pa_{O_2} (<75 mm Hg); *chest x-ray:* bilateral interstitial and alveolar infiltrates; restlessness; orthopnea; pallor; diaphoresis
Ineffective airway clearance related to hemoptysis	Complains of difficulty breathing	Crackles (rales), pallor, tachypnea, dyspnea, cough with bloody sputum
Fluid volume excess related to renal insufficiency	Reports a decline in urine output and inability to catch his breath	Peripheral edema; urinary output <30 ml/h; shortness of breath; respiratory rate >30; orthopnea; pulmonary infiltrates and congestion on x-ray; restlessness
Altered renal tissue perfusion related to changes in glomerular basement membrane	Complains of decreased urinary output and weight gain	Urinary output <30 ml/h; hematuria; proteinuria; 2 kg weight gain in 24 h; elevated BUN, creatinine, and potassium

Other related nursing diagnoses: Pain related to arthralgias; **Activity intolerance** related to fatigue; **Fatigue** related to anemia; **Ineffective breathing pattern** related to changes in pulmonary alveoli basement membranes and hemoptysis; **Anxiety** related to dyspnea and renal insufficiency; **Potential for aspiration** related to hemoptysis and changes in level of consciousness due to decreased oxygenation.

→ › ›

3   PLAN

Patient goals

1. The patient's gas exchange will be improved.
2. The patient's airways will remain patent.
3. The patient's respiratory pattern, oxygenation, and blood gas levels will be normal.
4. The patient will have a normal fluid volume status.
5. The patient will have improved renal tissue perfusion and cellular oxygenation.

4   IMPLEMENT

NURSING DIAGNOSIS	NURSING INTERVENTIONS	RATIONALE
Impaired gas exchange related to alveolar basement membrane changes	Auscultate lungs frequently to assess for crackles (rales), rhonchi, and decreased breath sounds at bases.	To assist in determining adequacy of gas exchange and to detect atelectasis.
	Assess respiratory rate and depth.	To determine amount of air being moved and work of breathing; increased respiratory effort may indicate hypoxia.
	Assess and monitor skin color and capillary refill to nail beds.	To determine circulatory adequacy.
	Assess and monitor level of consciousness, restlessness, and irritability.	To detect hypoxia.
	Assess and monitor ABGs.	To identify hypoxia and determine need for supplemental oxygen and acid-base balance.
	Administer oxygen as ordered, and monitor patient response.	To improve pulmonary gas exchange and decrease work of breathing.
	Assess and monitor Hct and Hb.	To detect amount of Hb available to carry oxygen; decreased Hct: <35% in men, <30% in women, <25% in children.
	Administer blood as ordered and monitor patient response.	To increase oxygen-carrying capacity.
	Assess and monitor changes in activity tolerance.	Routine activity may trigger dyspnea.
	Administer corticosteroids as ordered and monitor patient response.	To decrease inflammatory response in basement membrane of alveoli.
	Place patient in high Fowler's position.	To optimize breathing and decrease risk of aspiration.
	Instruct patient to stop smoking.	Nicotine causes vasoconstriction and reduces availability of oxygen.

NURSING DIAGNOSIS	NURSING INTERVENTIONS	RATIONALE
Ineffective airway clearance related to hemoptysis	Auscultate lungs for crackles, rhonchi, or wheezes.	To determine extent of airway obstruction by secretions.
	Assess and monitor sputum characteristics (color, quantity, and consistency).	To detect extent of bleeding (frank red, pink, or brown tinged) and possible infection (thick, tenacious, white, yellow, or green sputum with traces of blood).
	Assist patient with coughing, and teach him effective coughing techniques.	To help remove secretions from airway; ineffective coughing may tire patient.
	Perform nasal, oral, endotracheal, or tracheostomy suctioning as needed.	To stimulate cough reflex and help remove secretions.
	Place patient in high Fowler's position to optimize breathing and assist in removing secretions.	Elevating the head of the bed promotes movement of abdominal contents away from the diaphragm, enhancing diaphragmatic contractions and removal of secretions.
	Teach and assist patient in using incentive inspiratory (blow bottles).	To promote deep breathing and removal of secretions.
	Administer corticosteroids as ordered and monitor patient response.	To decrease inflammation of alveolar basement membrane.
	Provide oral hygiene daily and as needed.	To remove taste of bloody secretions; provide comfort.
Fluid volume excess related to renal insufficiency	Measure and monitor intake and output.	To obtain information on fluid balance status.
	Weigh patient daily.	To monitor changes in fluid status and to detect fluid gain or loss.
	Assess and monitor central venous pressure (CVP) or pulmonary capillary wedge pressure (PCWP).	Elevated pressure indicates increased intravascular fluid volume (normal: CVP, 2-6 cm H_2O; PCWP, 4-12 mm Hg).
	Assess and monitor pulmonary artery pressure (PAP).	To detect increase or decrease in pulmonary congestion (normal systolic PAP 20-30 mm Hg).
	Assess and monitor jugular vein distention.	To detect volume overload.
	Assess and monitor skin turgor and albumin levels.	Peripheral edema may indicate volume overload or decreased albumin.
	Restrict fluids and sodium as ordered.	To prevent accumulation of excess fluid.
Altered renal tissue perfusion related to changes in glomerular basement membrane	Assess and monitor fluid status (measure intake and output hourly, weigh daily, check for peripheral edema, auscultate lungs).	Increased fluid volume may indicate decreased renal function and kidneys' inability to handle excess volume.

→ → →

NURSING DIAGNOSIS	NURSING INTERVENTIONS	RATIONALE
	Administer diuretics as ordered and monitor patient response.	To remove excess fluid volume.
	Assess and monitor BP.	Hypertension may be the result of volume overload or a disruption in the renin-angiotensin mechanism.
	Assess and monitor urine for color and presence of blood and protein.	Proteinuria (>1 g/24 h) or hematuria may indicate changes in the glomerular basement membrane and renal function.
	Monitor urinary specific gravity (SpGr).	(Normal: 1.010-1.025); increased SpGr indicates kidneys' ability to continue to concentrate urine; this is a normal response to decreased renal perfusion. Decreased SpGr reflects kidneys' inability to concentrate urine and indicates renal insufficiency.
	Assess and monitor 24-h creatinine clearance (CrCl).	Decreased CrCl indicates changes in renal function (normal, 85-140 ml/min; mild dysfunction, 50-84 ml/min; moderate dysfunction, 10-49 ml/min; severe dysfunction, 0-10 ml/min).
	Assess and monitor BUN and serum creatinine (SCr).	Increases in BUN and SCr indicate changes in renal function (normal: BUN, 10-25 mg/dl; SCr, 0.5-1.5 mg/dl).
	Assess and monitor potassium (K^+).	Increased K^+ indicates kidneys' inability to excrete excess K^+; causes of elevated K^+ are decreased renal function with associated metabolic acidosis, bleeding, or blood transfusions (normal K^+, 3.5-5 mEq/L).
	Assess and monitor Hct and Hb.	These may be decreased in renal failure due to inadequate secretion of erythropoietin.
	Limit dietary protein to 0.6-1 g/kg/day; recalculate after the initiation of renal replacement therapy.	To decrease metabolic workload on kidneys and accumulation of hydrogen ions and uremic waste products.

5 EVALUATE

PATIENT OUTCOME	DATA INDICATING THAT OUTCOME IS REACHED
Gas exchange has improved.	Lungs are clear, anxiety is decreased, orthopnea and dyspnea have been reduced; respirations have improved; there is no hypoxia; Hb and Hct are normal to supply adequate oxygen carrying.

PATIENT OUTCOME	DATA INDICATING THAT OUTCOME IS REACHED
Blood gases are within normal limits.	Pao_2 is 80-100 mm Hg; $Paco_2$ is 35-45 mm Hg; arterial pH is 7.35-7.45.
Airways are patent.	Breath sounds are clear; breathing occurs without obstruction; chest x-ray is clear; and hemoptysis has subsided; patient demonstrates effective cough techniques.
Fluid volume is within normal limits.	CVP is 2-6 cm H_2O; PCWP is 4-12 mm Hg; breath sounds are clear; there is no evidence of jugular vein distention or peripheral edema; weight remains stable.
Renal tissue perfusion has improved (in severe cases is supported with some type of renal replacement therapy).	Laboratory values are within normal limits: BUN, 10-25 mg/dl; SCr, 0.5-1.5 mg/dl; CrCl, 80-140 ml/min; K^+, 3.5-5.5 mEq/L; urine output is adequate; weight is stable.

PATIENT TEACHING ▪▪▪▪▪▪▪▪▪▪▪▪▪▪▪▪▪▪▪▪▪▪▪▪▪▪▪▪▪▪▪▪▪▪

1. Explain all procedures and treatments as they occur.
2. Teach the patient and family about the disease and the purpose of all treatments.
3. Teach the patient the name, dosage, purpose, and side effects of all medications.
4. Teach the patient about the risks of smoking, and encourage him to avoid using nicotine.
5. Teach the patient effective deep-breathing and coughing techniques.
6. Instruct the patient to obtain a Medic-Alert bracelet if the disease is progressive.
7. In collaboration with the nephrology nurse, teach the patient and family about end-stage renal disease (ESRD), treatment options, and home management when appropriate (see teaching plan for ESRD, page 271).
8. Encourage the patient to obtain regular follow-up care with his health care provider after discharge.

Immune-Complex Glomerulonephritis

Immune-complex glomerulonephritis (ICGN) is caused by circulating antigen-antibody (immune) complexes that produce granular deposits in the glomerulus of the kidney, resulting in tissue damage, renal insufficiency, and subsequent renal failure.

Immune-complex glomerulonephritis is an inflammatory process that affects the glomerular capillaries of the kidneys. Primary ICGN is generally classified histologically according to the glomerular lesion (see Table 9-1). Secondary types of ICGN are those associated with systemic disease (e.g., systemic lupus erythematosus). Immunogenetic factors indicating an increased susceptibility to glomerular disease such as HLA-DR4 and HLA-Bw35 have also been associated with ICGN.

An increasing number of antigen-antibody systems have been identified in ICGN. However, in most cases the causative system is unknown, and testing for specific antigens is extremely difficult. The immune-complex systems that are known to cause ICGN can be characterized as exogenous (foreign) antigens or endogenous (self) antigens. Those considered exogenous include iatrogenic agents (e.g., drugs or foreign serum) and infectious agents (e.g., streptococci or hepatitis B).

Endogenous antigens include nuclear antigens, as in systemic lupus erythematosus; immunoglobulins, as in cryoglobulinemia; or the tumor antigens seen in various neoplasms (see box).

Approximately 75% of all glomerular diseases of the kidneys are the result of an immune-mediated mechanism. The most common antigenic cause of primary ICGN in the United States is acute poststreptococcal glomerulonephritis. It occurs predominantly during childhood and adolescence, with a greater incidence in young boys than girls. The onset usually occurs 1 to 2 weeks after a beta-hemolytic streptococcal infection of the throat or skin. Antistreptococcal antibodies are produced against the antigen and immune complexes formed and deposited in the glomerulus of the kidney. The prognosis often is good, especially for children; however, some patients do subsequently develop end-stage renal disease (ESRD).

PATHOPHYSIOLOGY

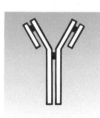 There are basically two types of immune mechanisms that contribute to immune-complex glomerular tissue damage. The first type is the deposition of circulating soluble antigen-antibody complexes in the glomerulus. This type of glomerular damage is the most prevalent, affecting more than 90% of individuals with immunologic glomerulonephritis. The second type of immune mechanism is the formation of antibodies specific for the glomerular basement membrane (circulating anti–glomerular basement membrane antibody), as in Goodpasture's syndrome; this type is responsible for approximately 5% of cases of immunologic glomerulonephritis. This discussion will focus on the first type of immune mechanism.

Soluble antigens that remain in the circulation can combine with antibody to form immune complexes (IC). Generally, immune complexes that demonstrate excess antigen form small immune complexes that are easily removed by the kidneys without harm. Immune complexes with an excess of antibody tend to be large, insoluble complexes that are rapidly removed from the circulation by the mononuclear phagocyte system. Immune complexes that escape clearance by either mechanism are deposited in the glomerular capillaries.

Because of its function as a filter, the glomerulus is highly susceptible to deposition of immune complexes. Factors that influence deposition of immune complexes in the glomerulus include changes in blood flow, systemic clearance of the immune complexes by the mononuclear phagocyte system, the duration of exposure to immune complexes, and the composition and location

(focal or diffuse) of the antigen-antibody complex. Factors within the glomerulus itself include permeability and the electrical charge of the glomerular membrane.

The primary immunoglobulin or antibody involved in immune-complex formation is IgG (sometimes IgA or IgM). The antibody binds with the offending antigen to form immune complexes that are then deposited in the glomerular capillaries. These immune complexes are deposited in a granular formation along the glomerular basement membrane, as seen on electron microscopy. The deposition of immune complexes activates the complement system, which generates the release of anaphylatoxins and chemotaxins; this in turn prompts polymorphonuclear cells (PMNs) to invade the region.

EXAMPLES OF ANTIGEN-ANTIBODY SYSTEMS THOUGHT TO CAUSE IMMUNE-COMPLEX GLOMERULONEPHRITIS

Suspected antigens	Clinical disease
Exogenous	
Iatrogenic causes	
Foreign serum, certain drugs, inoculations	Serum sickness
Bacterial causes	
Nephritogenic streptococci	Poststreptococcal GN
Staphylococcus aureus	Staphylococcal infection
Enterococci	Endocarditis
Alpha-hemolytic streptococci	
Salmonella typhosa	Typhoid fever
Mycoplasmata	Pneumonia
Parasitic causes	
Toxoplasma gondii	Toxoplasmosis
Fungal causes	
Candida albicans	Candidiasis
Viral causes	
Hepatitis B virus (HBsAg, HBcAg, HBeAg)	Hepatitis
Measles	Measles
Epstein-Barr virus (EBV)	EBV infection
Cytomegalovirus (CMV)	CMV infection
Endogenous antigens	
Nuclear (ANA)	SLE
Immunoglobulin	Cryoglobulinemia
Thyroid	Hashimoto's

From Wilson et al[192]; Brenner and Rector.[27]

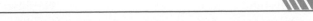

Table 9-1

MAJOR TYPES OF IMMUNE-COMPLEX GLOMERULONEPHRITIS

Glomerular lesion	Example of associated disease	Clinical symptoms
Membranous glomerulonephritis (GN)	Systemic diseases (e.g., SLE)	Proteinuria with nephrotic syndrome, generally associated with neoplasm; may progress to ESRD, predominantly in older adolescence or adults
Membranoproliferative GN	Renal vein thrombosis; nephrotic syndrome; cryoglobulinemia; sarcoidosis; hypocomplementemia	Proteinuria, hematuria, hypertension, generally progresses to ESRD
Diffuse proliferative GN	Poststreptococcal GN; nephrotic syndrome	Severe proteinuria, predominantly in children; usually resolves
	Nonstreptococcal GN	Hematuria, proteinuria; may progress to ESRD
Diffuse proliferative GN with crescent formation	Systemic diseases (e.g., SLE), cryoglobulinemia, Henoch-Schönlein purpura	Oliguria or anuria, rapid onset, progressive renal failure; hematuria; proteinuria; RBC casts in urine; appears predominantly in middle adulthood
Focal proliferative GN	IgA nephropathy, SLE, Henoch-Schönlein purpura	Hematuria, proteinuria; occurs in young adults, late adolescence; may progress to ESRD

From Wilson et al[192]; Brenner and Rector[27]; McCance and Huether.[113a]

Infiltration of PMNs into the area causes inflammation and tissue damage through the release of lysosomal enzymes.

Proliferation of the glomerular membrane cells and swelling of the glomerular capillary bed decrease renal blood flow, reduce glomerular filtration, and cause further tissue damage. Membrane damage and impaired glomerular filtration stimulate degranulation and platelet aggregation. Platelets release vasoactive amines, such as serotonin and histamine, which contribute to the already increased glomerular permeability, causing further impairment in filtration. With activation of the coagulation system, fibrin is deposited in Bowman's space, promoting crescent formation (crescents are discussed in the section on Goodpasture's syndrome, page 249).

Glomerular injury results in an increased permeability of the membrane, decreased filtration, and potential loss of the normal negative electrical charge across the membrane. The increased permeability of the glomerular filtration membrane and the loss of its electrical charge allow protein molecules and/or red blood cells to pass into the urine. This is demonstrated clinically as proteinuria or hematuria.

The immune-mediated inflammation caused by the deposition of immune complexes in the glomerular basement membrane results in a decreased glomerular filtration rate and subsequent renal insufficiency and failure.

IgA Nephropathy

IgA nephropathy is a type of glomerulonephritis. It is differentiated by the predominance of IgA immune-complex deposition in the glomerulus. IgA nephropathy occurs primarily in patients with focal glomerulonephritis. The onset frequently occurs after an infectious episode, usually in the oropharynx. Preformed antibodies to the microorganism are produced, and immune complexes are formed with the antibody excess and deposited in the glomerulus. Of the patients with IgA glomerular deposits, approximately 60% will have circulating IgA containing immune complexes.

CLINICAL MANIFESTATIONS

Immune-complex deposition in the glomeruli can produce all types of glomerulonephritis with varying clinical symptoms. The two major urinary manifestations of glomerulonephritis are hematuria with red blood cell

System	Clinical feature	Physiologic explanation
Cardiac	Hyperkalemia with ECG changes; peaked T waves, prolonged PR interval, depressed ST segment, progressing to loss of P wave, widening QRS complex, eventual ventricular fibrillation and cardiac standstill	Inability of kidneys to excrete potassium (K^+); increased dietary intake of potassium; blood transfusions and/or bleeding (RBC breakdown, releasing K^+); acidosis: causes an exchange of ions, the increasing extracellular hydrogen ions diffuse into cells as potassium ions diffuse into the extracellular fluid
	Hypertension	Volume overload; excessive circulatory fluid and sodium; alteration in the angiotensin system
	Congestive heart failure	Persistent volume overload; decreased urinary output
	Pericarditis	Seen in severe azotemia and uremia; uremic toxins accumulate in the pericardial sac, causing irritation and inflammation
Pulmonary	Pulmonary edema	Excessive intravascular volume and fluid overload
	Pleural effusions	Uremic toxins accumulate in the pleura; volume overload
	Pneumonia	Altered immune response
Hematologic	Anemia	Decreased erythropoietin production by the kidneys; RBCs' survival time half of normal due to uremia; GI bleeding due to uremic irritation of gastric membranes; frequent blood sampling (particularly in children)
	Platelet dysfunction and increased bleeding tendencies	Uremic toxins prevent platelet aggregation; loss of factors essential to convert prothrombin to thrombin
	White blood cell dysfunction	Decreased number and function of lymphocytes and decreased chemotactic response by PMNs and monocytes
Gastrointestinal	Anorexia, nausea, vomiting	Uremia, generally worse in the morning due to overnight dehydration and increased uremic toxins; increased urea irritates mucous membranes
	Fetor uremicus (urine smell to the breath)	Excessive salivary urea (converted by the enzyme urease from bacteria on the teeth to ammonia)
	Gum ulcerations; metallic taste in the mouth	Excessive urea accumulation in the mouth
	Gastritis with bleeding	Uremic irritation of gastric membrane
	Constipation	Caused by aluminum hydroxide gels used to bind excess phosphorus
Skeletal	Metastatic calcium/phosphorus calcifications; hyperparathyroidism; osteomalacia; osteoporosis; bone demineralization	Decreased glomerular filtration causes retention of phosphorus, $CaPO_4$ complexes are formed and deposited in various parts of the body; meanwhile, the kidneys are unable to activate vitamin D to its active form, thus interfering with absorption of Ca^{++} from the gastrointestinal tract. Parathormone is secreted in response to low serum Ca^{++}, causing absorption of calcium from the bone to the plasma; symptoms occur with a calcium/phosphorus product >70 mg/dl
Integument	Gray, bronze color	Accumulation of retained urochrome pigments not excreted by the kidneys
	Dry, scaly, and itchy	Decrease in activity of oil glands, size of sweat glands, and perspiration
	Ecchymoses, purpura	Increased capillary fragility due to uremia
	Nails: transverse bands, brittle, break easily	Seen in hypoproteinemic states, decreased albumin

---

Calculation of calcium (Ca^{++})/phosphorus ($PO_4^=$) product:

$$Ca^{++} \times PO_4^= = Ca^{++} PO_4^= \text{ product}$$

$$Ca^{++} (11) \times PO_4^= (8) = 88$$

$$Ca^{++} (10) \times PO_4^= (4) = 40$$

MAJOR MANIFESTATIONS OF CHRONIC RENAL FAILURE—cont'd

System	Clinical feature	Physiologic explanation
Integument —cont'd	Pallor	Anemia due to decreased erythropoietin synthesis
Neurologic	Mental and behavioral changes (shortened memory, decreased attention span, confusion, irritability, depression, delusions)	Encephalopathy due to accumulation of uremic toxins in the brain; stress of chronic illness
	Tremors, twitching, convulsions	Electrolyte disturbances; uremic encephalopathy
	Peripheral neuropathy, cramps, prickly feeling, burning sensation, pain	Decreased nerve conduction secondary to uremic toxins
Endocrine	Increased parathyroid function	Changes in calcium and phosphorus balance
	Increased renin production	Kidneys react to decrease in renal perfusion as a decrease in circulatory volume; renin production is increased as a compensatory mechanism
	Decreased or stunted growth in children	Mechanism is not completely clear (may be due to body's inability to utilize excess growth hormone); changes in protein metabolism; calcium/phosphorus imbalances and skeletal problems; anemia; acidosis
	Gonadal: *adults:* decreased libido; *women:* failure to ovulate, amenorrhea; *men:* decreased potency and testosterone levels, gynecomastia; *children:* failure to reach menarche, produce sperm, or develop secondary sex characteristics	Accumulation of uremic toxins
Metabolic	Carbohydrate and glucose intolerance	Slowed insulin degradation by the kidneys, increasing the half-life of insulin; insensitivity of peripheral tissues to insulin; delayed insulin production by the pancreas
	Hyperlipidemia; elevated triglycerides	Increased triglyceride production related to peripheral resistance to insulin; increased serum insulin causes increased hepatic output of glycerides and decreased activity of the enzyme lipoprotein lipase
	Elevated urea levels (BUN)	Accumulation of end products of protein metabolism and increased nitrogenous waste are reflected in increased BUN
	Metabolic acidosis (pH <7.35)	Kidneys' inability to excrete hydrogen ions; decreased ammonia production by the kidneys, which normally bind and excrete excess hydrogen; retention of acid end products of metabolism, which subsequently use available buffers; failure of the kidneys to produce bicarbonate

TYPES AND CHARACTERISTICS OF GLOMERULAR LESIONS
Focal: alterations in a few interspersed glomeruli while others remain normal
Segmental: alterations in sections of individual glomeruli while other parts remain unaffected
Diffuse: more than 95% of all glomeruli uniformly affected (most common)
Membranous: capillary wall of glomerulus thickens; more than 75% of glomeruli affected
Proliferative: increased number of glomerular cells
Sclerotic: scarring of glomerulus from previous injury
Crescentic: accumulation of proliferating cells in Bowman's space that appear in crescent formation
From Lancaster[96]; McCance and Huether.[113a]

casts and proteinuria, primarily albumin, of greater than 1 g/24 hours. These urinary characteristics are caused by the increased permeability of the glomerular basement membrane and the loss of its negative electrical charge. As a result, red cells, red cell casts, and protein leak through the glomerular membrane, giving the urine a smoky brown color. In contrast, bleeding from lower in the urinary tract produces a pink or red-tinged urine.

As the glomerular filtration rate (GFR) decreases, there is a concomitant decrease in urine output; this leads to progressive fluid retention and edema. Salt and water are reabsorbed, contributing to the increasing intravascular volume and eventual hypertension. As renal function deteriorates, clinical symptoms of chronic renal failure become more significant. The symptoms of chronic renal failure can affect all organs and are primarily due to progressive uremia and excess fluid volume (see box on pp. 260-261). The onset of symptoms related to chronic renal failure varies, but many symptoms are clinically evident when the creatinine clearance is less than 10 ml/min, the blood urea nitrogen is over 100 mg/dl, and the serum creatinine is greater than 10 mg/dl.

Uremia is the accumulation of toxic metabolic waste products that results in the constellation of symptoms related to renal failure.

The prognosis for ICGN varies considerably, depending on the histologic type. Diffuse proliferative types generally carry a worse prognosis than do proliferative or nonproliferative types and usually result in end-stage renal disease (Table 9-1).

COMPLICATIONS

End-stage renal disease (ESRD)
Severe hypertension
Severe proteinuria and hypoalbuminemia (causing extreme edema and anasarca)
Alteration in coagulation factors, leading to venous thrombosis or pulmonary embolism

DIFFERENTIAL DIAGNOSIS

The presence of proteinuria (>1 g/24 h) and urinary casts generally confirms glomerular disease. The differential diagnosis regarding the specific cause of glomerular disease is extensive and must include evaluation of systemic lupus erythematosus (SLE), hypertension, viral hepatitis (particularly hepatitis B), rheumatoid arthritis, cryoglobulinemia, recent streptococcal infection, and familial glomerular disease.

DIAGNOSTIC STUDIES AND FINDINGS

Diagnostic Test	Findings
Renal biopsy	
Immunofluorescence	Granular deposits of immunoglobulin in glomerular capillaries
Electron microscopy	Immune-complex deposition in glomerulus
Blood urea nitrogen (BUN)	Elevated with increased renal damage
Serum creatinine (SCr)	Elevated with increased renal damage
Creatinine clearance (CrCl)	Decreased (measure of GFR and glomerular damage)
Serum electrolytes	Potassium (K^+) may be elevated; bicarbonate decreased
Complete blood count (CBC)	May demonstrate decreased Hct secondary to reduced erythropoietin production and elevated WBC if infection is present, otherwise may be decreased
Serum complement	May be decreased
Urinalysis	Proteinuria, RBCs, WBCs, casts
Circulating IgA immunoglobulin	Elevated in IgA nephropathy
Antibodies for common infections	May be positive (e.g., hepatitis)
Antinuclear and anti-DNA antibodies	May be elevated (e.g., SLE, progressive sclerosis)
Rheumatoid factor	May be elevated with systemic disorder
Nephritic factor	May be elevated in membranoproliferative GN

MEDICAL MANAGEMENT

The goal of medical management is to preserve renal function, eliminate the source of antigen, and decrease the specific antibody production.

GENERAL MANAGEMENT

Treat the primary disease.

Monitor renal function and blood pressure: Increased serum creatinine and BUN with a decrease in creatinine clearance and elevated BP indicates progressive renal insufficiency.

Activity: Ensure bed rest during acute phase, with progressive increase in activity as tolerated.

Nutrition: Varies depending on renal function and type of renal replacement therapy (RRT); decreased renal function requires limited sodium and fluids with protein and potassium restrictions (protein: 0.6-1 g/kg/day [children may require slightly more for growth]; potassium should be limited in cases of hyperkalemia to approximately 20-50 mEq/day); after initiation of RRT diet should be reevaluated.

Fluid and electrolytes: Restrict fluids and sodium with decreasing renal function; use ECG monitoring if hyperkalemia is suspected; use chest x-ray to assess pulmonary congestion or edema.

DRUG THERAPY

Corticosteroids: To decrease antibody production and suppress inflammatory process.

Methylprednisolone: "pulse therapy," 7-15 mg/kg/day IV in divided doses for 3-7 days.

Prednisone, 1-2 mg/kg PO, tapering over 2-3 wk to maintenance dosage of 0.3-0.5 mg/kg/day.

Cytotoxic agents: To destroy and prevent lymphocyte proliferation.

Cyclophosphamide, 1-2 mg/kg/day PO; not to exceed 3 mo of therapy.

Azathioprine (Imuran), 1-2 mg/kg/day PO.

Continued.

Antibiotics: To treat underlying infections that may contribute to immune-complex responses.

Diuretics: (To promote diuresis and urine formation and flow) Lasix is the most commonly used diuretic in renal disease. It is classified as a loop diuretic, meaning it alters the sodium and water reabsorption from the ascending loop of Henle. Dosage varies according to the patient's size and the extent of renal damage (10 mg qd to 50 mg tid).

Antihypertensives: To treat blood pressure elevations that develop secondary to decreased renal function as a result of increased vascular volume or renin production.

Angiotensin inhibitors: enalapril (Vasotec), captopril (Capoten).

Vasodilators: *direct action:* hydralazine (Apresoline), nitroprusside (Nipride); *calcium channel blockers:* diltiazem (Cardizem), nifedipine (Procardia), verapamil (Isoptin).

Sympatholytics: *central acting:* clonidine (Catapres), methyldopa (Aldomet); *beta-adrenergic blockers:* propranolol (Inderal), nadolol (Corgard), metoprolol (Lopressor); *alpha-adrenergic blockers:* terazosin (Vasocard), prazosin (Minipress); *combined alpha- and beta-adrenergic blockers:* labetalol (Normodyne); *ganglionic blockers:* trimethaphan (Arfonad); *norepinephrine depletors:* reserpine (Serpasil).

Agents to treat hyperkalemia

Lasix is effective in treating mild hyperkalemia; sodium polystyrene sulfonate (Kayexalate) with 70% sorbital, 15 g qd-bid PO or enema, in 50 ml of palatable fluids; sodium bicarbonate, 2-5 mEq/kg IV, infuse over 4-6 h; glucose 50% 25-50 g IV and regular insulin 10-15 U IV (this often is only a temporary emergency measure and generally is followed with dialysis).

Erythropoietin: to stimulate red blood cell maturation (dose varies).

Anticoagulants: Used occasionally to control fibrin crescent formation.

ADJUNCTIVE THERAPY

Plasmapheresis.

Renal replacement therapy: dialysis (hemodialysis, peritoneal dialysis) or transplantation; acutely, continuous arteriovenous hemofiltration (CAVH) may be used.

1 ASSESS

ASSESSMENT	OBSERVATIONS
History	Recent infection (e.g., strep throat, hepatitis B), fever, chills; known systemic diseases (e.g., SLE); familial incidence of glomerular disease
General	Lethargy, malaise, fatigue
Renal	Proteinuria (>1 g/24 h); hematuria with red cell casts; decreased urine output (<0.5 ml/kg/h); increased BUN and serum creatinine; decreased creatinine clearance; weight gain (>2 kg in 24 h)

ASSESSMENT	OBSERVATIONS
Hematologic	Anemia; decreased Hct; pallor
Skin	Peripheral edema ($\geq$ +2), pallor, easy bruising, ecchymosis, increased dryness
Cardiovascular	Hypertension; elevated BP (infants <2 yr, $\geq$110/70; children, $\geq$120/78; adolescents, $\geq$130/80; adults, $\geq$140/90); ECG changes with peaked T waves, K^+ >5.5 mEq/L
Level of activity	Decreased, unable to perform routine activities
Psychosocial	Fear of chronic renal failure and dependency

2 DIAGNOSE

NURSING DIAGNOSIS	SUBJECTIVE FINDINGS	OBJECTIVE FINDINGS
Altered renal tissue perfusion related to immune-complex deposition in glomerulus	Complains of rapid weight gain and feeling weak	Fluid weight gain $\geq$2 kg/24 h; urine output <30 ml/h; microscopic hematuria +2; proteinuria >1 g/24 h; elevated BUN >25 mg/dl; elevated SCr >1.2 mg/dl; K^+ >5.5 mEq/L; decreased 24-hour creatinine clearance
Fluid volume excess related to decreased renal function	Complains of skin feeling tight and puffy and of decreased urine output	Fluid weight gain; decreased urine output; 2+ peripheral edema; elevated BP
Activity intolerance related to fatigue, generalized malaise, hyperkalemia, and/or anemia	Complains of inability to perform routine activities and decreased energy level	Hct decreased; K^+ elevated; patient is lethargic, listless, apathetic, and irritable and remains in bed more hours than usual
Altered nutrition: less than body requirements related to fatigue and progressive renal insufficiency	Reports inadequate intake and feeling too tired to eat	Body weight loss; inadequate intake; appears tired; poor muscle mass; albumin <3.5 g/dl; decreased triceps skin fold (men <16.5 mm, women <12.5 mm); decreased midarm circumference (men <29.3 cm, women <25.8 cm)
Anxiety related to threat of renal failure	Reports fear of impending renal failure and renal replacement therapy (RRT)	Appears worried, restless; shows facial tension; asks many questions about renal failure and RRT

Other related nursing diagnoses: Ineffective breathing pattern related to pulmonary edema due to volume overload and renal insufficiency; **Ineffective individual or family coping** related to potential life-style changes due to impending end-stage renal disease.

> > >

3 PLAN

Patient goals

1. The patient will have improved renal tissue perfusion and cellular oxygenation.
2. The patient will have a normal fluid balance.
3. The patient will have sufficient energy to engage in routine activities or will adapt to decreased energy levels.
4. The patient will maintain an adequate nutritional state.
5. The patient's anxiety will be relieved.

4 IMPLEMENT

NURSING DIAGNOSIS	NURSING INTERVENTIONS	RATIONALE
Altered renal tissue perfusion related to immune-complex deposition in glomerulus	Monitor and record weight daily.	Weight gain >2 kg or 2,000 ml/24 h may indicate decreased renal function and kidneys' inability to manage excess fluid.
	Monitor and record intake and output.	To avoid fluid overload.
	Assess and monitor BUN, creatinine, and CrCl (normal: BUN, 10-25 mg/dl; SCr, 0.5-1.5 mg/dl; CrCl, 85-140 ml/min).	These indicate degree of renal insufficiency; will assist in guiding therapeutic interventions and when to initiate renal failure education.
	Assess and monitor urine for color and the presence of blood and protein.	Brown-tinged urine with hematuria and proteinuria indicates glomerular damage.
	Limit protein and potassium intake based on renal function.	To decrease excretory load on kidneys and possible accumulation of urea, H^+, and K^+.
	Assess and monitor serum potassium and monitor ECG if potassium is elevated.	Increased K^+ indicates inability of the kidneys to excrete excess K^+, increased K^+ may interfere with cardiac contractility.
	Monitor specific gravity (SpGr).	(Normal 1.01-1.25); decreased SpGr indicates kidneys' inability to concentrate urine and demonstrates renal insufficiency.
	Assess and monitor Hct and Hb.	These may be decreased with progressive renal failure due to inadequate secretion of erythropoietin.
	In collaboration with the nephrology nurse, prepare patient and family for access (vascular or peritoneal) and renal replacement therapy.	To provide support and educate patient and family.
Fluid volume excess related to decreased renal function	Weigh patient daily (bid for pediatric patients).	To obtain information on fluid balance status.

NURSING DIAGNOSIS	NURSING INTERVENTIONS	RATIONALE
	Maintain accurate record of hourly intake and output.	To assess kidney function and avoid volume overload and to obtain information on fluid balance status.
	Assess and monitor central venous pressure (CVP).	(Normal, 3-6 cm H_2O); elevated CVP indicates increased intravascular volume.
	Assess and monitor pulmonary artery pressure (PAP).	To detect increase or decrease in pulmonary congestion.
	Assess jugular vein distention.	Distention indicates increased intravascular volume.
	Assess skin turgor.	Peripheral edema may indicate volume overload.
	Restrict sodium and fluids (fluid restriction is limited to 5-7 ml/kg/day plus urine output).	To prevent volume overload and pulmonary compromise.
	Administer diuretics as ordered and monitor response.	To remove excess fluid.
	Monitor BP.	Increased intravascular fluid may cause hypertension.
	Administer antihypertensive agents as ordered, and monitor BP.	To maintain normal BP.
	Auscultate lungs frequently for decreased breath sounds, crackles (rales), rhonchi, dyspnea.	To monitor for possible pulmonary congestion or edema.
Activity intolerance related to fatigue, generalized malaise, hyperkalemia, and/or anemia	Observe response to activity.	To determine extent of tolerance and to assist in guiding therapy.
	Perform activities for patient until he can perform them.	To meet patient's needs without causing him fatigue.
	Progressively increase activities as tolerated; consult exercise physiologist to develop an exercise plan.	To slowly increase endurance for activities.
	Plan rest periods between activities.	To reduce fatigue by providing periods of rest and sleep.
	Provide positive feedback about progress.	To motivate patient to continue progressive activity.
	Keep frequently used objects within reach.	To make them convenient for patient and to decrease oxygen demand.

NURSING DIAGNOSIS	NURSING INTERVENTIONS	RATIONALE
	Identify factors that may contribute to activity intolerance (e.g., hyperkalemia, anemia, stress, side effects of drugs, lack of sleep).	To guide selection of therapeutic intervention.
	Assess and monitor potassium.	Increased potassium can cause muscle weakness.
	Administer Kayexalate to decrease serum potassium as ordered, and monitor patient response.	Kayexalate is an exchange resin that works in the gastrointestinal tract to remove K^+ in exchange for sodium; elevated K^+ may cause fatigue.
	In collaboration with dietitian, teach patient and family about low-potassium diet.	To prevent indiscreet ingestion of excess potassium from the diet.
	Assess and monitor Hct and Hb.	Low Hct (anemia) due to reduced erythropoietin production may contribute to fatigue.
	Administer erythropoietin (Epogen), and monitor iron stores as ordered.	To stimulate RBC production to increase Hct; may decrease fatigue.
	Problem-solve with patient to identify methods of conserving energy while performing routine tasks (e.g., sit while bathing, rest for 15 min between activities).	To identify ways to conserve energy and minimize fatigue; incorporates patient into process and promotes self-care.
Altered nutrition: less than body requirements related to fatigue and progressive renal insufficiency	Assess dietary habits and needs by instructing patient in how to keep a diet diary.	To identify current dietary habits and assist in providing individual diet regimen.
	In collaboration with dietitian and patient, provide diet instruction using individualized plan.	To provide correct information about caloric needs and to incorporate patient into process, thus promoting self-care.
	Weigh patient weekly.	To obtain data on nutritional adequacy.
	Auscultate bowel sounds.	To document gastrointestinal peristalsis.
	Monitor albumin and lymphocytes.	These indicate visceral protein (albumin <3.5 g/dl; lymphocytes <2100 or 30% of leukocytes) and assist in assessment of adequate nutrition.
	Measure midarm circumference.	This is an indicator of protein stores.
	Measure triceps skin folds.	These indicate fat stores.
	Encourage rest before meals.	To decrease fatigue during meals.
	Encourage oral care before meals.	To reduce uremic taste that may alter appetite.

NURSING DIAGNOSIS	NURSING INTERVENTIONS	RATIONALE
	Administer zinc as ordered and monitor patient response.	May improve sensation of taste with severe renal insufficiency or failure.
	Offer small, frequent meals. Reevaluate after initiation of RRT.	To decrease fatigue and ensure adequate nutrition.
	Provide low-protein diet (0.6-1 g/kg/day). Reevaluate after the initiation of RRT.	To decrease metabolic stress on kidneys and production of uremic toxins that may cause anorexia.
	Provide high-carbohydrate diet.	To ensure adequate calories.
	Assess and monitor for nausea and vomiting.	Increasing uremic toxins irritate the gastrointestinal tract and can cause nausea and vomiting.
Anxiety related to threat of renal failure	Assess patient's level of anxiety (mild, moderate, severe, panic).	To determine type and extent of interventions required to reduce anxiety.
	Help patient identify coping skills that have been useful in the past.	To facilitate problem-solving and self-care.
	Encourage patient and family to ask questions and express feelings.	To relieve anxiety and help patient and family to put their feelings and thoughts into perspective.
	In collaboration with nephrology nurse, provide accurate, adequate information about renal insufficiency or failure, procedures, and treatment plan.	Knowledge may decrease anxiety.
	Remain with patient during procedures and if patient is very anxious; stay calm; use reassuring voice.	To provide support and comfort.
	Instruct patient in relaxation and stress-reduction techniques (e.g., visualization).	To facilitate relaxation and decrease anxiety.
	Provide patient with information about support groups and organizations available to patient and family (e.g., National Kidney Foundation, American Kidney Fund).	For long-term community-based support and ongoing education.

5 EVALUATE

PATIENT OUTCOME	DATA INDICATING THAT OUTCOME IS REACHED
Renal tissue perfusion has improved.	Urine output is normal; BUN, creatinine, and electrolytes are normal; creatinine clearance is normal; weight is stable; there is no peripheral edema; breath sounds are clear.
Fluid status is within normal limits.	Weight is stable; intake and output balance is stable; chest x-ray shows no evidence of excess fluid; breath sounds are clear; there is no evidence of jugular vein distention; CVP, PAP are within normal limits.
Patient's activity level has improved, or he has adapted to decreased energy level.	Patient engages in routine activities or is able to seek assistance independently; he reports a feeling of improved well-being.
Patient's anxiety has resolved.	Patient appears calm and demonstrates initial steps of acceptance regarding renal insufficiency.

PATIENT TEACHING

1. Teach the patient and family about both normal renal function and immune-complex glomerulonephritis.
2. Teach the patient and family about prescribed medications (e.g., corticosteroids, diuretics, antihypertensive agents): name, purpose, dosage, side effects, and administration.
3. Teach the patient and family the signs and symptoms of hyperkalemia and where and when to obtain medical assistance.
4. In collaboration with the dietician, teach the patient and family the dietary regimen, the rationale for dietary changes, and how to keep a diet diary.
5. Teach the patient how to monitor urine output, peripheral edema, and respiratory patterns.
6. Teach the patient and family the importance of checking his weight daily.
7. Teach the patient relaxation and stress-reduction techniques.
8. Inform the patient and family about community resources for further education and support.
9. Encourage regular follow-up care with the patient's primary health care provider.
10. Encourage the patient to obtain a Medic-Alert bracelet if renal failure continues to progress.
11. When appropriate, in collaboration with the nephrology nurse, teach the patient and family about end-stage renal disease and renal replacement therapies (see box, p. 271).

MAJOR COMPONENTS OF END-STAGE RENAL DISEASE (ESRD) PATIENT AND FAMILY TEACHING PLAN

Topic	Content
Introduction	Determine patient/family readiness; present purpose of the program; review patient's expectations and discuss patient's and family's feelings about ESRD.
Normal urinary tract and kidney Renal failure	Anatomy (structure); physiology (function); types (e.g., Goodpasture's syndrome, SLE, poststreptococcal infection, other infections); causes (e.g., autoimmune, immune-complex deposition, hypertension, drugs).
Interpretation of laboratory values	Normal renal and related laboratory values; significance of abnormal laboratory values.
Dietary regimen (varies with RRT)	Protein: 0.6-1 g/kg/day, slightly more for pediatric patients; potassium: 1-3 mEq/day; sodium: no added salt; fluids: 5-7 ml/kg in addition to urine output; calories: sufficient for normal body function (depends on size, gender, and age); develop individual dietary plan.
Medication regimen	For every drug review purpose, side effects, dosage, time and method of administration, financial resources.
Treatment options	
Hemodialysis	In center or home (assisted or total self-care).
Access for hemodialysis	External shunt; internal arteriovenous fistula; graft; double-lumen catheter.
Peritoneal dialysis	Peritoneal dialysis: continuous ambulatory peritoneal dialysis (CAPD); intermittent peritoneal dialysis (IPD); continuous cycling peritoneal dialysis (CCPD).
Access using a peritoneal catheter	Peritoneal catheter placement.
Principles of dialysis	Principles of hemodialysis and peritoneal dialysis; procedures for each type of dialysis; complications of peritoneal dialysis and hemodialysis.
Transplantation	Types: living related (LRT), cadaveric (CRT), living nonrelated (LNRT); basic principles; operative procedure; postoperative course and complications; long-term management.
Complications of ESRD	Review every organ system for cause of complication; signs and symptoms; diagnostic process; treatment; prognosis; prevention (e.g., hyperkalemia, pulmonary edema).
Available resources	Family, friends; health care community; financial; spiritual; organizations.
Program evaluation	

From Lancaster[96]; Lancaster[97]; Richards.[142a]

CHAPTER 10

Neurologic Disorders

Multiple Sclerosis

Multiple sclerosis (MS) is a chronic relapsing neurologic disease of unknown cause or cure. It is characterized by disseminating inflammatory demyelination in the central nervous system (CNS) thought to be caused by a defect in the immunoregulatory system.

ETIOLOGY

The etiology of MS is thought to be a defect in the immune-regulatory system. However, current understanding of the disease is continually being revised by new findings. To date there are four hypotheses of the etiology of MS: epidemiologic, genetic, viral, and immunologic.

Epidemiology Theory

The incidence of MS in the United States is 40 to 60 cases per 10,000 population. There is a higher prevalence in the Great Lakes region, the northern Atlantic states, and the Pacific Northwest. Worldwide the disease is seen more often in western Europe, southern Canada, southern Australia, and New Zealand. Because the prevalence of MS is low in warmer climates and higher in colder climates, geographic areas close to the equator have a lower incidence. Local epidemics have also been described, indicating the possibility of a transmissible cause. Geographic prevalence in certain areas of the world may indicate an epidemiologic relationship between individuals affected with MS and where they live.[79c]

Individuals who move from areas of higher MS prevalence to areas of lower prevalence after 15 years of age retain the risk of MS associated with their previous environment. However, individuals younger than 15 years of age acquire the risk of the new environment, an indication of a possible epidemiologic cause of MS.[79c]

Most individuals diagnosed with MS are women, with a male-to-female ratio of 1:2 to 1:3. MS occurs in all races but predominates among Caucasians. Clinical onset of the disease occurs between 20 and 40 years of age in 75% of cases. It is rare in childhood, and the incidence decreases significantly after age 55. This distribution in age may suggest that a critical event (e.g., possible viral exposure) occurs during adolescence and is a predisposing factor to the onset of MS.

Genetic Theory

MS does not clearly exhibit a defined genetic inheritance; however, it is 15 times more likely to occur in first-degree relatives of affected individuals than in the general population. Also, an individual who has an identical twin with MS has a 20% greater risk of acquiring the disease, which is 300 times greater than that of the general population.

MS has also been associated with specific HLA antigens that may indicate a link to an MS susceptibility gene. In the northern European and North American populations, a significant association has been demonstrated with HLA-A3 and HLA-B7, with higher associations to HLA DR2 and HLA-DQw1. According to the genetic theory of MS, the specific haplotype marker for the disease increases the risk of altering the immune response to a viral infection. This alteration causes an interaction between the central nervous system and the immune system that subsequently precipitates the demyelinating process.[79c,113a]

Viral Theory

A number of viruses have been implicated as possible causes of MS. It is thought that the virus is acquired early in life and causes a slow, progressive viral infection over time.

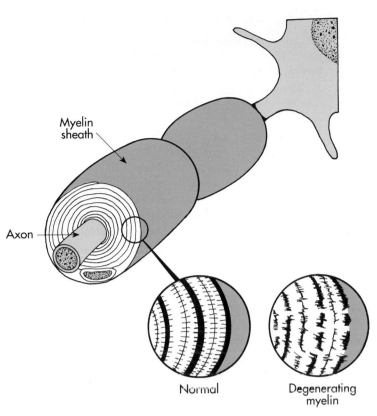

FIGURE 10-1
In multiple sclerosis the myelin sheath is progressively destroyed until the myelin is totally disrupted and the axon is nonfunctional.

Information that supports a viral etiology includes the presence of specific antibodies in the cerebral spinal fluid (CSF), viral DNA or RNA in brain tissue or mononuclear cells, and specific viral isolation. The most recent research has suggested a retrovirus, specifically the human T-cell leukemia/lymphoma virus, type 1 (HTLV-1), as a possible etiologic cause. However, further investigation needs to be done to confirm this possibility.[120]

Viruses or other antigens are thought to attack the myelin directly, causing a hypersensitivity reaction that destroys the myelin or the oligodendrogliocytes. This may or may not have an immunogenetic cause.

Autoimmune or Immunoregulatory Defects Theory

Defects in the immunoregulatory system suggest that MS is an immunologic disorder. It has been hypothesized to be a T cell–mediated autoimmune disease, primarily because suppressor T lymphocyte function is altered. This can be demonstrated by decreased suppressor T cell function during periods of exacerbation, accompanied by rebound elevation and function during remissions. Although the specific antigen is unknown, it is thought to be a component of myelin, possibly a protein.

The autoimmune theory is further supported by the response of the disease to immunosuppressive drugs (e.g., corticosteroids and alpha- and beta-interferons). These drugs are thought to inhibit the synthesis of gamma-interferon, thus altering its immunostimulatory effects. These medications may also be effective in preventing periods of exacerbation.

Findings that support an immunoregulatory hypothesis include the following:[79b,120]

1. Acute-stage plaques demonstrate lesions similar to those in cell-mediated immune responses.
2. Plasma cells that produce antibodies to myelin, as well as viral antigen, are present in the serum, cerebrospinal fluid, and plaques.
3. Activated macrophages are abundant in plaques; they release proteinases (enzymes) and phagocytize the myelin sheath.
4. Increased levels of IgG have been demonstrated in the cerebrospinal fluid.
5. T lymphocytes that react with viruses are present in the cerebrospinal fluid.
6. Several abnormalities in immunoregulatory T lymphocytes are noted in the serum and cerebrospinal fluid that may be responsible for the defective regulation of IgG synthesis in the nervous system (i.e., loss of CD4 suppressor-inducer cells; decreased CD8 T-cell subsets [inconsistent finding]; excessive numbers of activated T cells in the blood and cerebrospinal

fluid; absence of killer T-cell precursors in the cerebrospinal fluid that are specific for the measles virus [which are present in controls]; and abnormal suppressor T-cell function in the acute and chronic progressive phases).

PATHOPHYSIOLOGY

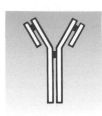

MS damages the myelin sheath of the body's central nervous system (CNS). The myelin sheath is a white fatty tissue that surrounds most of the axons of the nervous system; it acts as an insulator and promotes the conduction of nerve impulses. In MS only the white fibrous tracts of the central nervous system (the brain and the spinal cord) are affected. As the myelin is damaged, it is replaced first by lymphocytes and then by sclerotic tissue. Initially the myelin sheath continues to transmit impulses. However, as the disease progresses, the myelin sheath is permanently destroyed and replaced with scar tissue, resulting in significant interference in neural transmission.

The proposed pathologic features of MS include two processes: the interaction between the immune system and the central nervous system, and the formation of demyelinating lesions.

Interaction of the Immune System and the Central Nervous System

The immunoregulatory response that occurs in MS is not completely understood. It may be directed toward antigens of a virus infection or an unknown autoantigen of myelin or oligodendroglial cells. When the immune response is triggered, it causes a mild, recurrent inflammatory reaction. The inflammation causes a vasculitis that breaks down the blood-brain barrier. This allows B lymphocytes to enter the central nervous system during a period of exacerbation. When the inflammation subsides, the lymphocytes become trapped in the CNS. B lymphocytes then colonize within the central nervous system and secrete IgG antibody directed against the invading antigen (e.g., possible virus). Both central nervous system and systemic IgG can be detected on electrophoresis. Although useful in assisting with the diagnosis of MS, an elevated level of IgG in the cerebrospinal fluid and oligoclonal IgG bands are seen in other diseases as well and are not specific for MS.

The number of suppressor T cells in the serum of individuals with MS varies. The suppressor T-cell count tends to be depressed during periods of onset and exacerbation; otherwise, the count is normal.

Formation of Lesions of Multiple Sclerosis

It is unknown whether the lesions of MS are a cause or an effect of the interaction between the central nervous system and the immune system.

The pathology of plaque formation involves a number of processes, including breakdown of the myelin structure, lysis of oligodendrocytes, and activation of astroglial processes.

The plaques or lesions of MS involve the white matter of the central nervous system. These neuropathologic lesions are primarily confined to the CNS. They are multifocal plaques of demyelination that are distributed randomly within the white matter of the cerebrum, cerebellum, brainstem, and spinal cord. In the initial stages of the disease, these plaques consist of perivascular infiltrates of T lymphocytes and macrophages. Chronic lesions demonstrate further macrophage-mediated demyelination and increased reactive astrocytes. Plasma cells in the plaque lesions secrete oligoclonal IgG antibody into the extracellular fluid and cerebrospinal fluid.

Plaque formation has two stages, the acute (or early) stage and the chronic (or late) stage.

Acute stage. Plaque formation during the acute, or early, stage is the process of perivascular infiltration of T lymphocytes and macrophages. This occurs in conjunction with perivenular demyelination, primarily around the third and fourth ventricles. A mild lymphocytic meningitis accompanies these changes. The external surface of the brain appears normal, but the ventricles may be enlarged and brain weight may be diminished. The inflammatory edema in and around the plaque and partial demyelination are thought to cause the neurologic symptoms of MS.

Chronic stage. Plaque formation and the process of demyelination are characterized by a proliferation of astrocytic processes and degeneration of axons, which

---

Demyelination is the process whereby the myelin sheath and myelin sheath cells are destroyed. Demyelination causes four significant changes in the central nervous system: decreased nerve conduction velocity, nerve conduction block, differential rate of transmission of impulses, and complete failure of impulse transmission. These changes predispose the individual with MS to the numerous signs and symptoms of the disease. During a remission, demyelinated areas are healed with fibrotic tissue. If the nerve fiber is destroyed during the demyelination process, the symptoms are permanent.

lead to glial scarring. Plasma cells within the plaques secrete oligoclonal IgG antibody into the cerebrospinal fluid and extracellular fluid. Neurologic defects progress over years, with subsequent loss of function and increasing disability.

CLINICAL MANIFESTATIONS

The clinical manifestations of MS vary considerably and are characterized by periods of exacerbation and remission. How they manifest clinically depends on the area of CNS involvement. Initial symptoms generally manifest involvement of the cerebrum, the cerebellum, the brainstem, or the spinal cord. After several years, these patients show symptoms of mixed CNS involvement. Symptoms are caused by plaque formation and myelin loss in the white matter of the brain, usually in the periventricular area, which is thought to prevent conduction of nerve impulses.

Symptoms may develop acutely, with a rapid onset, or chronically, over several years. Acute exacerbations develop over a few days and persist for days or weeks, with eventual recovery. Chronic exacerbations develop at varying intervals, with less-than-complete recovery and decreasing function. The frequency of exacerbations varies considerably, depending on the individual. Generally the average rate of exacerbations is approximately one every other year. In some patients one or two exacerbations characterize the disease for a lifetime, whereas in others the course is a chronic progression of increasing disability. Approximately 60% of individuals with MS are fully functional at 10 years; 25% to 30% are functional 30 years after onset.[9]

Increased body temperature, infection, elevated serum calcium levels, and stress are factors that contribute to periods of exacerbation. Increases in body temperature and serum calcium levels cause leakage through the demyelinated neurons, aggravating the symptoms of MS. Infection tends to stimulate the immune system. Stress, both physical and emotional, can increase the symptoms of MS by imposing functional demands that may exceed the conduction capacity of the demyelinated neurons.

Increases in body temperature can be external (e.g., hot bath, sunbathing) or internal (fever). Although heat may exacerbate symptoms, it does not contribute to the disease process itself.

SIGNS AND SYMPTOMS OF MULTIPLE SCLEROSIS

Motor	Sensory	Cognitive	Psychologic
Muscle weakness (90%)	Numbness	Decreased short-term memory	Depression (30%-40%)
Muscle spasticity	Vertigo	Decreased ability to solve abstract problems	Anxiety
Nystagmus (70%)	Diplopia		Denial
Ataxia	Blurred vision	Poor judgment	Frustration
Intention tremor	Eyeball pain	Intellectual changes	Restlessness
Fatigue (>90%)	Scotomas	Inability to concentrate	Anger
Constipation	Impaired color perception	Confusion	Apathy
Bladder dysfunction (80%-90%) (urgency, hesitancy, incontinence)	Decreased hearing	Disorientation	Irritability
Dysarthria	Paresthesia		Instability, dementia, euphoria
Dysphagia	Loss of sphincter control		
Seizures	Facial sensory deficit		
Men: neurogenic impotence; premature, delayed ejaculation	Hemisensory loss, sexual dysfunction (90%)		
Women: diminished orgasmic response	Decreased libido, impaired genital sensation, sexual dysfunction (70%)		

BLADDER PROBLEMS ASSOCIATED WITH MULTIPLE SCLEROSIS

Problem	Cause	Symptom
Urgency	Decreased sensation of bladder fullness	Sensation of needing to empty bladder immediately
	Overstimulation of bladder with frequent messages	Inability to control or hold urine after sensation is felt
	Inability of bladder to suppress involuntary reflex contractions that normally occur	Intermittent expulsion of urine
	Spasticity (bladder contracts normally, but external sphincter does not relax)	Intermittent incontinence
Frequency	Same as in urgency	Increase in number of voids per day
Dribbling	Decreased external sphincter control; bladder fullness gives way to pressure	Frequent leakage of urine from bladder in small amounts
Hesitancy	Simultaneous bladder and external sphincter contraction	Difficulty in voiding after sensation to void is felt
Residual	Decreased bladder sensation of fullness with progressive loss of contraction reflex	Incomplete emptying of bladder
Incontinence	Simultaneous involuntary control of external sphincter and relaxation of bladder	Involuntary and unpredictable passage of urine

From Clark, 1991; Thompson et al, 1989; Kelly and Mahon, 1988.

COMPLICATIONS

Aspiration
Pneumonia
Respiratory failure
Infection
Contractures
Psychosis
Complications of immobility

DIFFERENTIAL DIAGNOSIS

CNS structural lesions
Neurosyphilis
Sarcoidosis
Systemic lupus erythematosus (SLE)
Sjögren's syndrome
Lyme disease

DIAGNOSTIC STUDIES AND FINDINGS

Diagnostic test	Findings
Lumbar puncture	
Cerebrospinal fluid specimen	
Electrophoresis	>90% have oligoclonal IgG bands
IgG antibody	75% have increased levels
Gamma globulin	Elevated
Protein	Normal or elevated

There is no single diagnostic test for MS. Diagnosis is based on a complete history and physical and a comprehensive neurologic examination, supported by information from the tests listed here.

Diagnostic test	Findings
White blood count (WBC)	Elevated
VDRL	Negative
Radioimmunoassay (RIA)	Myelin protein
Serum IgG antibody	Elevated
Serum antibody titers	Titers to many viruses may be elevated (e.g., herpes simplex type 1, parainfluenza, rubella, mumps, measles, Epstein-Barr virus)
Computed tomography (CT) scan	Areas of low attenuation around cerebral ventricles; may show ventricular enlargement and cerebral atrophy
Magnetic resonance imaging (MRI) studies	Visualization of plaques in cerebral white matter and brainstem lesions not detected by CT
Evoked response studies	Decreased conduction velocity in visual, auditory, and somatosensory pathways
Positron emission tomography (PET) studies	May show altered locations and patterns of cerebral glucose metabolism

MEDICAL MANAGEMENT

The goals of medical management are to preserve function and prevent complications.

GENERAL MANAGEMENT

Activity: Promote routine activity with a regular exercise program (consult with exercise physiologist or physical therapist); use braces, splints, cane, walker, or wheelchair when necessary to maintain optimum functioning.

Nutrition: Maintain optimum nutritional intake (consult dietician).

Promote independence: Consult occupational therapist and home nursing service and, when necessary, extended-care facilities.

Cognitive or psychologic support: Consult psychiatrist, assess medications, and refer patient to support groups.

Visual support: Teach use of aids and eye patch; refer patient to Association of the Blind.

Urinary impairment: Monitor for infection; institute bladder training program.

Dysphagia/dysphasia: Refer to speech therapist; with risk of aspiration, institute tube feedings when necessary to maintain nutritional intake.

DRUG THERAPY

Antiinflammatory drugs (used during periods of exacerbation and for maintenance therapy during remissions): corticosteroids: prednisone, 0.5-1 mg/kg/day in divided doses, taper to maintenance dosage; prednisolone, dexamethasone (Decadron), 0.75-9 mg/day, taper to maintenance dosage; methylprednisolone (Solu-Medrol), "pulse therapy" 1-2 mg/kg/day IV in divided doses for 3-7 days; adrenocorticotropic hormone (ACTH, Athcar), 40-50 U bid for 7-10 days.

Immunosuppressive drugs (currently under investigation): cyclophosphamide (Cytoxan), cyclosporine (Sandimmune), azathioprine (Imuran), alpha- and beta-interferons, monoclonal antibodies.

Continued.

MEDICAL MANAGEMENT—CONT'D

Antispasmodic drugs: Baclofen (Lioresal), 15-25 mg PO tid; diazepam (Valium), 5-10 mg PO qid; dantrolene (Dantrium), 25 mg PO qid maintenance dosage increased to 400 mg/day; cyclobenzaprine (Flexeril), 10mg tid.

Tremor-reducing drugs: Beta-adrenergic blocking agents; propranolol (Inderal), 40-240 mg/day PO; primidone (Mysoline), 100 mg qd, increase to 250 mg tid; isoniazid (INH), 5 mg/kg/day, maximum 30 mg qd; trihexyphenidyl (Artane), 1-15 mg qd; hydroxyzine (Vistaril), 50-100 mg qd in divided doses.

Drugs to minimize bladder dysfunction: Hyporeflexia causing urinary retention: cholinergic drugs: bethanechol (Urecholine), 10-50 mg tid. Hyperreflexia causing frequency and urgency: anticholinergics: propantheline (Pro-Banthine), 20-75 mg qd in divided doses; oxybutynin (Ditropan), 1-5 mg qid; imipramine (Tofranil), 50-150 mg qd.

Drugs to decrease fatigue: Amantadine (Symmetrel), 100-200 mg qd; methylphenidate (Ritalin) 20-60 mg qd in divided doses (should not be taken after 6 PM).

Drugs to decrease pain: Carbamazepine (Tegretol), 200 mg bid, increase to 800-1200 mg qd in divided doses; amitriptyline (Elavil), 25-150 mg qd in divided doses; imipramine (Tofranil), 100-300 mg qd in divided doses; antiinflammatory drugs (acetaminophen, aspirin, ibuprofen).

Antibiotics: To treat infections, particularly urinary tract infections.

ADJUNCTIVE THERAPY

Physical therapy; occupational therapy; hydrotherapy; speech therapy; sexual therapy; plasmapheresis.

SURGERY

Contralateral thalamotomy to relieve pain, tremors, and rigidity; rhizotomy to relieve intractable pain; penile implants for impotence; gastrostomy tube placement for nutritional support.

---

1 ASSESS

ASSESSMENT	OBSERVATIONS
History	Emotional or physical stress, recent infection, exposure to heat
Motor	Initial presentation demonstrates weakness in lower extremities; impaired motor function after a hot bath or shower (Uhthoff sign); uncoordinated movements, hyperactive reflexes; intention tremors of upper extremity; ataxia of lower extremities; staggering gait; intermittent spastic weakness of speech muscles; dysphasia and dysphagia; facial palsy; nystagmus; loss of sphincter control (urinary and later bowel incontinence)
Sensory	Numbness and tingling in involved extremity or the face; loss of joint sensation and proprioception; loss of sensation of position, shape, texture, and vibration (50%); eye pain and diplopia; vertigo; decreased libido
Psychologic/ cognitive	Emotional lability, irritability, depression, changes in memory

2 DIAGNOSE

NURSING DIAGNOSIS	SUBJECTIVE FINDINGS	OBJECTIVE FINDINGS
Impaired physical mobility related to muscle weakness and fatigue	Complains of difficulty walking and controlling movements	Spasticity and tremors; focal motor deficits; intention tremor with purposeful movements
Activity intolerance related to fatigue and CNS involvement	Reports inability to perform activities of daily living (ADLs), fatigue, and tremors with exertion	Progressive muscle atrophy, psychomotor incoordination, listlessness
Altered patterns of urinary elimination (functional, stress, and urge incontinence, and retention) related to altered nerve impulse transmission	Complains of urgency and intermittent urinary incontinence	Urinary incontinence, decreased bladder sensation, >150 ml residual urine after voiding
Potential for urinary tract infection related to catheterization and residual urine	Reports urinary frequency, dysuria	Residual urine >150 ml; *urinalysis:* bacteriuria; elevated WBC; microhematuria; cloudy, turbid urine; fever; serum WBC >10,000
Altered thought processes related to altered nerve innervation	Reports forgetfulness and memory loss	Slowness in thinking and problem solving, altered judgment, short-term memory loss
Impaired verbal communication related to speech disturbances	Complains of inability to express self and articulate words	Slurred, jerky speech pattern; slow speech with decreased fluency; tremors of lips, tongue, and jaw; faint voice with fluctuations in volume
Sensory-perceptual alterations (visual) related to optic nerve demyelination	Reports decreased vision in one eye; complains of seeing double (diplopia) and having blurred vision	Diplopia, nystagmus, optic neuritis; able to identify only large objects
Altered nutrition: less than body requirements related to decreased intake associated with dysphagia, tremors, and fatigue	Reports inability to eat due to shaking, lack of appetite, and fear of swallowing	Weight loss, albumin <3.5 g/dl, poor muscle mass, anorexia, dysphagia, and hand tremors
Potential ineffective individual coping related to multiple stressors	Reports feelings of uselessness and lack of control over life	Lack of social support systems and adequate resources

→ › ›

NURSING DIAGNOSIS	SUBJECTIVE FINDINGS	OBJECTIVE FINDINGS
Impaired home maintenance related to activity intolerance, inadequate finances, and lack of knowledge about resources	Reports inability to care for self	Lives alone with minimal or no help; has limited financial resources
Self-care deficit in all ADLs related to progressive dysfunction, mental changes, and neurologic impairment	Reports inability to care for self	Remains in bed much of the day; decreased participation in self-care activities; has neglected appearance
Sexual dysfunction related to altered nerve innervation	Reports difficulty with sexual function; decrease in libido and desire for intimacy; fatigue	

Other related nursing diagnoses: Altered family processes related to role changes; **Social isolation** related to deteriorating function; **Impaired swallowing** related to progressive dysphagia; **Body image disturbance** related to incontinence and ataxia; **Powerlessness** related to progressive debilitation and perceived lack of control over disease outcome and health care management; **Bowel incontinence** related to progressive neuromuscular impairment; **Chronic pain** related to altered nerve transmission.

3 PLAN

Patient goals

1. The patient will remain mobile without weakness or fatigue.
2. The patient will develop a pattern of activity and rest.
3. The patient will participate in energy-sparing activities.
4. The patient will obtain adequate sleep and rest.
5. Urinary incontinence and retention will be resolved, or the patient will develop strategies for management.
6. The patient will show no signs of urinary tract infection.
7. The effects of altered thought processes will have a minimal effect on the patient's life.
8. Communication will be maximized; the patient will develop strategies to improve speech or communicate needs by nonspeech methods.
9. The patient will demonstrate restored visual acuity or will develop strategies for coping with visual impairments.
10. The patient will have adequate caloric and nutritional intake to meet metabolic needs; her weight will remain stable or increase to optimum level.
11. The patient will develop methods of coping with multiple stressors.
12. The patient will identify factors that she can control and make informed decisions about health care needs and legal and financial support.
13. The patient will develop strategies for home maintenance and will maximize resources.
14. The patient will increase her ability to complete ADLs or develop strategies and explore resources to assist in coping with self-care and routine activities.
15. The patient and significant other will participate in satisfying sexual activities.

4 IMPLEMENT

NURSING DIAGNOSIS	NURSING INTERVENTIONS	RATIONALE
Impaired physical mobility related to muscle weakness and fatigue	Assess range of motion (ROM) and level of mobility.	To establish baseline and guide therapeutic interventions.
	Consult with exercise physiologist, physical therapist, and occupational therapist to develop daily exercise program in collaboration with patient.	Professional health team members provide an important service in complex care; a routine exercise program will assist in maintaining a maximum level of mobility.
	Encourage patient to participate in a routine exercise program.	Exercise may improve ROM, strengthen muscles, relieve spasms, increase coordination, and provide training to substitute nonaffected muscles for those that are impaired.
	Encourage patient to participate in an independent stretching program.	To temporarily relieve spasticity and promote muscle strength.
	Teach patient the importance of balancing periods of rest and activity, and ensure such balance.	Overwhelming fatigue occurs in over 85% of patients; balancing rest and activity decreases feelings of weakness and fatigue.
	Problem solve with patient to determine strategies for decreasing fatigue (e.g., fatigue occurs most often in the afternoon, so the most demanding activities should be performed in the morning).	To identify ways to conserve energy, thereby decreasing fatigue and weakness.
	Advise patient to avoid rigorous activity.	Rigorous activity increases fatigue and weakness and core body temperature, which could provoke an exacerbation.
	Turn or reposition patient q 2 h; provide support to back and joints.	To prevent complications of immobility.
	Provide passive ROM exercises.	To prevent contractures and temporarily relieve spasticity, which is the cause of an imbalance in muscle groups resulting in contraction and relaxation simultaneously; spasticity requires excess energy and causes weakness and fatigue.
	Provide hydrotherapy; use tepid water.	Water often permits movements that otherwise may be impossible; tepid water is used because hotter water may elicit an exacerbation.
	Do not use heat on affected muscles.	Heat may increase body's core temperature and cause an exacerbation of symptoms.
	Apply splints to affected extremities.	To maintain mobility and function of affected limb.

NURSING DIAGNOSIS	NURSING INTERVENTIONS	RATIONALE
	Administer antispasmodic medications as ordered and monitor patient's response.	To decrease spasticity and fatigue.
Activity intolerance related to fatigue and CNS involvement	Assess past and present activity pattern.	To assist in guiding therapeutic interventions.
	Monitor response to activity.	To determine extent of tolerance, which may vary at different times during the day.
	Help patient develop a daily schedule that balances activity with periods of rest.	Additional rest is necessary to prevent overwhelming fatigue.
	Encourage patient to exercise muscles not affected by MS.	To help decrease general fatigue.
	Provide care and perform activities that patient cannot perform.	Progressive debilitation may interfere with patient's ability to perform ADLs; patient's needs are met without contributing to fatigue.
	Structure nursing care to provide for periods of uninterrupted rest.	Increased rest is necessary to prevent fatigue.
	Encourage friends and family to support patient in efforts to perform ADLs and routine activities.	As the patient adjusts to a pattern of activity and rest in performing daily activities, the support of family and friends can help the patient avoid fatigue.
	Provide passive and ROM exercises to temporarily relieve spasticity.	Spasticity requires excess energy to perform activities.
	Administer Ritalin or Symmetrel as ordered and monitor patient response.	To decrease fatigue.
Altered patterns of urinary elimination (functional, stress, and urge incontinence, and retention) related to altered nerve impulse transmission	Identify the type of bladder condition by recording frequency and measuring urinary output, followed by residual checks for 48 hours.	To guide therapeutic interventions. Types of bladder conditions: spastic (urgency); flaccid (urgency, frequency, hesitancy, dribbling, incontinence); dyssynergia (hesitancy, incontinence).
	Assess current voiding pattern and factors associated with incontinence episodes.	To assist in guiding therapeutic interventions.
	Develop strategies with the patient to assist in restoring and maintaining continence.	To prevent urinary incontinence.
	Implement techniques to ensure complete bladder emptying (e.g., tapping or stroking bladder, Credé's maneuver [bladder massage], coughing, listening to running water, pouring lukewarm water over perineal area, stimulating anus digitally).	To ensure complete bladder emptying, prevent urinary incontinence, and decrease risk of infection from residual urine.

NURSING DIAGNOSIS	NURSING INTERVENTIONS	RATIONALE
	Establish a timed voiding schedule with fluid intake control (start with q 2 h voids).	To prevent urinary incontinence and gain control over urinary pattern.
	Instruct patient to control fluid intake and balance intake with voiding schedule; patient should receive 2,000-2,500 ml/day.	To assist in scheduling voiding times, to prevent incontinence and possible infection, and to ensure renal perfusion.
	Alter environment to provide accessible toilet facilities (e.g., bedside commode).	To facilitate urinary continence and provide patient with a sense of control.
	Teach patient to use urinary control devices as needed.	To control urinary leakage between toilet trips.
	Help patient and family formulate plans for bladder management during outings (e.g., urinate every hour, use of a diaper pad).	To prevent incontinence and embarrassment.
	If bladder regimen fails, institute clean intermittent catheterization and instruct patient and family in procedure.	To restore urinary continence; intermittent straight catheterization decreases the risk of infection compared to a permanent, indwelling catheter.
	Assess condition of perineal skin, and provide and teach patient routine hygiene.	To prevent irritation and breakdown of perineal skin.
	Administer drugs to minimize bladder dysfunction (e.g., Pro-Banthine) as ordered and monitor patient response.	To promote urinary continence and prevent bladder spasms.
	Teach patient perineal (Kegel) exercises.	To improve muscle tone of urinary sphincter.
Potential for urinary tract infection related to catheterization and residual urine	Assess for history of urinary tract infections (UTIs) and for presenting symptoms.	To assist in guiding therapeutic interventions.
	Assess and monitor patient and urinalysis (UA) for signs of infection (urgency, frequency, dysuria, incontinence, fever, elevated serum WBC; *UA:* bacteriuria; elevated WBC; turbid, cloudy, foul-smelling urine; microhematuria).	To prevent and detect UTIs and to institute appropriate therapy in a timely manner.
	Assess complete bladder emptying by measuring postvoid residual urine with straight catheterization.	To determine amount of residual urine and the need for strategies to ensure complete bladder emptying.
	Ensure complete bladder emptying using the Credé's maneuver, self-catheterization, or double voiding.	To prevent residual urine and the risk of UTI.
	Encourage adequate fluid intake (2,000-2,500 ml/day).	To flush urinary tract and prevent stagnation of residual urine in bladder, which may increase risk of infection.

→ > >

NURSING DIAGNOSIS	NURSING INTERVENTIONS	RATIONALE
	Teach female patients to wipe from front to back, especially after a bowel movement.	To decrease risk of fecal contamination (*Escherichia coli* is the most common cause of UTI and is a normal inhabitant of the intestinal tract).
	Teach patient to avoid synthetic underwear.	Synthetic underwear tends to collect and trap moisture, contributing to the risk of infection.
	Administer 1 g of vitamin C every day as ordered (cranberry juice does not significantly lower urinary pH).	To decrease the pH (acidity) of the urine; alkaline urine promotes infection.
	Administer antibiotics as ordered and monitor patient response.	Prophylactic antibiotics may be necessary with chronic urinary retention and frequent UTI.
Altered thought processes related to altered nerve innervation	Assess cognitive, emotional, and neurologic processes.	To establish baseline functioning and guide therapeutic interventions.
	Provide a structured environment with comfortable, familiar surroundings.	To minimize disorienting stimuli.
	Encourage patient to have familiar people and objects in her environment; reorient as indicated to new events (e.g., provide clocks, calendars, newspaper).	To provide tangible reminders as an aid to memory and to maintain orientation.
	Encourage patient to make a list or write things down.	To prevent or control forgetfulness.
	Develop an outline of daily activities, and structure time.	To provide a familiar routine and control forgetfulness.
	Encourage patient to attempt varying tasks in sequential steps; speak slowly, and offer simple, short instructions.	To ease demands on memory.
	Help patient arrange power of attorney as condition deteriorates.	To handle finances and legal matters.
Impaired verbal communication related to speech disturbances	Assess patient's verbal ability.	To establish baseline and guide therapeutic interventions.
	Advise patient to avoid fatigue and weakness.	Fatigue and weakness contribute to fluctuations in voice volume.
	Encourage proper posture.	To enhance voice volume.
	Encourage patient to speak slowly and to concentrate and stay focused on content of communication.	Slowed speech will increase diction and decrease slurring of words.

NURSING DIAGNOSIS	NURSING INTERVENTIONS	RATIONALE
	Allow patient adequate time to express herself.	To decrease frustration and promote communication.
	Teach patient jaw and facial exercises.	To reduce spasticity and tremors and strengthen unaffected muscle groups.
	Teach patient stress reduction and relaxation exercises.	Stress and tension may contribute to tremors of lips and tongue, thus impeding speech.
	Consult speech therapist.	To obtain help in developing strategies for communication.
	Provide alternative methods of communication (e.g., picture books, magnetic slate).	To provide a means for patient to communicate.
	Administer antispasmotic medications (e.g., Lioresal) as ordered and monitor patient response.	To reduce and control tremors and spasticity.
Sensory-perceptual alterations (visual) related to optic nerve demyelination	Assess degree of visual impairment.	To establish baseline and guide therapeutic interventions.
	Orient patient to environmental surroundings; encourage family and friends to stay with patient as much as possible.	To decrease anxiety and fear, promote independence, and decrease risk of injury.
	Speak to patient often.	To provide sensory stimulation and to improve patient's ability to locate a person in the room.
	Provide meaningful stimuli, and reduce extraneous stimuli in the environment.	To maintain orientation to environment.
	Identify yourself when entering the patient's room.	To promote orientation and decrease anxiety.
	Alternate patching patient's eyes q 2 h as ordered and monitor patient response.	To relieve diplopia; double vision stems from weakness in one or more eye muscles.
	Provide a safe environment.	To prevent injury caused by visual impairment.
	Refer patient with decreased visual acuity to the Association for the Blind or the National MS Society.	These organizations may send a representative to the home to teach the patient and family adaptive strategies.
	Administer tremor-reducing medications (e.g., Inderal) as ordered.	To decrease eye tremors.

NURSING DIAGNOSIS	NURSING INTERVENTIONS	RATIONALE
Altered nutrition: less than body requirements related to decreased intake associated with dysphagia, tremors, and fatigue	Assess dietary habits and needs; encourage patient to keep a diet diary.	To identify current dietary intake and assist in planning an individualized diet.
	Refer patient to nutritionist.	To obtain expert help in devising an individualized meal plan.
	Weigh patient weekly.	To help gauge nutritional adequacy.
	Monitor albumin.	Albumin level indicates visceral protein.
	Encourage rest periods before eating.	To reduce fatigue during meals.
	Provide small, frequent meals.	To decrease fatigue.
	Encourage patient to eat with others.	The support of others helps establish a positive environment for meals.
	Provide a high-protein diet.	To support the immune system.
	Provide a low-fat diet.	To decrease incidence of exacerbations.[172a]
	Encourage patient to use assistive devices (e.g., special eating utensils, plate guards).	To facilitate independent eating patterns.
	Assess availability of food in the home; loss of significant other(s), job, or income and inability to get to the store may be problems.	To identify problems with availability of food and guide appropriate interventions.
	Assess gag and cough reflexes and ability to swallow.	To prevent aspiration.
	Do not give liquids to patients who have difficulty swallowing (provide semisolid food).	Liquids may cause aspiration.
	With progressive difficulty in swallowing, assist with and teach home care and management of nasogastric or gastrostomy tubes.	To ensure optimum nutrition and prevent aspiration.
	Refer patient to speech therapist.	For expert help with strategies for coping with dysphagia.
Potential ineffective individual coping related to multiple stressors	Assess type, number, and degree of stressors.	To guide therapeutic interventions.
	Encourage patient to identify stressors and to verbalize feelings.	To help patient develop an awareness of emotional reactions to stress.
	Help patient set realistic goals for coping with stress.	To facilitate coping.

NURSING DIAGNOSIS	NURSING INTERVENTIONS	RATIONALE
	Help patient identify diversional activities.	To reduce anxiety and stress.
	Help patient identify past behaviors that were effective in coping with stress.	To facilitate patient involvement in problem solving.
Impaired home maintenance related to activity intolerance, inadequate finances, and lack of knowledge about resources	Assess family and home environment.	To establish baseline information and guide therapeutic interventions.
	Assess availability and adequacy of income for someone to come into the home to assist with direct care, housekeeping, shopping, meal preparation, and transportation.	Patient's disability may render her unable to continue home maintenance activities.
	For the hospitalized patient, identify appropriate referrals using the multidisciplinary team.	To reduce risk of readmission and promote independence at home.
	Obtain appropriate equipment to facilitate home maintenance and self-care (e.g., bedside commode, wheelchair ramps).	To facilitate adequate home maintenance and adapt home to promote maximum independence, health, and safety.
	Refer patient to home health nursing agency.	To ensure care and social stimulation.
	Provide patient and family with community resources.	To assist with home maintenance, direct care, financial support (e.g., food stamps), transportation, and social contacts.
	In cases of progressive cognitive disability, refer to halfway house, group home, or foster home.	To promote self care, independence, and social contact.
Self-care deficit in all ADLs related to progressive dysfunction, mental changes, and neurologic impairment	Assess patient's ability to perform ADLs; assess effort involved to complete task.	To establish baseline functioning and guide therapeutic intervention.
	Assist with self-care and ADLs until patient can perform them.	To meet patient's needs and conserve energy.
	Refer patient to occupational therapist for assistive devices and home maintenance equipment.	To encourage independence and self-care.
	Encourage patient to participate in a routine exercise program.	To increase strength of unaffected muscle groups and promote functional ability.
	Teach significant other to assist with or provide ADLs.	To maintain care at home for as long as possible.
Sexual dysfunction related to altered nerve innervation	Assess problem; obtain description of problem in patient's own words.	To clarify patient's perception and guide therapeutic interventions.
	Assess patient's knowledge of the effects of illness or treatment on sexual functioning.	To determine patient's knowledge base.

➜ ➜ ❯

NURSING DIAGNOSIS	NURSING INTERVENTIONS	RATIONALE
	Provide an atmosphere in which discussion of sexual problems is permitted and encouraged.	To facilitate problem solving.
	Discuss importance of open communication with significant other regarding sexual needs and concerns.	To help patient clarify needs and concerns with significant other and promote problem solving between them.
	Encourage patient to explore with significant other alternate methods of sexual gratification and pleasure.	To promote problem solving between the two and to encourage and provide permission to explore alternatives.
	Determine with patient strategies to promote sexual functioning (men: surgical intervention for impotence; women: taping indwelling catheter to abdomen; emptying bowel and bladder before sexual contact; planning sexual contact to minimize fatigue; using K-Y Jelly; using alternative positions; or taking medication before sexual contact to decrease spasticity).	To promote sexual enjoyment and provide strategies to maintain sexual contact with significant other.
	Refer patient for sexual counseling when appropriate.	To provide strategies for promoting sexual functioning.

5   EVALUATE

PATIENT OUTCOME	DATA INDICATING OUTCOME THAT IS REACHED
Patient maintains muscular functioning.	Patient participates in routine exercise program; satisfactory ROM is maintained; muscle mass without atrophy is maintained; and unaffected muscle groups have been strengthened.
Patient can independently perform ADLs or uses modified equipment, strategies, and resources for assistance.	Patient can perform routine ADLs without fatigue; she uses assistive devices to facilitate ADLs (e.g., specialized eating utensils); and she uses community resources to assist with ADLs (e.g., transportation services).
Urinary continence has been restored.	Regular, complete bladder emptying has been achieved; perineal skin is intact; there is no urinary leakage or dribbling; and patient demonstrates strategies for urinary continence (e.g., double voiding, voiding schedule, fluid control, access to toilet).
Urinary retention has been resolved, or patient has developed management strategies.	Less than 150 ml of residual urine is present after voiding; patient demonstrates double-voiding technique and can perform intermittent catheterization.
Patient has no urinary tract infection.	Urine is clear, yellow or amber, without bacteria or elevation in white cells; serum WBC is <10,000; and patient is afebrile.

PATIENT OUTCOME	DATA INDICATING OUTCOME THAT IS REACHED
Effects of altered thought processes on patient's life and routine activities are minimized.	Patient can participate and complete ADLs without evidence of frustration and depression; she has arranged assistance with personal, financial, and legal matters.
Communication with patient is maximized.	Patient can communicate feelings and needs without excess frustration.
Patient's visual capacity has increased, or patient has developed strategies with decreased vision.	No injury ensues related to impaired vision; patient can perform routine activities; and nystagmus is controlled.
Nutritional status has improved.	Food and fluid intake is adequate for metabolic needs; weight has increased and is stable at optimum level; albumin is 3.5-4.5 g/dl; muscle mass has increased; triceps skin fold and midarm circumference have increased.
Patient can cope with and respond to stressful events.	Patient recognizes source of stress and demonstrates effective skills for coping with stress; patient uses resources for help in coping with stress.
Patient participates in self-care activities as possible.	Patient can participate in ADLs and has assistance with shopping, meals, and transportation; she develops a routine of daily activities to promote an optimum living situation (e.g., cleans one room a day, shops one morning a week, does laundry one day a week)
Patient and family are knowledgeable about community and health care resources and services.	Patient and family can describe resources available in the community and how to use them.
Patient's sexual needs are met.	Patient reports plans with significant other to improve sexual activity and describes methods of satisfying sexual expression.

PATIENT TEACHING

1. Instruct the patient and family about the disease, diagnostic procedures, treatments, supportive functional activities, and medications.
2. Teach the patient and family about medications: purpose, dosage, route and time of administration, and side effects.
3. Encourage the patient to keep a diary of her illness (i.e., symptoms, medications, and treatments used).
4. Stress the importance of paced and structured routine activities.
5. Teach the patient to adhere to her activity and rest schedule to prevent overwhelming fatigue.
6. Instruct the patient and family in passive and active ROM exercises.
7. Teach the patient to monitor her response to activity and to alter her activity when the signs and symptoms of excessive fatigue develop.
8. Emphasize the importance of diversional activities to reduce stress and fatigue.
9. Instruct the patient and family in visualization and stress-reducing exercises to prevent overwhelming fatigue and potential periods of exacerbation.

10. Teach the patient and family to clean toiletry device regularly; white vinegar may be used to clean and deodorize the receptacle.
11. Teach the patient and family the Credé method of bladder emptying (apply pressure on the lower abdominal wall, manually compressing the bladder and allowing expulsion of urine).
12. Instruct the patient and family in intermittent catheterization and how to use clean technique at home.
13. Stress the importance of speech therapy to assist with communication.
14. Teach the patient and family forms of communication other than speaking (e.g., pictures, magnet drawing board, using objects to point to, signaling with eye movements).
15. Instruct the family to provide a safe environment to prevent injuries caused by visual impairment.
16. Teach the patient the importance of a balanced diet and to eat after resting.
17. Teach the patient about factors that may cause an exacerbation of symptoms: overexertion, hot baths, excessive sun exposure, fever, emotional or physical stress, high humidity, extreme hot or cold weather, and pregnancy.
18. Instruct the patient in community resources and services and how to use these programs.
19. Instruct the patient in strategies for simplifying ADLs (e.g., allow for periods of rest, develop a routine and schedule, use assistive devices, maximize resources).
20. Teach the patient and significant other methods of achieving sexual satisfaction, or refer to sex counselor.
21. Refer the patient and family to the MS Society.

Myasthenia Gravis

The name **myasthenia gravis (MG)** comes from the Greek words meaning "grave muscle weakness." Myasthenia gravis is a disease of neuromuscular transmission in which autoantibodies are directed against the acetylcholine receptor. It is characterized by abnormal motor weakness of the skeletal muscles that is exacerbated by effort and improves with rest.

EPIDEMIOLOGY

The incidence of myasthenia gravis is approximately 2 to 10 cases in every 100,000 individuals. It occurs at all ages with two distinct age subgroups, 20 to 30 years of age and after age 40 (see box). It is not considered a hereditary disorder; however, 19% of infants born to mothers with MG demonstrate transitory symptoms lasting from 7 to 14 days after birth.[57a] There have also been associations with other autoimmune diseases such as systemic lupus erythematosus (SLE), rheumatoid arthritis, polymyositis, and thyrotoxicosis.

PATHOPHYSIOLOGY

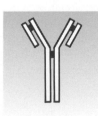

The exact cause of myasthenia gravis is unknown, but it is thought to be an autoimmune disorder. The basic physiologic defect is the inability of the nerve impulses to pass into the skeletal muscle at the myoneural junction. This defect may result from a deficiency in the release of acetylcholine from the presynaptic terminals or from a deficiency in the postsynaptic membrane receptor sites. It is thought characteristically to produce circulating antibodies against acetylcholine receptor host antigen.

Normally acetylcholine attaches to its receptors at the myoneural junction. This attachment changes the electrical potential of muscle cells. The change in electrical potential (depolarization) induces transmission of impulses, which subsequently results in a muscle contraction. This is followed by release of the enzyme cholinesterase, which breaks down the acetylcholine, and the process is terminated.

In myasthenia gravis, anti-acetylcholine receptor antibody is produced and binds to acetylcholine receptors at the postsynaptic membrane of the neuromuscular junction. This blocks the reception of nerve impulses that normally are carried across the junction by acetylcholine molecules. Immune complexes are formed and bind complement, further damaging the postsynaptic membrane site. With fewer functional receptor sites available, impulse conduction is diminished and muscle contraction is impaired.

No evidence has emerged that myasthenia gravis is a disease of the central or peripheral nervous systems, and generally no loss of sensation results.

CLINICAL MANIFESTATIONS

Myasthenia gravis has an insidious onset. Initial symptoms often appear during pregnancy, post partum, in

```
┌─────────────────────────────────────────────────────────────┐
│         SUBGROUPS OF MYASTHENIA GRAVIS                       │
└─────────────────────────────────────────────────────────────┘
```

	Onset at 20-30 years of age	Onset after 40 years of age	
Gender predominance	Women	No sex link	Men
Thymus involvement	Not present	Present	Not present
HLA association	HLA-A1, HLA-B8, HLA-DR3	No HLA link	HLA-A3, HLA-B7, HLA-DR2

From Hillel et al [79c]; Thompson et al. [178]

conjunction with the use of anesthetic agents, or during physical or emotional stress. Weakness of the voluntary muscles with repetitive use is the most common clinical feature. The muscles most often affected include the proximal skeletal muscles and the oculomotor, facial, laryngeal and pharyngeal, and respiratory muscles. The clinical course of the disease varies considerably, depending on what muscle groups are affected. Generally weakness begins in the extraocular muscles with ptosis and diplopia and progresses over time to involve other muscle groups. Most symptoms are more prominent at the end of the day when the patient tends to be more fatigued.

The disease is characterized by periods of exacerbation and remission. Exacerbations may be triggered by emotional or physical stress, infection, ultraviolet light, menstruation, or pregnancy. During an acute exacerbation, symptoms often progress quickly and can be life threatening.

The exact function of the thymus gland in myasthe-

```
┌─────────────────────────────────────────────────────────────┐
│      EXAMPLES OF CLINICAL MANIFESTATIONS                    │
│            OF INVOLVED MUSCLES IN MG                         │
└─────────────────────────────────────────────────────────────┘
```

Proximal skeletal muscles (affects approximately 60%)
Lower extremities
Difficulty climbing stairs, rising from a chair or toilet, prolonged walking, getting out of bed

Upper extremities
Difficulty combing or brushing hair, brushing teeth, lifting objects (children, boxes, groceries), reaching for objects (items in a cupboard), pushing objects (vacuum cleaner, lawn mower)

Head *(affects approximately 60%)*
Bobbing of the head up and down, inability to hold head up

Oculomotor muscle (affects approximately 90%)
Ocular palsy, ptosis, diplopia, fatigue with driving or reading

Facial muscles (affects approximately 80%-90%)
Changes in expression, impaired facial mobility, drooling

Pharyngeal/laryngeal muscles (affects approximately 60%)
Dysphagia, nasal speech, slurred speech, weak voice (whisper), choking, aspiration

Respiratory muscles (affects approximately 10%; increases with exacerbation)
Dyspnea, breathlessness, decreased respirations, respiratory failure, decreased tidal volume (V_T) and vital capacity (VC)

Other
Urinary stress incontinence, anal sphincter weakness (diarrhea, constipation)

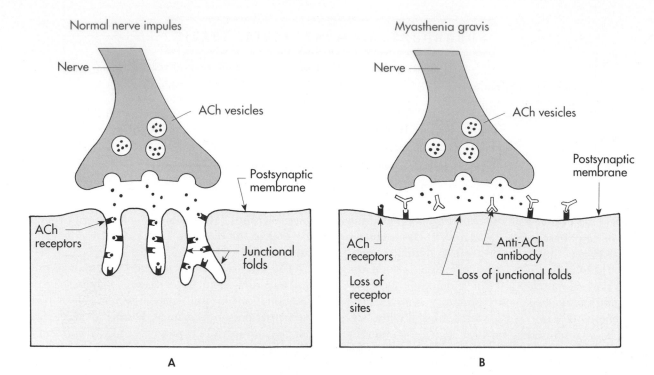

FIGURE 10-2
A, Normally acetylcholine (Ach) is released from the nerve terminal and taken up by the receptors on the junctional folds on the postsynaptic membrane. **B,** In myasthenia gravis anti-acetylcholine receptors (anti Ach R), antibodies, and immune complexes induce complement-mediated destruction of the postsynaptic membrane and loss of junctional folds and receptor sites, reducing the effect of each vesicle.

MYASTHENIA GRAVIS CRISIS

Myasthenia gravis crisis is a medical emergency that is thought to occur when there is a severe decrease in the amount of acetylcholine available or in the postsynaptic membrane receptor sites.

Symptoms associated with a myasthenia gravis crisis

Respiratory distress	Impaired anal sphincter	Ptosis
Tachypnea	Diarrhea/constipation	Diplopia
Tachycardia	**Positive response to Tensilon**	Ocular palsy
Restlessness	**test**	Increased muscular weakness
Elevated blood pressure	Dysphagia	Proximal muscle weakness
Fear	Inability to chew	Apprehension
Restlessness	Gag reflex absent	Extreme fatigue
Anxiety	Speech impaired	Facial/head weakness
Stress incontinence	Fever	Masklike expression

CHOLINERGIC CRISIS

Cholinergic crisis is a medical emergency that occurs when excessive amounts of anticholinesterase medications are administered, resulting in an accumulation of acetylcholine.

Symptoms associated with a cholinergic crisis

Respiratory distress
Dyspnea
Bradycardia
Hypotension
Dysphagia (difficulty swallowing)
Dysarthria (impaired speech articulation)
Negative response to Tensilon test

Sweating
Anorexia
Apprehension
Salivation
Nausea/vomiting
Abdominal cramps
Diarrhea

Generalized weakness
Vertigo
Blurred vision
Lacrimation
Diplopia
Muscle spasms
Muscle cramps

nia gravis is unknown. However, approximately 75% of patients with the disease have an enlarged thymus gland, caused by either hyperplasia or a thymoma. Currently 90% of patients who undergo a thymectomy in conjunction with other types of treatments can expect improvement or complete remission within 5 years. This seems to imply that the involvement of the thymus gland may somehow be linked to MG.[79a,79c,136a]

COMPLICATIONS

Respiratory insufficiency and failure
Pulmonary infections from aspiration
Myasthenic crisis (see box)
Cholinergic crisis (see box)
Complications related to immobility

MG: FACTORS THAT MAY EXACERBATE SYMPTOMS

Anticholinesterase therapy
   Cholinergic crisis
   Myasthenic crisis
Extreme hot or cold temperatures
Aerosol cleaner
Quinine water
Excessive alcohol intake
Ultraviolet light
Emotional or physical stress
Hormonal changes (pregnancy, postpartum, menstruation)
Certain medications
   Antibiotics (aminoglycosides)
   Paralytic agents (succinylcholine and curare)
   Analgesics (morphine and meperidine)
   Antiarrhythmics (quinine, quinidine, procainamide)
   General anesthetics (ether)

From Bell[17a], George.[66a]

DIAGNOSTIC STUDIES AND FINDINGS

Diagnostic test	Findings
Edrophonium (Tensilon) test (performed by a physician) (2 mg of Tensilon is injected intravenously, and patient is monitored for improved or progressive muscle weakness and tone; if muscle tone does not change, an additional 8 mg is injected, and changes in muscle tone and weakness are again monitored)	Within 30 sec to 1 min, patients with MG will have a marked increase in muscle tone that lasts about 4-6 min; patients with *known* MG who demonstrate a decrease in muscle tone generally are diagnosed with an anticholinesterase overdose
Serum anti-acetylcholine receptor antibodies	Present in 90% of patients
Anti–striated muscle antibodies	Present; significance is undetermined
Electromyogram (EMG)	Amplitude of action potential of stimulated muscles decreases quickly (muscle fiber contraction with progressive decremental response)
Chest x-ray; computed tomography (CT) scan of chest	May detect thymoma or hyperplasia of thymus gland

MEDICAL MANAGEMENT

GENERAL MANAGEMENT

Activity:　Bed rest during acute phase; refer patient to an exercise physiologist and/or physical therapist for a routine exercise program; encourage a balance between rest and activity.

Nutrition:　Ensure maintenance of an adequate diet; if necessary, implement nasogastric or gastrostomy tube feedings or hyperalimentation in acute situations; consult dietician to optimize dietary intake.

Respiratory support:　With respiratory distress, bronchoscopy, intubation, and mechanical ventilation may be necessary.

Ocular support:　Patch alternating eyes to decrease diplopia and ocular fatigue.

Stress management:　Consult occupational therapist or psychiatrist; encourage patient to participate in a stress-management program.

Speech therapy:　Refer patient for management of dysphagia and speech strengthening to prevent aspiration and improve communication.

DRUG THERAPY

The goal of drug therapy is to increase and enhance the action of acetylcholine by suppressing cholinesterase, the enzyme that degrades the neurotransmitter.

During periods of exacerbation, medications are determined according to the patient's degree of fatigue and weakness. Specific assessment includes ability to swallow, grip strength, and subjective sense of fatigue based on a scale of 1-10 (1, no fatigue to 10, maximum fatigue).

First-line medications

Anticholinesterase/cholinergic agents: neostigmine bromide (Prostigmin), 20 mg q 4 h; pyridostigmine bromide (Mestinon), 60 mg q 6 h (60-600 mg qd in divided doses based on individual need); ambenonium chloride (Mytelase) (helpful in patients who also report GI symptoms), 10-25 mg PO tid or qid.

Anticholinesterase antidote for overdoses: atropine.

Second-line medications:　Corticosteroids, 1-2 mg/kg/day and taper to maintenance; azathioprine (Imuran), 1-2 mg/kg/day and taper; cyclophosphamide (Cytoxan), 1-5 mg/kg/day and taper.

ADJUNCTIVE THERAPY

Plasmapheresis (a process of separating blood into various components so that circulating anti-acetylcholine receptor antibodies can be removed; the blood is then replaced with donor plasma or another colloidal substance).

SURGERY

Thymectomy (to improve symptoms related to MG); tracheotomy (for pulmonary support in severe cases)

1 ASSESS

ASSESSMENT	OBSERVATIONS
History	Current medications (how long these drugs have been taken, amount, last dose); currently pregnant, early postpartum; recent surgery requiring anesthetic; recent infection; emotional or physical stress; sun exposure
Ocular muscles	Ocular palsy, double vision (diplopia), ptosis (drooped eyelids)
Facial muscles	Facial expression distorted as a result of weak oropharyngeal and facial muscles (smile appears as a snarl); palsy affecting half of face; ineffective chewing
Pharyngeal/laryngeal muscles	Dysphagia, difficulty chewing and speaking; choking; drooling; weak voice (whisper); nasal speech
Musculoskeletal	Generalized weakness, particularly in proximal muscle groups (e.g., quadriceps, biceps, and neck/head); slow gait; difficulty lifting legs (unable to climb more than three stairs); difficulty holding head up; unable to hold arms overhead for longer than 5 sec
Respiratory muscles	Dyspnea, breathlessness, weak respiratory muscles; decreased V_T and VC; increased respiratory exertion; restlessness; irritability
Reflexes	Normal or brisk
Psychosocial	Anxiety, apprehension, fear

2 DIAGNOSE

NURSING DIAGNOSIS	SUBJECTIVE FINDINGS	OBJECTIVE FINDINGS
Ineffective breathing pattern related to respiratory muscle weakness	Complains of difficulty breathing and inability to expand chest	Decreased breath sounds bilaterally; decreased V_T and VC; minimal use of accessory respiratory muscles; short, shallow respirations with increased rate; dyspnea; restlessness; confusion; arterial oxygen (Pao_2) <80 mm Hg
Ineffective airway clearance and Potential for aspiration related to muscle weakness of the pharynx/larynx	Complains of difficulty breathing and inability to cough	Depressed gag and cough reflexes; choking; difficulty swallowing; drooling; dyspnea
Impaired swallowing related to muscle weakness of the pharynx/larynx	Complains of difficulty swallowing oral secretions, food, and fluids	Depressed gag reflex; choking; stasis of food in oral cavity
Impaired physical mobility related to generalized weakness	Complains of profound weakness	Unable to keep head upright, climb more than one stair or step onto a step stool, brush hair or teeth or hold arms above head; has shuffling gait, trips while walking

→ ＞ ＞

NURSING DIAGNOSIS	SUBJECTIVE FINDINGS	OBJECTIVE FINDINGS
Impaired verbal communication related to pharynx/larynx muscle weakness	Reports difficulty speaking	Fluctuations in voice tone and quality; whispers when speaking; has slurred speech, drooping mouth
Sensory/perceptual alterations (visual) related to impaired ocular neurotransmission and ocular muscle weakness	Complains of seeing double and not being able to keep eyes open	Eyelids drooping (ptosis); diplopia; ocular palsy in one eye
Anxiety related to difficulty breathing and disease process	Complains of difficulty breathing and expresses concern about condition	Dyspnea; tachycardia; appears scared, apprehensive, and tense

3 PLAN

Patient goals

1. The patient's breathing pattern will be effective with diminished or no accessory muscle weakness.
2. The patient's airway will remain patent.
3. The patient will not aspirate.
4. The patient will demonstrate effective swallowing to ensure adequate nutrition and hydration and prevent choking or aspiration.
5. The patient will participate in energy-sparing activities.
6. The patient will maintain an adequate balance between rest and activities.
7. Communication will be maximized.
8. The patient will demonstrate improved visual perception.
9. The patient's environment will remain safe.
10. The patient's anxiety will be relieved.

4 IMPLEMENT

NURSING DIAGNOSIS	NURSING INTERVENTIONS	RATIONALE
Ineffective breathing pattern related to respiratory muscle weakness	Assess and monitor respiratory strength and rate.	To establish baseline, monitor respiratory changes, and guide therapeutic intervention.
	Auscultate lungs frequently.	To monitor for decreased breath sounds and pulmonary congestion.
	Assess and monitor respiratory rate and VC (during a period of exacerbation, q 15 min).	To determine progressive muscle weakness, which can result in sudden respiratory failure when the diaphragm and intercostal muscles become affected (VC $<$1,200 ml often requires intubation and ventilatory support).
	Assess for changes in orientation, behavior, affect, and awareness.	Alteration may indicate hypoxia (Pa_{O_2} $<$80 mm Hg; O_2 saturation $<$80%).

NURSING DIAGNOSIS	NURSING INTERVENTIONS	RATIONALE
	Position patient in semi-Fowler's position for optimum body alignment.	To maximize diaphragmatic contraction and decrease respiratory effort.
	Instruct patient in the use of relaxation techniques.	To decrease anxiety and work of breathing.
	Encourage the use of blow bottles.	To promote deep breathing and assist in monitoring respiratory strength.
	Teach patient abdominal breathing exercises.	To decrease work of breathing.
Ineffective airway clearance and Potential for aspiration related to muscle weakness of the pharynx/larynx	Assess and monitor gag and cough reflexes.	To monitor patient's control of airway, to prevent aspiration, and to determine need for airway placement or intubation.
	Evaluate chest x-rays.	To monitor for aspiration pneumonia.
	Assess and monitor vital signs q 4-6 h.	Fever may indicate aspiration pneumonia.
	Assess and monitor breath sounds q 4-6 h.	To determine adequacy of gas exchange and degree of airway obstruction by secretions.
	Provide regular chest physiotherapy and coughing exercises.	To promote removal of secretions.
	Teach patient effective coughing techniques.	Ineffective coughing increases fatigue and weakness, rendering patient susceptible to aspiration.
	Provide adequate hydration and humidification.	To keep secretions thin and easier to expectorate.
	Position patient on side.	To encourage drainage of secretions from oral cavity.
	Position patient in semi-Fowler's position, particularly when eating and for 30 min to 1 hour after meals.	Secretions move by gravity; elevating head of bed moves abdominal contents away from diaphragm to enhance diaphragmatic contractions; this position also decreases risk of aspiration.
	Assess patient's ability to manage food and fluids.	To establish baseline of functional ability, prevent aspiration, and promote nutritional intake.
	Monitor and remove from oral cavity any accumulation of secretions or food.	To prevent aspiration.
	If gag reflex is depressed, provide foods that form a small ball in the patient's mouth (e.g., bread, pasta, cheese), and avoid liquids and high-fiber foods (e.g., steak).	To prevent aspiration, facilitate swallowing, and provide adequate nutrition; high-fiber foods require increased chewing, which may promote fatigue and increase the risk of aspiration.

→ › ›

NURSING DIAGNOSIS	SUBJECTIVE FINDINGS	OBJECTIVE FINDINGS
	Have suction equipment at bedside.	In case patient chokes or aspirates.
	Administer anticholinesterase drugs as ordered, and monitor response.	To increase amount of acetylcholine at the neuromuscular junction and to improve muscle weakness.
Impaired swallowing and potential for aspiration related to muscle weakness of the pharynx/larynx	Assess and monitor gag and swallowing reflexes.	To prevent aspiration; reflexes may be absent when muscles that are innervated by the cranial bulbar nerve are affected.
	Provide oral hygiene before meals.	To stimulate salivation and promote swallowing.
	For meals, position patient in an upright position with head tilted slightly forward; keep upright for at least 30 min after eating.	To enhance swallowing and prevent aspiration.
	Provide a semisolid diet; avoid foods that require increased chewing (e.g., fibrous meats [steak]; certain vegetables [e.g., celery, carrots]).	Semisolid diet requires less chewing, is easier to swallow, and decreases risk of aspiration; it also ensures adequate nutrition.
	Do not give patient hot foods.	Heat aggravates muscle weakness and impairs swallowing.
	Place food in unaffected side of mouth.	To facilitate movement of food into back of mouth and to promote chewing and swallowing.
	Encourage patient to eat slowly and to rest before meals.	Overtiredness may aggravate weakness and impair swallowing.
	Administer feedings via a nasogastric or gastrostomy tube.	To ensure optimum nutrition despite decreased or absent gag reflex.
	Administer anticholinesterase drugs as ordered, and monitor their effectiveness and side effects (e.g., sweating, abdominal cramps, nausea, bradycardia).	If these drugs are given 20-30 min before meals, they provide smoother sustained muscle strength and chewing and swallowing are enhanced; they also decrease the risk of aspiration and help ensure adequate nutritional intake.
	Teach family members the Heimlich maneuver for emergencies.	To prevent aspiration if the patient chokes.
	Have suction available at bedside, particularly when patient is eating and for 1-2 hours after meals.	To provide emergency suctioning in case of choking or aspiration.

NURSING DIAGNOSIS	NURSING INTERVENTIONS	RATIONALE
Impaired physical mobility related to generalized weakness	Assess patient's functional status and ability to complete activities of daily living (ADLs).	To establish a baseline and guide therapeutic interventions.
	Encourage patient to develop a routine of rest and activity.	Overwhelming weakness occurs in more than 90% of patients; periods of rest minimize weakness.
	Encourage patient to participate in a regular exercise program; consult physical therapist and exercise physiologist to develop individual exercise program.	A paced exercise program minimizes weakness and maintains patient's functional status.
	Work with patient to identify methods of conserving energy (e.g., place objects low in cupboard, plan menus before going to store, use a chair with good support, avoid hot baths).	To facilitate problem solving with the patient and conserve energy, thus decreasing weakness.
	Instruct patient to use assistive devices (e.g., use extended handles to avoid bending, use a long-handled shoe horn).	To minimize energy expenditure and prevent weakness.
	Teach patient to break up ADLs into short activities and to rest in between.	To prevent fatigue and weakness.
	Administer anticholinesterase drugs as ordered and monitor response.	To enhance neurotransmission and decrease muscle weakness.
Impaired verbal communication related to pharynx/larynx muscle weakness	Assess muscle strength and speech.	To establish a baseline of speech effectiveness and to guide therapeutic intervention.
	Consult with speech therapist.	For help with developing an individualized plan of communication.
	Encourage slow-paced speech with rest periods.	To minimize weakness, decrease fluctuations in voice strength, reduce whispering, and enhance verbal communication.
	Minimize extraneous stimuli during periods of communication, and maintain eye contact.	Distractions require additional energy and may induce weakness and reduce verbal communication.
	Position patient in semi- or high Fowler's position.	Proper positioning may enhance voice volume.
	Allow patient sufficient time to express himself.	To decrease frustration and promote verbal communication.
	Employ other methods of communication (e.g., magic slate [easier to use than a pen or pencil], picture boards, letter boards).	To facilitate and maintain communication.

→ ⟩ ⟩

NURSING DIAGNOSIS	NURSING INTERVENTIONS	RATIONALE
Sensory/perceptual alterations (visual) related to impaired ocular neurotransmission and ocular muscle weakness	Assess degree of visual impairment.	To establish a baseline of visual perception and to guide therapeutic interventions.
	Place patch on one eye, alternating eyes q 2 h as ordered.	To minimize double vision.
	Encourage patient to close his eyes and relax ocular muscles for a few minutes at a time, particularly when reading or after driving.	To minimize muscle weakness and promote relaxation of eye muscles; may decrease blurred vision.
	Provide a safe environment; orient patient to environment and changes in the environment.	To prevent injury related to impaired vision.
	Encourage friends and family to stay with patient whenever possible.	Familiar individuals may provide support and decrease anxiety related to impaired vision.
	Help patient identify alternative methods of completing ADLs when vision is impaired (e.g., keep objects in the same place and within reach, obtain necessary articles for patient, use guard bars in the bath or shower).	To promote independence and control over one's environment.
Anxiety related to difficulty breathing and disease process	Assess patient's level of anxiety.	To establish baseline state of anxiety (mild, moderate, severe, or panic) and to guide therapeutic interventions.
	Provide rest periods between activities.	To decrease weakness and reduce respiratory rate, thus decreasing anxiety.
	Provide comfort measures (e.g., foot and back massage).	To promote relaxation and decrease respiratory effort.
	Problem solve with patient to identify coping mechanisms that have been used successfully in the past.	To facilitate problem solving with the patient; may decrease respiratory effort.
	Encourage patient to express his feelings and ask questions.	Helps patient put thoughts into perspective; correct answers to questions may relieve anxiety.
	Stay with patient during acute episodes of dyspnea and anxiety.	To decrease anxiety and fear and provide support.

5   EVALUATE

PATIENT OUTCOME	DATA INDICATING THAT OUTCOME IS REACHED
Respiratory pattern is effective.	Patient uses accessory respiratory muscles adequately; V_T and VC are optimum for patient's status; breath sounds are clear; there is no aspiration.

PATIENT OUTCOME	DATA INDICATING THAT OUTCOME IS REACHED
Airways are patent.	Breath sounds are clear; breathing occurs without obstruction; patient can manage secretions; arterial blood gases are within normal limits; there is no aspiration.
Patient can swallow safely.	Patient can consume adequate nutritional and fluid intake (>2,000 ml/day); patient swallows safely without gagging, choking, or aspirating; family members can perform the Heimlich maneuver.
Patient participates in energy-sparing activities.	Patient has an established routine of activity and rest; ADLs are scheduled with rest periods; demonstrates use of various assist devices to conserve energy; utilizes stress-reduction tactics (e.g., self-hypnosis and visualization).
Physical mobility is maintained with adequate periods of rest and activity.	Patient is able to complete ADLs without weakness, demonstrates a daily routine that incorporates periods of rest and activity.
Communication is maximized.	Patient can communicate needs and express thoughts and demonstrates effective verbal and nonverbal communication techniques.
Patient's visual capacity has improved.	No injury occurs related to impaired vision; diplopia has been controlled; patient demonstrates strategies to relax eye muscles.
No injury occurs as a result of decreased visual acuity and neuromuscular weakness.	Frequently used items remain within reach; no changes are made in the environment without patient's knowledge of change; persons entering the room announce themselves; patient demonstrates use of side bars in the bathroom and other assist devices.
Patient's anxiety has been relieved.	Patient reports decreased anxiety with return of adequate breathing pattern and knowledge of disease process and management.

PATIENT TEACHING

1. Instruct the patient and family about the disease, treatments, and home management.
2. Instruct the patient and family in all medications, their purpose, dosage, route and time of administration, and side effects.
3. Instruct the patient not to take over-the-counter medications without consulting his primary care provider.
4. Stress the importance of activity and exercise only to tolerance.
5. Emphasize the importance of an adequate diet.
6. Teach the patient stress-reduction and relaxation exercises (e.g., visualization; self-hypnosis).
7. Emphasize the importance of diversional activities.
8. Provide information on organizational resources and support.
9. Teach the patient and family the signs and symptoms of a myasthenia gravis crisis and a cholinergic crisis (see boxes, pages 292 and 293); advise the patient to seek immediate medical care if these symptoms arise.
10. Teach the patient and family the symptoms of an exacerbation and when to seek medical assistance.
11. Teach the patient to monitor for an upper airway infection (chills, fever, cough) and to seek medical care when symptoms arise.
12. Instruct the patient to report changes in or progression of symptoms to his health care provider.
13. Teach the patient and family to avoid conditions that may precipitate an exacerbation when possible (see Box, p. 293).
14. Instruct the patient not to use alcohol for at least 1 hour after taking anticholinesterase medication; it tends to speed up absorption of the drug.
15. For emergency situations when the patient has an obstructed airway (e.g., aspiration of food), instruct family members how to perform the Heimlich maneuver, insert an airway, perform oral and nasal-oral suctioning, and use an Ambu bag.
16. Instruct the patient in the importance of wearing a Medic-Alert bracelet.
17. Teach the patient the importance of follow-up care.

CHAPTER 11

Endocrine Disorders

Hashimoto's Disease (Chronic Thyroiditis)

Hashimoto's disease is a form of chronic thyroiditis characterized as an inflammatory disorder with progressive destruction of the thyroid gland.

EPIDEMIOLOGIC AND GENETIC CONSIDERATIONS

The etiology of Hashimoto's disease is unknown, but it is thought to be an autoimmune disorder. It can appear in any age group and either sex but tends to be more common in women between 40 and 75 years of age. No clear genetic connection has been associated with Hashimoto's disease, but in families where one member has an autoimmune thyroid disorder, the likelihood of another family member developing Hashimoto's disease is increased. Thyroid antibodies are found in 50% of siblings of patients with the disorder.[180a] Although HLA-DR4 and DR5 have been demonstrated in individuals with Hashimoto's disease, the associations have been inconsistent. There is no geographic or racial predisposition.

Hashimoto's disease is often observed in association with other autoimmune diseases, most frequently Graves' disease, systemic lupus erythematosus (SLE), chronic active hepatitis, and scleroderma. It is responsible for more than 45% of cases of individuals initially diagnosed with hypothyroidism.

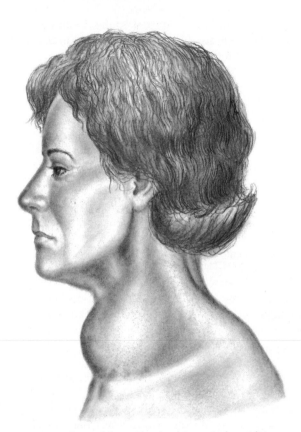

Enlarged thyroid in hashimoto's thyroiditis

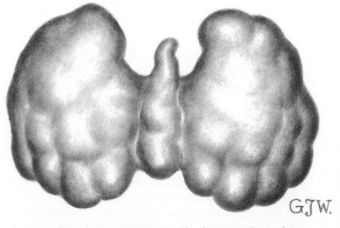

Pseudopodia-characteristic in hashimoto's thyroiditis

PATHOPHYSIOLOGY

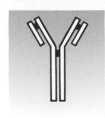 Hashimoto's disease is thought to be an autoimmune disorder with autoantibodies produced against the thyroid gland (thyroglobulin, thyroid peroxidase, thyroid growth-stimulating immunoglobulin, and thyrotropin-binding inhibitory immunoglobulin). Characteristically it manifests as a lymphocytic infiltration of primarily B and T lymphocytes into the thyroid gland. Phagocytic macrophages also invade, resulting in an abundance of dead thyroid cells. If left untreated, this infiltrative and phagocytic process disrupts the entire architectural structure of the thyroid, causing severe damage and dysfunction.

During the onset of Hashimoto's disease, patients commonly are euthyroid. However, hyperthyroidism is also common in the early stages of the disease. This hyperthyroidism is secondary to the inflammatory process, causing a breakdown of the thyroid follicles and increased secretion of thyroid hormones into the circulation. As the disease progresses and the gland is further damaged, hypothyroidism results. This hypothyroidism is due to glandular damage and the thyroid's inability to manufacture thyroid hormones.

CLINICAL MANIFESTATIONS

The onset of Hashimoto's disease usually is insidious, without well-defined symptoms or pain. Occasionally the patient will complain of fullness in the back of the throat, hoarseness, dysphagia, or a feeling of tracheal compression.

The main clinical manifestation of Hashimoto's disease is an enlarged thyroid gland, which is particularly common in children with this disorder. The enlarged thyroid gland, or goiter, typically is firm, freely movable, nontender, and without evidence of local inflammation. It generally is diffusely enlarged and nodular and may be either symmetric or asymmetric in shape.

If thyroid-stimulating hormone (TSH) is measured routinely to determine the need for hormone replacement therapy, the prognosis for Hashimoto's disease typically is excellent. If the hypothyroidism is not diagnosed and treated, myxedema coma may develop. Myxedema coma generally is seen in the elderly who have not had medical care; it occurs more often during the winter months, suggesting that exposure to cold may be a precipitating factor. Myxedema coma is characterized by coma, hyperthermia, cardiovascular collapse, hypoventilation, and severe metabolic changes (hyponatremia, hypoglycemia, and lactic acidosis). The risk of mortality from myxedema coma is approximately 50%.

CLINICAL MANIFESTATIONS OF HYPOTHYROIDISM

Skin: pale, dry, cold, flaky, and coarse skin; coarse, thin, brittle hair, decreased nail and hair growth; hair loss; periorbital and peripheral edema

Neurologic: confusion, vertigo, slurred and slowed speech, memory loss, lethargy, fatigue, headaches, deafness, night blindness, slow or clumsy gait, decreased reflexes

Hematologic: normocytic and normochromic anemia; pallor

Cardiovascular: cold intolerance, bradycardia, hypertension, decreased cardiac output, increased peripheral vascular resistance, pericardial effusions

Renal: alterations in renal blood flow secondary to hemodynamic changes

Pulmonary: dyspnea, pleural effusions

Upper respiratory: hoarseness

Gastrointestinal: anorexia, thickened tongue, constipation, weight gain, fluid retention

Musculoskeletal: weakness, myalgias, arthralgias, aching and stiff joints, slow movement, slowed reflexes

Reproductive: changes in menstruation, decreased libido; impotence and oligospermia in men

---

COMPLICATIONS

Severe hypothyroidism (see box above)
Myxedema coma
Thyroid lymphoma
Hyperthyroidism (p. 306)

DIFFERENTIAL DIAGNOSIS

Thyroid cancer or lymphoma

NURSING CARE

See pages 309 to 313.

DIAGNOSTIC STUDIES AND FINDINGS

Diagnostic test	Findings
Autoantigens and autoantibodies (using enzyme-linked immunosorbent assay [ELISA] method)	Present in varying levels
Thyroid peroxidase (microsomal antigen)	Present in >90% of cases
Thyroglobulin	Present in >50% of cases
Thyroid-stimulating hormone (TSH)	Slightly elevated
Serum thyroxine (T_4)	Usually normal but may be elevated or depressed
Serum triiodothyronine (T_3)	Usually normal but may be elevated or depressed
Thyroid scan	Diffuse or patchy pattern; cold nodules occasionally are seen
Surgical or needle biopsy of thyroid	Intrathyroidal lymphocytes, plasma cells, and autoantibodies
Computed tomography (CT) or magnetic resonance imaging (MRI) studies	To rule out cervical adenopathy and risk of malignancy

MEDICAL MANAGEMENT

The main goal of medical management in Hashimoto's disease is to keep the patient in a euthyroid state.

GENERAL MANAGEMENT

Thyroid function: monitor serum thyroxine (T_4) and thyroid-stimulating hormone (TSH) to prevent a hypothyroid crisis.

Monitor for signs or symptoms of hypothyroidism and hyperthyroidism (as a side effect of excess thyroid replacement) (see Boxes, pp. 303 and 306).

DRUG THERAPY

The goal of drug therapy is thyroid hormone replacement. If a symptomatic goiter is present, thyroid hormone may be administered to suppress TSH secretion to reduce the gland's size.

Natural thyroid hormone

Thyroid USP (Delcoid, Thyrar, Thyroxine, Thyroid-Teric), 60-180 mg daily PO for adult maintenance; initial dosage is 15 mg daily; if patient is unresponsive, increase the dose by 15 mg double dose every 2 weeks until maintenance dose or a good response is achieved (contains T_3 and T_4 replacement).

Thyroglobulin (Proloid), 32-180 mg daily PO for adult maintenance; initial doses are low with gradual increase to maintenance (contains T_3, T_4, and iodine compounds).

Synthetic thyroid hormones

Levothyroxine sodium (Cytolin, Levied, Levothyroid, Synthroid Sodium), 150-200 µg daily PO for adult maintenance; initial dose with 100-200 µg IV daily; initial doses are low with gradual increase to maintenance; IV form is used for myxedema coma, 400 µg for adults (contains chemically pure T_4 with mannitol [Synthroid] and without Levothyroid).

Liothyronine sodium (Cytomel, Cytosine), 25-75 µg daily PO for adult maintenance; initial doses are low with gradual increase to maintenance (chemically pure form of T_3).

Liotrix (Euthroid, Thyrolar), 30 µg T_4, with 7.5 µg T_3, or 25 µg T_4, with 6.25 µg T_3 PO for adults; doses may be gradually increased (chemically pure T_3 and T_4 administered in a ratio of 4:1).

MEDICAL MANAGEMENT—cont'd

Adenohypophyseal hormones

Thyroid-stimulating hormone (Thytropar), 10 IU IM or SC qd or bid (contains a natural peptide extract from bovine anterior pituitary gland); side effects include cardiovascular symptoms and allergic reactions; these may cause the release of thyroid hormones and precipitate an adrenal crisis in patients with secondary adrenal insufficiency.

Thioamides (to lower thyroid hormone levels)

Propylthiouracil (PTU), 50-300 mg daily in divided doses for adults (inhibits thyroid hormone synthesis but not release).

Methimazole (Tapazole), 5-20 mg daily PO in divided doses for adults (inhibits thyroid hormone synthesis but not release).

SURGERY

Thyroidectomy for a large or painful thyroid gland.

Graves' Disease

Graves' disease is a multisystem autoimmune disorder of unknown origin characterized by a diffuse goiter and thyrotoxicosis.

Graves' disease is a multisystem autoimmune disorder that manifests one or more of the following symptoms: hyperthyroidism, diffuse thyroid enlargement, ophthalmopathy, dermopathy, or thyroid acropathy.[55a]

The incidence of Graves' disease in the United States is 0.1% to 0.5% with a greater prevalence among women at a ratio of 7:1. The disorder usually appears in the third or fourth decade, but it has also been known to develop later in life. It rarely occurs in children.

HEREDITARY AND GENETIC CONSIDERATIONS

There is strong evidence that heredity and genetic factors predispose an individual to the development of Graves' disease. HLA haplotype associations have shown a predominance of DR3 in whites and Bw35 and Bw47 in Asians.[169] Family members of patients with Graves' disease have demonstrated thyroid antibodies, abnormalities in thyroid regulation, and thyroid-stimulating immunoglobulins (TSIs). Increasing evidence suggests that other autoimmune disorders such as

Hashimoto's disease and pernicious anemia also affect these patients and their families.

PATHOPHYSIOLOGY

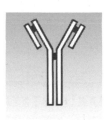

The exact cause of Graves' disease and the accompanying ophthalmopathy, dermopathy, and thyroid acropathy is unknown. The thyroid abnormalities that occur are thought to result from the action of autoantibodies against components or regions of the thyroid plasma membrane related to the thyroid-stimulating hormone (TSH) receptor. These autoantibodies are identified as thyroid-stimulating immunoglobulins (TSIs) of the IgG class and are found in approximately 90% of patients with Graves' disease. The TSIs bind to the thyroid cells and activate the TSH receptors. This action stimulates thyroid growth and function. The increased function of the thyroid gland is demonstrated by an increase in iodine uptake and the rate of thyroid gland metabolism. These actions may contribute to the increased vascularity and enlargement of the thyroid gland.[13a, 113a]

On pathologic examination, the thyroid gland appears uniformly enlarged. The gland has increased vascularity and often varying degrees of both CD4 and CD8 T lymphocytes and plasma cells. Immunofluorescent studies have also shown thyroid cells to express HLA-DR antigens on their surface.[13a,178]

Mechanisms implicated as possible causes of TSI production are thyroid injury, infection and other agents that stimulate autoantibody production, suppressed B lymphocytes, and abnormal T lymphocyte regulation of B lymphocytes.

CLINICAL MANIFESTATIONS

In Graves' disease the excess production of thyroid hormones causes a state of hypermetabolism. The action of the thyroid hormones generally is stimulatory; therefore the clinical features of Graves' disease and hyperthyroidism reflect the increased efforts of several organs and tissues to meet the increasing metabolic demands.

Graves' disease usually manifests as a diffuse goiter and **thyrotoxicosis,** a condition caused by the excess quantities of thyroid hormone presented to the body tissues. Graves' disease is characterized by one or several of the following conditions: diffuse thyroid enlargement (goiter), hyperthyroidism, ophthalmopathy, dermopathy, or thyroid acropathy (hypertrophic osteoarthropathy).

The major clinical manifestations of **hyperthyroidism** include heat intolerance, increased neuromuscular activity, and hyperactivity of the sympathetic nervous system. This can be seen clinically as warm, moist skin; nervousness; irritability; reflex alterations; weight loss; hyperdefecation; tachycardia; the characteristic "stare"; and changes in mental status.

The **compensatory mechanisms** that attempt to meet the increasing metabolic demands are reflected as increased cardiac output; increased peripheral blood flow with dilation of superficial skin capillaries; increased core body temperature; increased oxygen consumption with an elevated respiratory rate; increased absorption of glucose by the gastrointestinal tract; increased cellular use of glucose; hyperinsulinism; decreased availability of fats and carbohydrates; increased vitamin metabolism, possibly leading to vitamin deficiencies; increased bone mobilization, increasing the individual's susceptibility to hypercalcemia; and increased secretions of adrenocorticotropic hormone (ACTH) and melanocyte-stimulating hormone (MSH), causing changes in skin pigmentation.

Hyperthyroidism usually is tolerated fairly well, particularly in younger patients; it tends to be more debilitating in the elderly. An apathetic or masked hyperthyroidism often is seen in elderly patients with Graves' disease whose hyperthyroidism is demonstrated mainly by cardiac failure, atrial fibrillation, muscle weakness, and weight loss. These patients generally do not manifest the clinical symptoms commonly seen in younger patients (e.g., nervousness, heat intolerance, increased appetite, and hyperactivity).

Endocrine, eye, and skin disorders often accompany Graves' disease. They may appear in combination or independently and may have varying clinical courses in the same patient. **Ophthalmopathy** occurs in approximately 20% to 40% of patients with Graves' disease. Ocular manifestations are divided into two categories: (1) functional changes, which result from hyperactivity of the sympathetic nervous system, and (2) infiltrative changes, which are the result of lymphocytic infiltration and fibrosis of the extraocular muscles and eyelid retractors. Clinical manifestations of functional abnormalities include lid lag and proptosis; neither vision nor ocular function appears to be affected. The problem resolves with treatment for hyperthyroidism. Infiltrative ophthalmopathy occurs in 2% to 7% of patients with

---

CLINICAL MANIFESTATIONS OF HYPERTHYROIDISM

Skin: diaphoresis, flushing; very warm skin; heat intolerance; hair loss (temporary); fine, soft, thin, straight hair

Neurologic: restlessness, irritability, inability to concentrate, hyperactivity, brisk reflexes, tremors, emotional lability

Cardiovascular: palpitations, tachycardia, hypertension

Renal: increased renal perfusion with corresponding polyuria

Pulmonary: rapid, shallow respirations; hyperventilation

Upper respiratory: hoarseness

Gastrointestinal: weight loss, either anorexia or increased food intake, diarrhea

Musculoskeletal: muscle weakness, loss of muscle mass, hyperactive reflexes, tremor

Endocrine: enlarged thyroid gland in 90% or more of cases (goiter)

Ocular: lid lag and retraction, proptosis, startled look

Reproductive: decreased libido, amenorrhea, impotence

THYROID FUNCTION STUDIES

Study	Normal values
Thyroxine (T_4) total	5-10 µg/dl
Triiodothyronine (T_3) total	110-230 ng/dl
Triiodothyronine resin uptake (RT_3U)	25%-35%
Thyroid-stimulating hormone (TSH)	1-4 µU/ml
Thyroxine-binding globulin (TBG)	12-28 µg/ml
Antithyroglobulin antibody	Titer <10

Graves' disease. It is characterized by orbital edema and protrusion, optic neuropathy, and retinal damage. These changes may result in exophthalmos; weakness of the extraocular muscles, causing diplopia; orbital irritation and pain; photophobia; and blurred vision. Rarely changes in visual acuity may progress to blindness.[33a]

Infiltrative dermopathy is seen in 5% to 10% of patients with Graves' disease. It usually is manifested as myxedema with swelling in the pretibial area, the feet, hands, and face, with an accompanying induration and erythema.

Thyroid acropathy generally is seen in patients who have been previously treated for hyperthyroidism, localized dermopathy, and ophthalmopathy. Although typically no symptoms or deformities are seen, thyroid acropathy may produce contractures.

The prognosis for Graves' disease is generally good once thyroid function has been brought under control. The most serious problems are caused by ophthalmopathic and dermopathic complications, which may not respond to treatment.

COMPLICATIONS

Thyroid storm
Severe hyperthyroidism
Visual impairment and blindness as a result of ophthalmopathy
Bulbous or ulcerated lesions as the result of dermopathy
Toxic nodular goiter

DIFFERENTIAL DIAGNOSIS

Hashimoto's disease
Pituitary tumors
Thyroid adenomas

DIAGNOSTIC STUDIES AND FINDINGS

Diagnostic test	Findings
Autoantigen and autoantibodies (using enzyme-linked immunosorbent assay [ELISA] method)	
Thyroid-stimulating immunoglobulin (TSI)	Present in 50%-90% of cases
Thyroid peroxidase (microsomal antigen)	Present in 50%-80% of cases
Thyrotropin-binding inhibitory immunoglobulin (TBII)	Present in 50%-80% of cases
Thyroid growth-stimulating immunoglobulin (TGSI)	Present in 20%-50% of cases
Thyroglobulin	Present in 20%-70% of cases
Thyrotropin-releasing hormone (TRH) stimulation test	Minimal or no response of TSH to TRH stimulation
Serum thyroxine (T_4)	Elevated
Serum triiodothyronine (T_3)	Elevated
Radioactive (T_3) uptake (RT_3U)	High
Thyroid radioiodine uptake and scan	Increased uptake

MEDICAL MANAGEMENT

GENERAL MANAGEMENT

Optical: Monitor eye involvement; encourage routine ophthalmologic checkups.

Activity: Encourage regular exercise program.

Nutrition: Encourage a balanced, nutritional diet and increased carbohydrate intake; provide supplemental vitamins.

Cardiac: Institute ECG monitoring; observe for dysrhythmias; monitor for signs of congestive heart failure, particularly in the elderly.

Skin: Monitor skin changes; facilitate optimum skin care.

Thyroid: Monitor thyroid function studies.

Autoantibodies: Monitor function of autoantibodies, since this may correlate with clinical course of disease.

Psychotherapy: Institute psychotherapy as appropriate; short-term therapy may be indicated for behavioral changes, anxiety neurosis, or other mental alterations.

DRUG THERAPY

Beta-adrenergic blockers: Initial treatment used to inhibit symptomatic beta-adrenergic hyperstimulation.

Propranolol (Inderal), 40-240 mg daily PO in divided doses for adults; IV 0.5-1 mg/min, maximum 5 mg; controls symptoms of hyperthyroidism by blocking beta-adrenergic receptors; does not lower T_3 and T_4 levels and causes a 10%-20% reduction in serum T_3 concentration.

Antithyroid drugs: Thioamides: These drugs may also inhibit production of thyroid hormones, minimize hyperthyroidism, decrease the size and vascularity of the goiter, and alter the autoimmune process.[13a]

Propylthiouracil (PTU), 50-300 mg daily PO in divided doses for adults; initial dosage is 300-600 mg daily, tapered to maintenance dosage.

Methimazole (Tapazole, MMI), 5-20 mg daily PO in divided doses for adults; initial dosage is 30-60 mg daily PO in divided doses.

Oral cholecystographic agents: Ipodate, experimental dosage is 1.5-3 g qd PO in adults; inhibits extrathyroidal T_3 production and may be useful for short-term therapy when antithyroid drugs or iodine is contraindicated.

Iodine: Potassium or sodium iodide (Strong Iodine or Lugol's solution), 0.1-1.3 ml PO tid for adults; 250-500 mg daily for adults in thyrotoxic crisis; causes short-term inhibition of thyroid hormone synthesis by direct action on the thyroid; often used as a presurgical medication to decrease the size of the thyroid gland after thioamide therapy.

Immunosuppressive agents (used to treat ophthalmoplegia, mild optic neuropathy, or severe optic pressure effects): Corticosteroids, azathioprine (Imuran), cyclosporine (Sandimmune), cyclophosphamide (Cytoxan).

Lubricating eye drops: 0.5% methylcellulose eye drops prn for irritation and pain.

Topical agents: 0.2% fluocinolone or other corticosteroid creams prn to treat dermopathy.

ADJUNCTIVE THERAPY

Radioactive iodine (^{131}I NaI or ^{125}I NaI), total dose: 6,000-8,000 rad over approximately 6 mo; used to destroy thyroid tissue without surgery for control of Graves' disease.

MEDICAL MANAGEMENT—CONT'D

Radiation of the eye orbit.

SURGERY

Subtotal thyroidectomy; surgical orbital decompression; surgical correction of orbital muscle imbalance.

1 ASSESS

	OBSERVATIONS	
ASSESSMENT	HASHIMOTO'S DISEASE	GRAVES' DISEASE
Endocrine	Thyroid may be enlarged	90% have enlarged thyroid
Skin	Cool, pale, dry, coarse, yellow skin; rough, scaly, puffy, masklike face; hyperthermia; myxedema; hair loss; decreased hair and nail growth	Warm, moist, smooth texture; erythema; increased sweating; increased diffuse pigmentation; localized myxedema; hyperthermia; increased body temperature ($>37.8°$ C [$100.4°$ F]); slight hair loss
Ocular	Periorbital edema	Proptosis; lid lag and retraction; conjunctival irritation; lacrimation; characteristic wide-eyed, frightened look
Cardiovascular	Bradycardia, dysrhythmias, decreased BP, cold intolerance, decreased exercise tolerance	Tachycardia, palpitations, dysrhythmias, increased systolic BP, wide pulse pressure
Pulmonary	Hypoventilation, hoarseness, slight dyspnea	Increased rate of respiration, hyperventilation, restlessness
Gastrointestinal	Anorexia, slight weight gain, constipation, fecal impaction, abdominal distention	Weight loss or slight weight gain, anorexia or increased food intake, diarrhea
Musculoskeletal	Fatigue, weakness, slow movements, delayed relaxation of tendon reflexes, stiff joints, arthralgias	Muscular wasting, weakness, hyperactive deep tendon reflexes, tremor
Nervous system	Slowing of intellectual function and speech; impaired memory; diminished hearing; lethargic, somnolent, apathetic demeanor	Restlessness, irritability, decreased ability to concentrate, memory loss, insomnia
Renal	Decreased urine output, mild reduction in ability to concentrate	Polyuria, urgency, polydipsia
Reproductive	Decreased libido, failure to ovulate, amenorrhea, impotence	Amenorrhea and hypomenorrhea, decreased libido and potency, gynecomastia
Psychosocial	Depression, agitation, paranoia; family reports behavioral changes	Restlessness, irritability, agitation, emotional lability, manic behavior; family reports behavioral changes

→ > >

2 DIAGNOSE

NURSING DIAGNOSIS	SUBJECTIVE FINDINGS	
	HASHIMOTO'S DISEASE	GRAVES' DISEASE
Altered cardiac output (decreased in Hashimoto's disease and increased in Graves' disease) related to changes in thyroid function	Complains of fatigue; weakness; decreased ability to participate in routine activities; bradycardia; weak, thready pulse; hypotension; pallor; diaphoresis; decreased cardiac output (COP)	Reports feeling "hyper"; increased systolic BP; tachycardia; bounding pulse
Ineffective breathing pattern related to changes in thyroid function	Complains of shortness of breath; raspy, hoarse voice; decreased breath sounds at bilateral bases; hypoventilation	Complains of shortness of breath; agitation; shallow, rapid respirations; decreased breath sounds at bilateral bases; hyperventilation
Impaired skin integrity related to changes in peripheral blood flow due to altered thyroid function	Complains of feeling cold and that skin is itchy; hypothermia; dry, scaly skin and rough periorbital edema; slight peripheral edema	Complains of feeling hot and diaphoretic; elevated temperature (≥37.8° C [100.4° F]); pretibial edema; moist, erythematous skin
Altered bowel elimination (diarrhea in Graves' disease, constipation in Hashimoto's disease) related to changes in metabolism	Complains of constipation; stools hard, no bowel movement reported in 3 days, hypoactivity bowel sounds	Complains of diarrhea or frequent, watery, loose stools; hyperactive bowel sounds
Altered thought processes related to changes in metabolism	Complains of depression and feelings of paranoia; withdrawn; distorted thinking and sequencing of thought; unable to focus attention; appearance demonstrates neglect of personal hygiene; appears preoccupied; loss of short-term memory	Complains of inability to think clearly and insomnia; intermittent disorientation; easily distracted; appearance demonstrates neglect of personel hygiene; unable to concentrate; impaired judgment; appears agitated and restless

Other related nursing diagnoses: Altered nutrition: less than body requirements related to hypermetabolic state of Graves' disease; **Potential for hyperthermia** related to hypermetabolism of Graves' disease; **Body image disturbance** related to lid lag and characteristic masklike expression.

3 PLAN

Patient goals

1. The patient will demonstrate improved and stable cardiac output.
2. The patient's breathing will be effective without dyspnea, fatigue, or excess expenditure of energy.
3. The patient's skin will remain intact.
4. The patient will have a regular pattern of bowel elimination.
5. The patient will demonstrate an improved ability to define and communicate reality and relate to others.

4 IMPLEMENT

NURSING DIAGNOSIS	NURSING INTERVENTIONS	RATIONALE
Altered cardiac output (decreased in Hashimoto's disease and increased in Graves' disease) related to changes in thyroid function	Assess pulse, BP, skin color, and temperature.	To determine cardiac stability and guide interventions.
	Assess resting or sleeping pulse.	To more accurately monitor for tachycardia or bradycardia.
	Monitor intake and output.	To evaluate fluid status and prevent overhydration or underhydration.
	Monitor effects of medications (lower doses should be used in Hashimoto's disease).	To identify cardiac depression caused by drug accumulation that may result from hypometabolism in Hashimoto's disease.
	Monitor hemodynamic parameters as ordered: mean arterial pressure (MAP), central venous pressure (CVP), pulmonary capillary wedge pressure (PCWP).	To evaluate patient's volume status.
	Monitor ECG for dysrhythmias and report change.	Changes in thyroid function can cause dysrhythmias (Hashimoto's disease: bradycardia, severe heart block; Graves' disease: tachycardia).
	Monitor COP as ordered; restrict activities, and provide for periods of rest between activities.	To evaluate cardiac function, minimize energy expenditure, and decrease metabolic and oxygen demands.
Ineffective breathing pattern related to changes in thyroid function	Assess and monitor rate, depth, and character of respirations.	To identify respiratory depression and adequacy of breathing pattern.
	Assess and monitor breath sounds and vital signs and report changes.	To monitor for hypoventilation and early signs of possible pulmonary congestion; increased temperature is a sign of infection.
	Provide for periods of rest between activities.	To maximize energy for respirations.
	Measure vital capacity (VC) and tidal volume (V_T); elevate head of bed to semi-Fowler's position.	To monitor volume of air movement, improve diaphragmatic contraction and ventilation, and minimize work of breathing.
Impaired skin integrity related to changes in peripheral blood flow due to altered thyroid function	Assess skin daily, and monitor changes.	To detect and prevent breakdown, increased edema, erythema, and signs of infection.
	Provide daily skin care: use mild soap, dry thoroughly, and lubricate skin with lanolin-based lotion bid.	To maintain skin integrity and avoid breakdown and infection.
	Regulate environmental temperature (warmer with Hashimoto's disease, cooler with Graves' disease).	To provide comfort and prevent overdrying of skin or excess moisture.

→ ❭ ❭

NURSING DIAGNOSIS	NURSING INTERVENTIONS	RATIONALE
	Instruct patient with Hashimoto's disease to wear warm clothing in cool weather.	To prevent skin from becoming chapped and cracked to minimize risk of infection and discomfort.
	Assess skin and body temperature.	To prevent hypothermia or hyperthermia related to changes in metabolism.
Altered bowel elimination (diarrhea in Graves' disease, constipation in Hashimoto's disease) related to changes in metabolism	Auscultate bowel sounds tid.	To detect peristalsis, hypermotility, hypomotility, and possible need to defecate.
	Assess frequency, color, consistency, and amount of stool.	To confirm change in bowel function.
	Observe and monitor for blood in stool.	Blood in stool indicates rectal bleeding, possibly as a result of forced bowel movement or irritation from frequent diarrhea.
	Assess and monitor intake and output; encourage adequate fluid intake.	To establish adequate fluids, prevent dehydration, and promote adequate stool evacuation.
	Encourage patient to increase fiber in diet (cereals, bran, wheat).	To promote normal stool formation and regulation of bowel habits.
	Assess effectiveness of antidiarrheal and anticonstipation aids (medications, enemas).	To identify resolution of diarrhea or constipation and the need for alternative measures.
	Implement bowel training program.	To repattern bowel habits.
Altered thought processes related to changes in metabolism	Assess orientation to person, place, and time.	To establish baseline orientation and guide therapeutic interventions.
	Use reality orientation as indicated; orient to person, place, and time, and avoid generalizations and vagueness.	To assist patient in reality identification.
	Provide a physically and emotionally safe environment.	To prevent injury.
	Explain all procedures and events slowly, concisely, and clearly.	If the patient's ability to concentrate and memory are impaired, simple and slow explanations will facilitate understanding.
	Provide and maintain a regular schedule of activities.	To prevent further disorientation.
	Decrease unnecessary external stimuli (loud noises, numerous visitors); provide patient with a private room if possible.	To minimize distraction and increase hyperactive patient's inability to concentrate.
	Encourage patient to express feelings, express needs, and interact with others.	To promote patient's ability to relate to herself and others positively.

NURSING DIAGNOSIS	NURSING INTERVENTIONS	RATIONALE
	Administer thyroid hormone replacement drugs or antithyroid drugs as ordered, and monitor patient's response.	To obtain optimum thyroid function and promote resolution of distorted thought processes.

5 EVALUATE

PATIENT OUTCOME	DATA INDICATING THAT OUTCOME IS REACHED
Cardiac output has improved, and cardiovascular function is stable.	Patient is normotensive and is resting quietly; COP is 4-5 L/min; there are no dysrhythmias on the ECG; skin is warm and dry; urine output is ≥30 ml/h.
Breathing pattern is effective and patient shows no dyspnea or hypoventilation.	Patient demonstrates adequate rate and depth of respirations; V_T and VC are normal for patient; behavior has been modified to conserve energy; patient has no dyspnea or restlessness.
Skin integrity is maintained.	Skin shows no signs of breakdown; edema has resolved; skin is warm and dry, with normal turgor; patient can demonstrate daily skin care.
Bowel elimination has been regulated.	Patient's bowel movements are regular according to her usual frequency; she has no diarrhea or constipation.
Patient has a model of reality and can relate positively to others.	Patient is oriented to person, place, time, and environment; her statements are reality based; she is able to concentrate, and her memory has improved; she has increased her interaction with others.

PATIENT TEACHING

1. Teach the patient and family the signs and symptoms of hyperthyroidism and hypothyroidism to facilitate early recognition and treatment.
2. Teach the patient the importance of wearing Medic-Alert identification, and tell her where it can be obtained.
3. Prepare the family members and patient for possible emotional outbursts as a result of patient's altered thyroid function.
4. Teach the patient about her disease and its management.
5. Teach the patient about her medications: name, dosages, time, side effects, and the importance of taking medications on schedule.
6. Teach the patient that thyroid medications are essential for life and that treatment is lifelong.
7. Teach the patient the importance of eating a balanced diet high in fiber and of drinking adequate fluid.
8. Stress the importance of balancing rest with activity to prevent overexhaustion or excess expenditure of energy.
9. Teach the patient the importance of follow-up evaluations and care with her primary health provider.

CHAPTER 12

Transplantation and Therapeutic Procedures

Bone Marrow Transplantation

Until recently most bone marrow transplants have involved donors of two types, an identical twin (syngeneic transplant) or an HLA-matched, mixed lymphocyte culture (MLC)–compatible sibling (allogeneic transplant). A syngeneic (identical twin) transplant is ideal, because the donor is matched with the recipient at all genetic loci.

A transplant using bone marrow from anyone other than an identical twin or the patient himself is called an allogeneic transplant. In most allogeneic bone marrow transplants, a sibling who matches at HLA-A, HLA-B, HLA-C, and HLA-D loci is the donor. The HLA loci are on a small region of chromosome 6, and these loci usually are inherited as a unit, known as a haplotype. Each parent has two haplotypes, and a child inherits one haplotype from each parent. A 25% probability exists that two siblings will be HLA identical.

An unrelated HLA-identical donor may also be used when no related donor is available. There is a 1 in 25,000 chance that two unrelated individuals will be HLA identical. A number of centers worldwide perform unrelated transplants, and the International Bone Marrow Registry is available to try to match donors and recipients. Initial reports on the use of unrelated donors are available; however, results have been poor, and further research is needed.

A partially matched donor, such as a sibling, parent, or uncle, may be selected when no HLA-identical sibling is available. Preliminary reports on the use of par-

tially matched donors are encouraging, but further investigation is needed.

Another form of bone marrow transplantation (BMT), the autologous graft, involves the use of the patient's own bone marrow. As with identical twins, no clinically significant graft-versus-host disease (GVHD) will occur. However, with autologous grafts, tumor cells may be present in the marrow harvested during remission; therefore attempts to purge the marrow of occult tumor cells before cryopreservation (freezing of the marrow) are being studied. Autologous bone marrow transplantation currently is under investigation as a treatment for a variety of malignancies.

INDICATIONS

Allogeneic bone marrow transplantation is the treatment of choice for patients with aplastic anemia who are under 50 years of age and who have an HLA-identical donor. It is also a treatment for severe immunodeficiency disorders, acute leukemias, myelodysplastic syndromes, chronic myelogenous leukemia, multiple myeloma, and hematopoietic defects.

Autologous bone marrow transplantation is being used with increasing success to treat acute leukemia, multiple myeloma, lymphoma, both Hodgkin's and non-Hodgkin's disease, and responsive solid tumors, including neuroblastomas, cancers of the breast and testes, and small cell lung cancer.

HARVEST

With both allogeneic and autologous transplants, marrow is harvested in the operating room with the donor under general or spinal anesthesia. About 100 aspirations are obtained from the posterior iliac crest (if necessary the anterior iliac crest may also be used) (Figure 12-1). Because children require a smaller amount of marrow, fewer aspirations are necessary than for an adult. A small amount of bone marrow (20 ml) is collected with each aspiration and placed in a tissue culture medium containing heparin. This solution is filtered through a stainless steel screen to remove bone chips, fat globules, and clots. The marrow is filtered initially through a large-screen filter and again through a smaller screen filter. The marrow is then transferred to a blood transfusion bag. The amount of bone marrow aspirated depends on several factors: the donor's weight, the concentration of cells in the donated marrow, and the processing procedure used before the marrow is transfused. If no special processing is done, the amount of marrow obtained is approximately 10 to 15 ml/kg of the recipient's body weight. Some of the cells are destroyed when the marrow is processed, leaving fewer cells for infusion. In a typical adult, a unit of 500 to 750 ml of blood and bone marrow contains 10 billion to 20 billion nucleated marrow cells.

ADMINISTRATION OF MARROW

After harvesting, the marrow is administered intravenously through a central venous access device (such as a Hickman or Cook catheter) or frozen in liquid nitrogen. If the marrow is to be purged either with a chemotherapeutic agent (e.g., 4-HC-4 hydroperoxycyclophosphamide) or a monoclonal antibody, this is done before cryopreservation. Purging eliminates any occult tumor

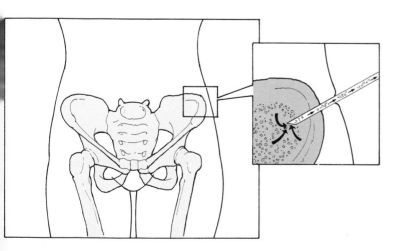

FIGURE 12-1
Bone marrow harvest.

cells in the marrow. Cell volume and viability are also evaluated before cryopreservation.

In the stem cell disorders, bone marrow transplantation is used to replace defective or missing hematopoietic stem cells with healthy ones. In the treatment of hematogenously spread malignant diseases, transplantation is done after chemotherapy to replace defective stem cells with healthy ones. In the treatment of solid tumors, transplantation is done after high-dose chemotherapy has eradicated the marrow. The high-dose chemotherapy destroys normal bone marrow, and transplantation is done to repopulate or rescue the patient's own hematopoietic system.

COMPLICATIONS: GRAFT-VERSUS-HOST DISEASE

Graft-versus-host disease (GVHD) is a major cause of mortality following allogeneic transplantation, with an incidence as high as 45%. GVHD results when the mature lymphocytes in the marrow (graft) recognize the recipient (host) as foreign. Since most patients are HLA-A, HLA-B, and HLA-D/DR identical to their donors, minor antigenic differences are thought to cause GVHD. In any mismatch transplants, the probability of GVHD developing increases with the degree of mismatch. A number of factors increase the probability of GVHD, as shown in the box below.

Clinical Presentation

In GVHD, the lymphocyte in the graft attacks the patient's skin, liver, and gastrointestinal tract. With acute GVHD, peak onset occurs 30 to 50 days after transplantation, although the disorder may start as early as day 10 and last up to day 100. The median duration of onset is 25 days. Patients may manifest symptoms in one or all three systems. Skin GVHD usually starts as a fine maculopapular rash on the trunk, palms, soles, and ears; this may progress to generalized erythroderma with desquamation of the skin. The major complaints associated with gastrointestinal involvement are abdominal pain, nausea, vomiting, and diarrhea. The diarrhea

---

FACTORS INCREASING THE PROBABILITY OF GVHD

Recipient over 30 years of age
Advanced disease
Donor of the opposite sex
High degree of mismatch
Diagnosis other than acute lymphocytic leukemia

From Gale et al, 1987.

usually is watery and may amount to as much as several liters in a 24-hour period. GVHD involving the liver is characterized by an increase in liver enzymes and alkaline phosphatase. Patients may complain of pain in the right upper quadrant, and hepatomegaly may develop.

Chronic GVHD has an onset of 100 days after transplantation, although in rare cases it has been diagnosed at 1 year afterward. The disease occurs as an extension of acute GVHD (progressive-type onset), subsequent to a period of resolution of acute GVHD (quiescent onset), or without preceding acute GVHD (de novo onset). The signs and symptoms of chronic GVHD in the skin are itching and burning, particularly on the palms and soles; patchy hyperpigmentation that may appear mottled; erythema; rough, flaky bronze-colored hyperpigmentation; and possibly contractures.

The incidence of chronic GVHD affecting the liver may be as high as 90%. Symptoms reported by Corcoran-Buchsel[46] include increases in alkaline phosphatase, serum glutamate oxaloacetate transaminase (SGOT), and bilirubin.

Other manifestations of chronic GVHD include involvement of the oral mucosa and ocular lining, esophageal abnormalities, vaginal problems, and immunodeficiencies.

Diagnosis and Treatment

The diagnosis usually is made by biopsy of the skin or gastrointestinal tract. GVHD may be treated with cyclosporin A, prednisone, methotrexate, monoclonal antibodies, and antithymocyte globulin. Investigational agents include thalidomide and xomazyme. These agents may be used individually or in combination, and a number of studies are attempting to determine the best combination for treatment and prophylaxis.

The diagnostic tests for chronic GVHD include skin and oral mucosa biopsies, liver and pulmonary function tests, the Schirmer tear test, and autoimmune blood tests (Table 12-1). Therapy for chronic GVHD includes immunosuppressive agents and antibiotics to prevent infection. Immunosuppressive agents include prednisone, procarbazine, cyclophosphamide, and azothioprine. Vogelsang[184] has reported that the transplant group at Johns Hopkins is using thalidomide to treat chronic GVHD. The antibiotic most commonly used to prevent infection is trimethoprim-sulfamethoxazole (Bactrim), and acyclovir is given for prophylaxis against recrudescence of the herpes virus.

Tables 12-2 and 12-3 present two systems for clinical staging of GVHD. In about 40% of patients, acute GVHD is mild and limited to the skin. Vogelsang[184] noted that 15% to 20% of allograft recipients had severe multiorgan disease, which may be fatal.

CONDITIONING REGIMEN

The purposes of conditioning are to eliminate defective stem cells; to provide immunosuppression, thereby minimizing the possibility of rejection; and to eliminate any residual malignant cells.

The conditioning regimen used before bone marrow transplantation depends on the disease being treated.

Table 12-1

DIAGNOSTIC STUDIES AND FINDINGS IN GRAFT-VERSUS-HOST DISEASE

Diagnostic test	Findings	
	Acute GVHD	Chronic GVHD
Biopsy of skin, gut, or oral mucosa	Infiltration of T cells into skin or gastrointestinal tract	Infiltration of lymphocytes and T cells into skin and oral mucosa
Liver function test	Elevated bilirubin, alkaline phosphatase, and SGOT	Elevated bilirubin, alkaline phosphatase, and SGOT
Pulmonary function test	Decreased diffusion capacity and lung capacity	Decreased diffusion capacity and lung capacity
Schirmer tear test	Dry eyes with increased risk of corneal abrasions and ulcerations	Dry eyes with increased risk of corneal abrasions and ulcerations
Autoimmune blood test	Not applicable	Positive test result; patient may have patchy dispigmentation and lichen planus–like papules on the skin and may have salivary changes similar to those in Sjögren's syndrome

Table 12-2

SEVERITY OF ACUTE GRAFT-VERSUS-HOST DISEASE

Stages of GVHD according to organ system

Skin		*Liver*		*Gastrointestinal*	
Stage		Stage		Stage	
+1	Maculopapular eruption involving less than 25% of the body surface	+1	Moderate increase in SGOT (150 to 170 IU) and bilirubin (2 to 3 mg/dl)		Diarrhea, nausea, and vomiting are also grade +1 through +4 in severity. The severity of GI
+2	Maculopapular eruption involving 25% to 50% of the body surface	+2	Rise in bilirubin (3 to 5.9 mg/dl) with or without an increase in SGOT		involvement was assigned to the most severe of the three involvements noted. It is difficult
+3	Generalized erythroderma	+3	Rise in bilirubin (6 to 14.9 mg/dl) with or without an increase in SGOT		to quantitate most of these manifestations, except diarrhea.
+4	Generalized erythroderma with bulbous formation and often with desquamation	+4	Rise in bilirubin (15 mg/dl) with or without an increase in SGOT (increases in SGOT are temporarily related to either onset or worsening of the skin rash)	+1	500 ml of stool/day
				+2	1,000 ml of stool/day
				+3	1,500 ml of stool/day
				+4	2,000 ml of stool/day

Adapted from Thompson et al.[178]

Table 12-3

CLINICAL GRADING OF GRAFT-VERSUS-HOST DISEASE

Grade	Degree of Organ Involvement
I	+1 to +2 skin rash; no gut involvement; no liver involvement; no decrease in clinical performance
II	+1 to +3 skin rash; +1 gut involvement or +1 liver involvement (or both); mild decrease in clinical performance.
III	+2 to +3 skin rash; +2 to +3 gut involvement or +2 to +3 liver involvement, or both; marked decrease in clinical performance
IV	Similar to grade III with +2 to +4 organ involvement and extreme decrease in clinical performance

From Thomas ED: Reprinted by permission of the New England Journal of Medicine 292:896, 1975.

Conditioning regimens include high-dose chemotherapy with or without radiotherapy.

The patient, family, donor, and significant others are provided with instructions about the procedure, its course, and complications.

Radiation

Typical side effects of total body irradiation include nausea and vomiting, which may be severe; diarrhea; erythema of the skin; and parotitis. These side effects usually are of short duration when moderate fractionated radiotherapy is used. Except for erythema of the skin, these side effects usually resolve within 7 days.

Cyclophosphamide

Cyclophosphamide may cause hemorrhagic cystitis. This may be counteracted by inserting a three-way Foley catheter and providing continuous saline irrigation at the rate of 1 L/hour. The Foley catheter remains in place for 24 hours after the last dose of cyclophosphamide. Removal of the catheter is delayed because of the prolonged half-life of cyclophosphamide (21 hours). Uric acid is released as cells are destroyed, resulting in deposition of uric acid crystals in the kidneys. This can be decreased by providing an alkaline environment. Maintaining a urine pH above 6.5 reduces the potential for uric acid nephropathy. Allopurinol may be used to prevent the formation of uric acid from cell byproducts. Cardiotoxicity is another problem with cyclophosphamide, yet it is found in fewer than 5% of the patients receiving this drug.

Busulfan

Because busulfan is available only in 2 mg tablets, the patient must swallow a significant number of pills for each dose. The tablets should not be swallowed all at once, since this increases the risk of emesis. The patient should be instructed to take five to eight of the tablets at a time. The dose should be taken over a period no longer than 30 minutes.

The toxicities associated with busulfan include severe pancytopenia, potential pulmonary toxicity, severe nausea and vomiting (at high doses), and skin alterations such as ulcerations and erythema of the palms, soles, axillae, and groin. Busulfan also has been reported to lower the seizure threshold, and grand mal seizures have been reported. The toxicities most often seen in transplant recipients are nausea, vomiting, and skin alterations. Appropriate skin care measures should be instituted to prevent infection in the affected areas.

Etoposide (VP-16)

Fever and chills usually are noted within a few hours of starting etoposide. Acetaminophen is given to control the fever, and if the chills progress to rigors, meperidine (25-50 mg IV) may be used to diminish the shaking. Metabolic changes include acidosis, which may be noted by a decreasing carbon dioxide level within 24 hours after administration. Significant mucositis is noted within 5 to 7 days after completion of the therapy. Significant skin toxicity is also seen within 1 week of completion of therapy and may last for 3 weeks. Hypotension, dysrhythmias, hepatic toxicity, and neurotoxicity have also been reported with use of this drug in high doses.

ADMINISTRATION

The goal of BMT is to restore defective or missing stem cells. For autologous marrow, blood bags containing approximately 50 ml of cryopreserved marrow are thawed quickly, one at a time, in a basin of warm water at approximately 37.7° C (100° F). The contents of the bag are removed with a 50-ml syringe and a 16-gauge needle and then administered rapidly through a central

---

PREPARATIVE SCHEDULES FOR BONE MARROW TRANSPLANT

The days before transplant are indicated by negative numbers, with day 0 being the day of transplant.

An allogeneic conditioning regimen:

Wednesday	Day −8	Admission
Thursday	Day −7	Cyclophosphamide, Foley catheter, continuous bladder irrigation
Friday	Day −6	Cyclophosphamide, Foley catheter with continuous bladder irrigation
Saturday	Day −5	Removal of Foley catheter; rest
Sunday	Day −4	Rest
Monday	Day −3	TBI, fractionated bid
Tuesday	Day −2	TBI (as above)
Wednesday	Day −1	TBI (as above)
Thursday	Day 0	Marrow infusion

An autologous conditioning regimen:

Wednesday	Day −8	Admission
Thursday	Day −7	Busulfan PO
Friday	Day −6	Busulfan PO
Saturday	Day −5	Busulfan PO
Sunday	Day −4	Busulfan PO
Monday	Day −3	Etoposide (VP-16) IV
Tuesday	Day −2	Rest
Wednesday	Day −1	Rest
Thursday	Day 0	Marrow infusion

line (double-lumen Cook or Hickman catheter). A solution of 0.9% normal saline is infused during the procedure. Before the infusion the patient usually is given diphenhydramine (50 mg), acetaminophen (650 mg), and hydrocortisone (50 mg). Because the patient may react to the preservative dimethylsulfoxide (DMSO) used in the marrow bags, epinephrine, diphenhydramine, and hydrocortisone are kept at the bedside. The patient may experience fever, chills, rash, chest pain, bradycardia, heart block, and nausea and vomiting. Major hemolytic reactions, along with elevated serum creatinine, have also been reported.

For a syngeneic or allogeneic donation, a standard-type blood bag containing fresh bone marrow just obtained from the donor and appropriately filtered is transported from the operating room. After the recipient is given diphenhydramine (50 mg) and acetaminophen (650 mg), the donated marrow is administered (over a period of no more than 4 hours) through a Hickman catheter without a filter. Patients receiving the marrow may have some chest pain, shortness of breath, or flushing, but these symptoms usually subside with appropriate intervention. The usual interventions for any side effects of marrow infusion are steroids, oxygen, and nitroglycerin tablets.

MEDICAL MANAGEMENT (PHYSICIAN'S ORDERS)

GENERAL MANAGEMENT

Physical therapy: Activate referral on admission; daily exercise program.

Vital signs: Check q 4 h or more frequently as necessary.

Diet: Regular diet as tolerated; calorie count when unable to eat; obtain orders for hyperalimentation (hyperalimentation usually lasts for at least 3 weeks).

IV therapy: To maintain hydration and renal perfusion.

Pain management: Intermittent use of narcotics for pain control, followed by continuous infusion via patient-controlled analgesia as needed.

Antiemetic therapy: Used to decrease nausea from conditioning regimen and results of alteration in gastrointestinal tract from chemotherapy: metoclopramide, lorazepam, diphenhydramine, dexamethasone, ondansetron.

Skin care management: To decrease effects of toxicity from combination chemotherapy and/or radiation therapy (see the following box): Aquaphor, Burow's solution, Silvadene (for those not allergic to sulfa).

Treatment for rigors: Meperidine, 25-50 mg IV, to control rigors from preparative regimen or reaction to blood products and/or antifungal agents.

PROPHYLACTIC DRUG THERAPY

Antibiotics: Usually given for prophylaxis after right atrial catheter is placed; trimethoprim-sulfamethoxazole (Bactrim) is given to prevent *Pneumocystis carinii* pneumonia; often started when absolute neutrophil count drops below 500/mm^3.

Antiviral drugs: Acyclovir to prevent recrudescence of herpes virus.

Antifungal drugs: To prevent fungal infections (e.g., fluconazole, amphotericin).

CONDITIONING REGIMEN

Chemotherapy: Usually given for 2-6 days, depending on protocol.

TBI: Dosage varies from 800 to 1,200 rad (e.g., 1,200 rad given in fractionated doses of 200 rad two times per day).

Continued.

MEDICAL MANAGEMENT (PHYSICIAN'S ORDERS)—cont'd

DRUG THERAPY—CONDITIONING REGIMEN

Cyclophosphamide: Usually given for 2-4 days.

Busulfan: Usually given over 4 days at dosing interval of q 6 h.

Etoposide (VP-16): Can be given over 2-4 days or as a single large dose.

Methotrexate: 12 mg intrathecally for leukemic patients or those with lymphoma; for CNS prophylaxis.

DRUG THERAPY—GVHD PROPHYLAXIS (ALLOGENEIC TRANSPLANT ONLY)

Cyclosporin A; prednisone; methotrexate; gamma globulin: given on a regular basis to provide antibodies that were ablated during preparative regimen; antipyretics: for fever.

UNIVERSITY OF CALIFORNIA—SAN FRANCISCO SKIN CARE PROGRAM

1. Wash affected areas tid with water, no soap.
2. Apply Aquaphor cream tid to erythematous areas without skin breakdown.
3. For skin breakdown other than on the scrotum or in the pubic area, use Burow's soaks (one capful of solution in 1 quart of water) for 20 minutes, followed by application of Silvadene cream. (**Silvadene cream should not be used if the patient is allergic to sulfa.**) Wrap the affected areas with Kerlix. Repeat the procedure tid until all areas have healed.
4. For skin breakdown on the scrotum and in the pubic area, apply soda bicarbonate soaks to decrease the irritation; then apply Aquaphor or nystatin cream to affected areas.

NURSING CARE OF THE BONE MARROW TRANSPLANT PATIENT

NURSING DIAGNOSIS

Altered nutrition: less than body requirements related to nausea and vomiting, indigestion, and loss of appetite from chemotherapy.

NURSING INTERVENTIONS AND RATIONALE

1. Administer antiemetic drug before treatment and at frequent intervals afterward as ordered to relieve nausea and anxiety related to nausea, and monitor patient response.
2. Consider using behavioral relaxation techniques to reduce the onset and duration of nausea.
3. Instruct patient to avoid quick movements while nauseated. Quick movements can trigger the gag reflex and increase nausea.
4. Encourage patient to eat slowly and chew thoroughly to aid digestion.
5. Instruct patient to avoid lying flat for at least 1 h after eating to aid digestion.
6. Encourage patient to drink liquids (clear, cool beverages or soups) slowly through a straw before, not during, meals to maintain adequate fluid intake.
7. Provide carbonated beverages, dry crackers or toast, tart foods (e.g., lemons or sour pickles), ice pops, and gelatin desserts to curb nausea.
8. Suggest high-protein, high-calorie diet and small, frequent meals to ensure adequate nutrient intake and curb nausea.
9. Maintain optimum nutritional status; check weight daily; monitor calorie counts; arrange dietary consultation; administer TPN as ordered to maintain adequate nutritional intake.
10. Monitor serum electrolytes daily, and check urine for glucose, ketones, and protein to identify electrolyte accumulations.

NURSING DIAGNOSIS
Pain related to parotitis.

NURSING INTERVENTIONS AND RATIONALE

1. Encourage increased fluid intake to provide adequate hydration and to compensate for lack of saliva.
2. Encourage frequent oral hygiene to eliminate bad taste in patient's mouth.
3. If xerostomia is present, suggest hard candies, sugarless gum, or a commercial product such as Xero-Lube or Orabase to increase salivary secretion.
4. Administer medications as ordered to alleviate pain, and monitor patient response; narcotic analgesics may be required.
5. Tell patient to avoid using irritants such as alcohol or tobacco to prevent further discomfort.

Table 12-4

NURSING ASSESSMENT FOR THE BONE MARROW TRANSPLANT PATIENT

Assessment	Observations
Volume status	Anxiety; tachycardia; cool, moist skin; cyanotic lips and nail beds; if edema worsens, confusion and stupor appear; dyspnea and air hunger are accompanied by a productive cough and frothy, blood-tinged sputum; rales and rhonchi are also heard on examination
Pulmonary	Dyspnea; rapid, shallow respirations; shortness of breath; chest pain; cyanosis; increased heart rate; diaphoresis
Reaction to white cells in marrow	Chills, fever, rash, urticaria, chest pain, malaise, hypotension, shortness of breath
Renal	Grossly red urine and Hemastix-positive urine (normal for 24 hours after transplant)
Bacterial contamination of marrow	Hypotension, fever, rigors, diaphoresis, shaking chills, shortness of breath
Engraftment	Hematologic recovery, increasing neutrophil count within 10-14 days after marrow infusion, granulocytes, platelets, and erythrocytes within normal limits (normal time period, 21-160 days)
Rejection/failure to engraft	Marrow function does not return; obligatory 7 to 10 days for marrow recovery or to engraft after a period of recovery
Infection	Fever, chills, rigors, redness, swelling of any site, skin rash, wound drainage, cough, dyspnea, sore throat, mucositis, headache, dysuria, frequency, urgency, diarrhea, hypotension, positive blood cultures, spontaneous bacterial peritonitis, change in mental status
Anemia	Decreased RBCs, decreased Hct (<25%), decreased Hb (<8.2), excessive fatigue, dyspnea on exertion, shortness of breath, pallor, tachycardia, palpitations
Stomatitis	Oral soreness, pain, burning or tingling in mouth, thick secretions, inability to swallow, erythema, ulceration, pseudomembrane formation, taste changes, oozing from oral membranes
Thrombocytopenia	Petechiae, purpura, bleeding from any body orifice or site of catheter, epistaxis, hemoptysis, hematemesis, hematuria, hematochezia, change in mental status (e.g., headache, confusion, lethargy, nausea, change in pupil size, seizures)
Nutritional status	Anorexia, weight loss (>2 kg/wk), decreased albumin (<3.5), nausea, vomiting, diarrhea, fluid imbalance
GVHD	Mild maculopapular rash, generalized erythroderma that may progress to desquamation, increase in serum bilirubin, increase in SGOT, or alkaline phosphatase, abdominal cramping, diarrhea (green and watery), hematochezia
Venooclusive disease (VOD)	Sudden weight gain, increasing abdominal girth, right upper quadrant pain, jaundice, hepatomegaly, ascites, encephalopathy; elevated SGOT, alkaline phosphatase, and bilirubin; coagulation abnormalities (PT, PTT, fibrinogen)
Interstitial pneumonitis	Dry cough, dyspnea, nasal flaring, tachypnea (40-60 beats/min), rales; diffuse pulmonary infiltrates on chest x-ray; hypoxemia at room air (Pao_2 <70 mm Hg)
Cardiac toxicity	Dyspnea on exertion, orthopnea, weakness, fatigue, peripheral edema, chest pain, syncope, dysrhythmias, pericardial effusion, and tachypnea; changes noted on ECG and echocardiogram
Renal insufficiency	Decreased urine output; marked increase in body weight (>2 kg); peripheral edema; postural changes in BP (>20 mm Hg); thirst; complaints of dizziness; flat, distended neck veins; changes in specific gravity (<1.005) and urine electrolytes
Psychosocial status	Fear, anger, depression, anxiety, remorse, acting out, inappropriate behavior

NURSING DIAGNOSIS

Hyperthermia related to total body irradiation.

NURSING INTERVENTIONS AND RATIONALE

1. Maintain adequate hydration to compensate for dryness of mucosa caused by irradiation.
2. Administer antipyretics as ordered, and monitor patient response.
3. Alleviate patient's concern by informing him that fever usually disappears 4 to 6 days after TBI.
4. Monitor temperature every 2 to 4 hours to detect persistent or resolving hyperthermia.
5. Monitor intake and output and daily weights to ensure optimal fluid balance and prevent dehydration.
6. Adjust environmental temperature to patient's comfort (e.g., remove excess clothing and bedding). Body heat is lost through convection and evaporation of sweat.
7. Administer acetaminophen rather than aspirin to children, since aspirin has been implicated in Reye's syndrome in children.

NURSING DIAGNOSIS

Diarrhea related to effects of total body irradiation on gastrointestinal mucosa.

NURSING INTERVENTIONS AND RATIONALE

1. Administer antidiarrheal agents as ordered to prevent and control diarrhea, and monitor patient response.
2. Maintain adequate fluid intake to prevent dehydration.
3. Suggest a bland, low-residue diet high in potassium to provide adequate potassium from food that can be digested easily (irradiation can increase transit time in the colon).
4. Instruct patient in meticulous perianal skin care; tell him to use sitz baths after each bowel movement and to apply a soothing lubricant to the perianal area to prevent infection and alleviate pain and discomfort.

NURSING DIAGNOSIS

High risk for impaired skin integrity related to erythema of skin from irradiation.

NURSING INTERVENTIONS AND RATIONALE

1. Instruct patient to keep skin clean and dry before irradiation. Use mild soap such as Dove or Dial for bathing, rinse skin well, and pat dry, because irradiation dries and irritates the skin at the level of the dermis and epidermis.
2. Instruct patient to avoid using perfumed powders or lotions and extremes of temperature to skin (e.g., hot or cold baths, ice packs, and heating pads) to prevent further skin irritation.
3. Use lubricated cream (Aquaphor, Nutriderm) tid after irradiation to increase patient's comfort and minimize itching.

NURSING DIAGNOSIS

Altered bladder tissue perfusion (hemorrhagic cystitis) related to local effects of cyclophosphamide.

NURSING INTERVENTIONS AND RATIONALE

1. Begin IV hydration 4 h before cyclophosphamide administration, and continue for 24 h after therapy as ordered (IV fluids should be administered 1½ to 2 times maintenance rates) as a cleansing measure, because cyclophosphamide metabolites can destroy the uroepithelial lining of the bladder.
2. Perform continuous bladder irrigation using a three-way Foley catheter if ordered (not needed if patient can void qh) to eliminate toxic products of cyclophosphamide that irritate the bladder lining.
3. Monitor urine for blood q 4 h to identify destruction of bladder lining.
4. Maintain accurate intake and output records to detect altered fluid status.

NURSING DIAGNOSIS

Altered renal tissue perfusion related to potential toxicity from chemotherapy.

NURSING INTERVENTIONS AND RATIONALE

1. Maintain adequate hydration, check urine output hourly, and administer furosemide (Lasix) as ordered to prevent interference with renal function and damage to renal tubules that sometimes occurs with chemotherapy. Monitor patient response.
2. Check urine pH q 4 h; maintain at or above 7, and monitor BUN/creatinine to determine adequacy of renal function.
3. Administer allopurinol as ordered, and monitor patient response. Allopurinol may increase the incidence and degree of bone marrow suppression by prolonging the half-life of cyclophosphamide, which may cause further insult to the kidneys.

NURSING DIAGNOSIS

Decreased cardiac output (potential) related to cardiotoxicity from chemotherapy.

NURSING INTERVENTIONS AND RATIONALE

1. Check results of ECG to detect alterations indicating damage to myocardial muscle or the presence of a cardiomyopathy (ECG is obtained daily while patient is being treated with high-dose cyclophosphamide).
2. Monitor patient's level of consciousness, changes in baseline vital signs, and ECG. Changes in clinical status may indicate decreased cardiac output.
3. Monitor heart rate and rhythm to identify dysrhythmias.

NURSING DIAGNOSIS

High risk for infection related to leukopenia.

NURSING INTERVENTIONS AND RATIONALE

1. Maintain protective environment to reduce the risk of infection (reverse isolation protocols vary among centers).
2. Monitor WBC and absolute granulocyte count daily to detect evidence of infection induced by prolonged leukopenia.
3. Monitor vital signs q 4 h, and check skin and mucous membranes; inspect all body orifices daily for redness, swelling, and pain, and inspect insertion site of venous access device for redness, swelling, pain, and drainage, to detect infection early.
4. Auscultate lungs q 8 h for increased or decreased breath sounds, rhonchi, and rales to determine adequacy of gas exchange and detect presence of possible infection.
5. Maintain meticulous mouth care to prevent infection and eliminate bad taste in patient's mouth.
6. Use strict aseptic technique when changing dressings and in IV preparation and administration to prevent infection.
7. Avoid bladder catheterization, except when necessary; avoid administering enemas and suppositories and taking rectal temperatures to prevent introduction of bacteria.
8. Encourage patient to use deodorant rather than antiperspirant to avoid blocking axillary sweat glands, which may promote infection.
9. Obtain surveillance cultures of throat, urine, stool, skin, or other areas as ordered to detect colonization before infection spreads.
10. Do not allow fresh-cut flowers or plants in patient's room, and eliminate stagnant water to prevent colonization of bacteria.
11. Limit the number of visitors, and screen them for infection, recent vaccinations (e.g., oral polio vaccine is shed in the stool), or exposure to communicable diseases (especially children) to protect patient from exposure to communicable diseases.
12. Provide mask for patient when he leaves his room (isolation protocol varies) to protect him from infection.
13. Administer antibiotics on schedule per physician's orders to control proliferation of infection. Monitor patient response.
14. Patient's CMV status should be determined before transfusions. If the patient is CMV negative, administer only CMV-negative blood to prevent serious illness that can be caused by the virus, especially in organ transplant patients.

NURSING DIAGNOSIS

Alteration in protection related to decreased function of hemopoietic system (platelets).

NURSING INTERVENTIONS AND RATIONALE

1. Monitor platelet count regularly (the risk of bleeding is high when platelet count is $<10,000$ cells/mm^3) to prevent increased risk of bleeding caused by prolonged thrombocytopenia.
2. Monitor skin and mucous membranes for increased tendency to bruise, petechiae, bleeding gums, and epistaxis; test stool, urine, and emesis for occult blood to detect bleeding early.
3. Look for any changes in patient's vital signs, behavior, or pupil size to detect intracranial hemorrhage.
4. After invasive procedures such as bone marrow aspiration and biopsy, monitor site frequently to detect any oozing of blood.
5. Do not take rectal temperatures or administer rectal suppositories and enemas, to avoid irritating the rectal tissue and to decrease the risk of bleeding.
6. Encourage adequate fluid intake and use of stool softener to prevent constipation and straining, which may increase the risk of bleeding.
7. Place a sign indicating bleeding precautions over patient's bed to alert others to the potential for bleeding.
8. Administer medroxyprogesterone acetate as ordered to control menses, and monitor patient's response.
9. Apply topical agents (e.g., topical thrombin, ϵ-aminocaproic acid, topical cocaine, tranexamic acid, or Gelfoam) to bleeding sites per physician's order to control bleeding. Monitor patient response.
10. Administer irradiated platelet transfusions rapidly as ordered (families are encouraged to find donors for blood products), and monitor platelet count 1 h after transfusion to prevent further bleeding.

NURSING DIAGNOSIS

Activity intolerance related to anemia, nutritional status, disruption of sleep, anxiety, or depression.

NURSING INTERVENTIONS AND RATIONALE

1. Administer irradiated RBC transfusions as ordered to counteract fatigue and decreased activity tolerance caused by BMT process. Monitor patient response.
2. Check Hb levels and Hct values regularly to assess the need for more blood.
3. Maintain optimum nutritional status to improve strength and minimize fatigue.
4. Arrange nursing care so that patient has uninter-

rupted periods of rest and sleep, especially during the night, to relieve fatigue.

5. Encourage patient to discuss his feelings and concerns to alleviate or minimize anxiety or depression, which may contribute to persistent fatigue.

6. Encourage a progressive activity program as tolerated to prevent adverse effects of bed rest and increase activity.

NURSING DIAGNOSIS

Altered oral mucous membrane related to conditioning regimen or infection.

NURSING INTERVENTIONS AND RATIONALE

1. Implement nursing care related to stomatitis, based on assessment using grading system developed by Capizzi (see the box on page 326), to care for patient's mucositis/stomatitis.

NURSING DIAGNOSIS

Altered protection related to graft-versus-host disease (occurs only in allogeneic BMT).

NURSING INTERVENTIONS AND RATIONALE

1. Assess skin integrity each shift; assess level of pain and pruritus, and administer analgesics and antihistamines as needed, because donor T cells destroy host in areas of skin, gastrointestinal tract, and liver. Monitor patient response.

2. Provide meticulous skin care, including daily bath with povidone-iodine and normal saline or other antibacterial solution. Oatmeal or baking soda baths may be indicated for pruritus to prevent infection and to help healing.

3. Apply creams or lotions (Aquaphor or A&D Ointment with mineral oil) on intact skin to minimize breakdown of healthy skin and to promote healing of affected skin.

4. Apply mixture of silver sulfadiazine and nystatin on open areas of skin (other creams and ointments such as fluocinonide, hydrocortisone, and petroleum gauze may be used) to promote healing of affected skin.

5. Explain need to prevent scratching. Use mittens if necessary on infant or child. Use KenAire, Mediscus, or other flotation-type bed for patient with extensive skin involvement to prevent further irritation of skin.

6. Use bed cradle to prevent linens from touching skin, to alleviate pressure.

7. Assist patient frequently with active and passive range-of-motion exercises to prevent adverse effects of bed rest.

8. Note character and quantity of stool; test stool for occult blood to monitor blood loss.

9. Administer antidiarrheal agents as ordered (usually not helpful in controlling diarrhea with GVHD) to control diarrhea. Monitor patient response.

10. Provide meticulous perianal skin care to prevent infection.

11. Permit nothing by mouth as ordered to allow bowel to rest.

12. Reinstate oral feedings with isosmotic, low-fat, lactose-free beverages as ordered; increase diet as tolerated to provide adequate nutrients. Monitor patient response.

13. Monitor closely for dehydration, electrolyte imbalance, and weight change to monitor hydration and nutrition.

14. Ausculate bowel sounds q 8 h to monitor for development of ileus.

15. Check bilirubin and SGOT levels regularly to monitor for development of acute liver disease.

16. Measure abdominal girth twice a day to evaluate for ascites, hepatomegaly, or splenomegaly.

17. Position patient on left side to decrease pressure on liver.

18. Administer drugs to decrease the effects of GVHD (e.g., steroids, cyclosporin A, methotrexate, and antithymocyte globulin) as ordered according to protocol, and monitor patient response.

NURSING DIAGNOSIS

Altered protection related to venoocclusive disease stemming from fibrous obliteration of small hepatic venules.

NURSING INTERVENTIONS AND RATIONALE

1. Assess and monitor for sudden weight gain, right upper quadrant pain, ascites, jaundice, and disorientation, and measure abdominal girth twice a day at the level of the umbilicus with patient supine to de-

tect fibrotic obliteration of hepatic venules and alterations in hepatic function sometimes created by chemotherapy and irradiation.
2. Restrict sodium intake as ordered, and administer all intravenous medication in minimum volume of fluid to prevent fluid retention.
3. Monitor urine sodium levels and BP daily for orthostatic changes and to assess for fluid accumulation.
4. Monitor patient closely for toxic side effects of medication, which can be caused by impaired liver function.
5. Monitor liver function tests frequently to assess and monitor liver function.

NURSING DIAGNOSIS

Body image disturbance related to alopecia, weight loss, and sterility.

NURSING INTERVENTIONS AND RATIONALE

1. Encourage patient and significant others to express their feelings and concerns, and help them explore perceived meaning of loss, to facilitate recognition of body image changes.
2. Help minimize anxiety and promote adjustment of patient and significant others by informing them that alopecia and weight loss are temporary.
3. Help patient find ways to improve appearance (use of clothing, scarves, hats, or hairpieces) to enhance healthy self-image.
4. Convey an attitude of acceptance and understanding to enhance patient's feelings of self-worth.
5. Emphasize that negative reactions to altered body image are normal and expected, to minimize or alleviate patient's concern and anxiety.
6. Refer patient to community resources, organizations, and peer support group information. Shared experiences and methods of improving self-image may promote a positive body image and an improved sense of self.

NURSING DIAGNOSIS

Fear related to uncertain outcome of treatment, threat of death, isolation, and treatment protocols.

NURSING INTERVENTIONS AND RATIONALE

1. Encourage patient and significant others to express feelings and concerns and to ask questions, to facilitate recognition of fear and uncertainty.
2. Help patient decrease feelings of isolation through use of radio, television, tape recorder, or video cassette recorder.
3. Reinforce and restate information given to patient and significant others, to promote understanding of procedures and treatments.
4. Encourage patient and significant others to discuss hopes for positive outcome, to promote positive thinking, which generates energy and decreases feelings of fear and loneliness.

5. Consult other health care providers in planning a comprehensive approach to patient's care, to ensure that patient's needs are met and questions answered.

PATIENT TEACHING

Preparation for discharge includes teaching the following:

1. Teach the patient daily care for the central venous access device to maintain the patency of the catheter and prevent infection and bleeding.
   a. Cleanse area around catheter regularly and follow with povidone-iodine; cover with a gauze square and apply plastic dressing or paper tape.
   b. Monitor for signs of redness, pain, or swelling at catheter exit site.
   c. Heparinize line daily, according to the specific instructions given by your nurse.
   d. Contact your doctor if you experience chills, fever, or rigors (shaking chills after you flush the catheter).
2. Explain diet needed for optimum nutritional status (ideally the patient should be able to tolerate 1,000 calories a day to be discharged). All fresh fruits and vegetables should be thoroughly washed. Do not eat from salad bars or eat any raw food in restaurants. Make sure all your food is cooked and served at the appropriate temperature. Try to drink at least 2 quarts of fluid a day.
3. Teach the patient measures for preventing infection. Precautions are more rigid during the first 3 months after bone marrow transplantation and are relaxed as the year progresses.
   a. Monitor your temperature daily for the first month after discharge. Take your temperature in the late afternoon; it usually is highest at this time. If your temperature is over 38.5° C (101° F) call your doctor. Do not take medication to lower your temperature without first checking with your physician.
   b. Wear a face mask when you are out in crowds.
   c. Avoid contact with anyone who has had a cold or the flu or who has been exposed to such diseases as measles, mumps, or chickenpox.
   d. Avoid contact with young children who attend school. If you have young children and they are exposed to someone who has been ill, try to decrease your close contact for at least 24 hours.
   e. Make sure to wash your hands well before eating, after using the toilet, and after contact with anyone who might have a cold.
   f. Avoid crowds for the first 3 months; go grocery shopping and to theaters and restaurants during off peak hours.

ORAL CARE FOR STOMATITIS

For grade 1 or grade 2 stomatitis

1. Perform oral hygiene regimen every 2 hours while patient is awake and every 6 hours during night as follows:
   a. Use normal saline mouthwash if crusts are absent (1 teaspoon of salt in 1 L of sterile water may be used). If crusts and debris are present, use sodium bicarbonate solution (1 teaspoon in 8 ounces of water). Perform mouth care every 2 hours while patient is awake. Alternate bicarbonate solution with normal saline. Rinse with normal saline after bicarbonate.
   b. Floss gently with unwaxed dental floss every 24 hours if platelet count is above $50,000/mm^3$.
   c. Brush after each meal and before sleep, using a soft toothbrush and nonabrasive toothpaste such as Colgate.
   d. Remove dentures or partial plates; replace only for meals.
   e. Apply lip lubricant (e.g., Vaseline, Blistex, or K-Y Jelly) four times a day and as needed.
2. Measures for oral care include routine culture of mouth for bacteria, fungus, and virus. If these are present, use the following:
   a. For bacteria: Peridex, 15 ml bid.
   b. For fungus: nystatin, 15 ml qid; clotrimazole troche, 1 tablet 5 times a day; ketoconazole, 200 mg bid.
   c. For virus: acyclovir, 200 mg tablet 5 times a day, or 5 mg/kg IV q 8 h.
3. Suggestions for control of mouth pain:
   a. Initiate low-dose narcotics on a prn schedule; if necessary, proceed to continuous infusion (morphine, 2-4 mg q 2-4 h prn). If required more than q 2 h, switch to continuous infusion. If patient has problems with morphine, use Dilaudid, 0.5-1.5 mg q 2-4 h prn. If required more than q 2 h, change to continuous infusion. Patient-controlled analgesia may also be used at this time.
4. Implement dietary measures, including the following:
   a. Instruct patient to avoid abrasive foods such as toast, apples, and celery.
   b. Encourage intake of pureed, bland foods.
   c. Instruct patient to avoid tart or acid foods such as pickles or tomatoes.
   d. Instruct patient to avoid spices and vinegar.
   e. Instruct patient to avoid alcohol.
   f. Arrange for dietary consultation.
5. Discourage smoking.
6. Recommend use of artificial saliva for xerostomia. No comparative research on various agents is available.

For grade 3 or grade 4 stomatitis

1. Obtain sample from suspicious area and culture for bacteria, fungus, and virus per physician's order.
2. Institute oral hygiene regimen:
   a. Alternate antifungal or antibacterial suspension with warm saline mouthwash q 2 h while patient is awake and q 4 h during night.
   b. Do not floss.
   c. Brush gently with toothettes or cotton-tipped applicators.
   d. Remove dentures or bridge; do not replace for meals.
   e. Apply lip lubricant q 2 h.
3. In addition to local measures indicated for grades 1 and 2 stomatitis, systemic analgesics may be indicated, especially before eating.
4. Liquid diet may be indicated. If not, use pureed diet. See other measures as indicated in no. 3 for grade 1 and grade 2 stomatitis.
5. Discourage smoking.

   g. Avoid uncooked or rare meat for the first 3 months.
   h. Children who have had a bone marrow transplant should not attend school for 1 year.
   i. Do not swim in a private or public pool for 1 year after a bone marrow transplantation.
4. Teach the patient about contact with pets.

   a. Avoid contact with pets for the first 3 months after transplantation. Do not clean litter boxes or come in contact with animal feces.
   b. If you have an indoor/outdoor cat, do not allow the cat in your bedroom for the first 3 months. Cats carry organisms and may transmit diseases obtained while outdoors.

5. Instruct the patient about contact with plants and flowers.
   a. Do not garden for at least 3 months after transplantation.
   b. Do not cut fresh flowers or change their water; the water has bacteria that may cause infection.
   c. Try to decrease your contact with dirt and dust for at least 3 months after transplantation.
6. Instruct the patient in the importance of strict dental hygiene.
   a. See your dentist regularly.
   b. Brush your teeth at least twice a day.
   c. Continue your mouth care for the first month after discharge from the hospital.
   d. Floss your teeth daily if your platelet count is above 50,000/mm³.
   e. Do not use toothpicks.
   f. Use a soft-bristled toothbrush. If your platelet count is below 20,000/mm³, use a toothette instead of a toothbrush.
   g. Do not have elective dental work done during periods of thrombocytopenia, since it increases the risk of bleeding. Platelets must be above 50,000/mm³ before any dental work can be done.
   h. Do not use aspirin or products containing aspirin.
   i. If bleeding in your mouth occurs, control it with iced saline mouth rinses.
7. Provide the patient with information about immunizations.
   a. Do not have immunizations without your physician's approval.
   b. Avoid coming in contact with individuals who have recently been immunized with live viruses (e.g., measles, mumps, rubella, and oral polio).

8. Discuss sexuality with the patient.
   a. You may resume your normal sexual function when your platelets are above 50,000/mm³ and your energy level is sufficient.
   b. Avoid anal intercourse for at least 3 months after transplantation.
9. Discuss with patient necessary changes in activities of daily living.
   a. Take prophylactic antibiotics as prescribed.
   b. Take your temperature daily, and notify the physician of any elevation 2 degrees above baseline.
   c. Eliminate sharp objects in your environment (e.g., shave with an electric razor rather than a hand razor).
   d. Wear shoes or slippers at all times—no bare feet while walking.
   e. Do not use any beverages containing alcohol.
   f. Avoid blowing your nose or sneezing forcefully.
   g. Avoid bruising or bumping yourself.
   h. If epistaxis occurs, stay in a sitting position and apply ice to constrict small blood vessels. Applying pressure to your nose may control bleeding.
10. Teach the patient to call the doctor if:
    a. His temperature is over 38.5° C (101° F).
    b. He notices any rash, change in the color or consistency of his stool, change in the color of his urine, nausea or vomiting, pain, dryness of the mouth, difficulty swallowing, or change in skin color.
    c. He has a cough or shortness of breath.
    d. He notices any physical change that concerns him.

Transplant Immunology

Transplantation of organs and tissues has been performed for more than 5,000 years. Ancient records indicate that Hindus and Egyptians attempted skin transplantations to replace noses destroyed by syphilis. Celsus and Galen wrote of successful attempts to transplant tissue from one part of the body to another. Over the past 25 years, thousands of organs have been transplanted, with improving graft and patient survival, and many of these transplantations were performed for end-stage disease secondary to an immune disorder.

GENETIC FACTORS RELATED TO TRANSPLANT IMMUNOLOGY

Every human ovum and spermatozoan has 23 chromosomes. With the union of the ovum and the sperm, the unpaired chromosomes are brought together through the process of fertilization. After fertilization a total of 46 chromosomes is present, representing both maternal and paternal chromosomes. These 46 chromosomes are the new individual's total chromosomal inheritance.

Table 12-5

ORGAN TRANSPLANTATION PERFORMED BECAUSE OF IMMUNE DISORDERS

Disorder	Organ transplanted
Systemic lupus erythematosus (lupus nephritis)	Kidney
Autoimmune chronic active hepatitis	Liver
IgA nephropathy	Kidney
Primary biliary cirrhosis	Liver
Immune-complex glomerulonephritis	Kidney
Primary sclerosing cholangitis	Liver

A successful transplantation depends on the body's *inability* to recognize the graft as foreign.

Genes are a structural component of the chromosome and represent the functional sites of heredity. They carry the genetic code for unique protein and enzyme synthesis. All characteristics of the individual that eventually develop are influenced by the combination of genes carried by the ovum and sperm. The nucleus of a human cell has approximately 30,000 gene pairs, implying an almost infinite combination. However, because these chromosomes and genes are inherited, there are familial similarities (Figure 12-2).

On each chromosome a given gene is located in a specific position, known as a **locus.** Each of the two genes at the same locus of the chromosome is an **allele.**

Homozygous: Having a pair of identical alleles at a specific locus.
Heterozygous: Having different alleles at a specific locus.

The expression of a specific allele of the genotype depends on the recessive or dominant nature of the allele and whether it is homozygous or heterozygous. No two individuals have the same genotype, except for identical twins. Dominant traits are the physical expression of heterozygous alleles, and recessive traits are expressed only when the dominant allele is absent. Codominance refers to the expression of both alleles of the heterozygote.

Genes contain the code for specific cell surface antigens that influence transplantation. Two antigen systems that are important when considering transplantation are the ABO blood group and the major histocompatibility complex (MHC).

ABO Blood Group Antigens

ABO antigens are present in most body tissues and on the surfaces of red blood cells. They are serologically identified and form the classification system of human blood. ABO compatibility depends on whether antigens are present on the donor red blood cells, and whether antibodies develop in the recipient's serum. Three possible alleles can determine blood type for this genetic locus: A and B, which are codominant, and O, which is recessive and has no antigens. Anti-ABO antibodies are IgM class antibodies and typically cause agglutination, complement fixation, and hemolysis.

ABO typing is always performed before blood transfusions and organ transplantation to ensure compatibility between the recipient and the donor organ. If an ABO-incompatible donor organ is transplanted, hyperacute rejection generally occurs, with the possible exception of an ABO-incompatible liver transplantation.

Natural antibodies to blood group antigens also exist and may be responsible for hyperacute rejection in kidney transplantation involving ABO incompatibility.

Major Histocompatibility Complex

Another important antigen system is the major histocompatibility complex (MHC). This system has been

---

Genotype: An individual's genetic composition; refers to the polymorphic combinations of alleles on a chromosome.
Phenotype: The physical expression of the genotype as morphologic, biochemical, or physiologic characteristics.
Haplotype: A group of alleles made up of a set of closely linked genes that form a locus.

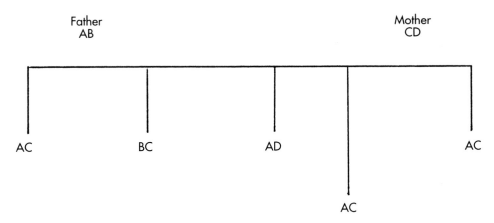

FIGURE 12-2
The principle of **genetic inheritance** states that every individual inherits one HLA region, a haplotype (A, B, C, D, gene coding for specific antigens), from each parent. Every offspring will have two haplotypes. Siblings with the same parents have a 25% chance of being HLA identical. Among family members, HLA-identical siblings provide the best match for transplantation.

identified in a number of different species. In humans it is called the human leukocyte antigen (HLA) system.

The HLA region and the genes that encode it are grouped into three categories, class I, class II, and class III. Three genetic loci code for class I antigens, which are HLA-A, HLA-B, and HLA-C. Class I antigens are located on virtually every nucleated cell in the body and are the main antigens recognized by the host during graft rejection.

Three genetic loci also code for class II antigens, which are HLA-DR, HLA-DP, and HLA-DQ. These antigens are located primarily on cells of the immune system, including B cells, macrophages, and activated T cells. Class II antigens can initiate a mixed lymphocyte response when allogeneic cells are cultured together, causing helper T-cell proliferation; activation of cytotoxic T cells; and production of antibody-secreting plasma cells. Class II antigens also participate in antigen presentation to T cells.

Class III antigens are the early components of the complement pathway. They are located between class I and class II antigens on chromosome 6. These genes code for factors C2, C4a, C4b, and Bf of the classic and alternative pathways.

HLA antigens are thought to play a major role in transplant rejection and are involved in various aspects of immunologic recognition and reaction. (Histocompatibility testing is discussed in Chapter 3.)

OVERVIEW OF THE IMMUNOLOGIC WORKUP FOR TRANSPLANTATION

In summary, immunologic workups for organ transplantation vary, depending on the center's protocol and the organ being transplanted.

Kidney Transplantation (Figure 12-3)

ABO testing is performed on all recipients and potential donors to prevent a hyperacute rejection caused by preformed isohemagglutinins; isohemagglutinins can damage the vascular endothelium, causing coagulation and subsequent graft loss. Individuals and their donors preparing for a living related kidney transplant should also have completed testing for HLA-A, HLA-B, HLA-C, HLA-DR, and HLA-DQ antigens. Generally the haplotype can be determined for each antigen identified. Haplotype matching is beneficial because the better the match (two haplotypes), the better the chances of graft survival. Cross-matching is done to

---

ABO BLOOD GROUP ANTIGENS

AB is the universal recipient; O is the universal donor.

The nomenclature of the **HLA system** is developed by the HLA Nomenclature Committee of the World Health Organization. Every HLA antigen is identified by a letter and a number. The letter indicates the genetic locus coding for the antigen, and the number designates order of discovery. The "w" means "workshop" and is dropped when worldwide agreement is attained, with the exception of Cw antigens, which will maintain the w to prevent confusion with complement. Further specificities are shown in parentheses.

A	B		C	D	DR	DQ
A1	B5	B51(5)	Cw1	Dw1	DR1	DQw1
A2	B7	Bw52(5)	Cw2	Dw2	DR2	DQw2
A3	B8	Bw53	Cw3	Dw3	DR3	DQw3
A9	B12	Bw54(w22)	Cw4	Dw4	DR4	DQw4
A10	B13	Bw55(w22)	Cw5	Dw5	DR5	DQw5(w1)
A11	B14	Bw56(w22)	Cw6	Dw6	DRw6	DQw6(w1)
Aw19	B15	Bw57(17)	Cw7	Dw7	DR7	DQw7(w3)
A23(9)	B16	Bw58(17)	Cw8	Dw8	DRw8	DQw8(w3)
A24(9)	B17	Bw59	Cw9(w3)	Dw9	DR9	DQw9(w3)
A25(10)	B18	Bw60(40)	Cw10(w3)	Cw10	DRw10	
A26(10)	B21	Bw61(40)	Cw11	Dw11(w7)	DRw11(5)	
A28	Bw22	Bw62(15)		Dw12	DRw12(5)	
A29(w19)	B27	Bw63(15)		Dw13	DRw13(w6)	
A30(w19)	B35	Bw64(15)		Dw14	DRw14(w6)	
A31(w19)	B37	Bw65(14)		Dw15	DRw15(2)	
A32(w19)	B38(16)	Bw67		Dw16	DRw16(2)	
Aw33(w19)	B39(16)	Bw71(w70)		Dw17(w7)	DRw17(3)	
Aw34(10)	B40	Bw70		Dw18(w6)	DRw18(3)	
Aw36	Bw41	Bw72(w70)		Dw19(w6)		
Aw43	Bw42	Bw73		Dw20		
Aw66(10)	B44(12)	Bw75(15)		Dw21	DRw52	
Aw68(28)	B45(12)	Bw76(15)		Dw22	DRw53	
Aw69(28)	Bw46	Bw77(15)		Dw23		
	Bw47					
Aw74(w19)	Bw48			Dw24		
	B49(21)	Bw4		Dw25		
	Bw50(21)	Bw6		Dw26		

TYPES OF GRAFTS

A graft is a tissue or organ that is removed from a donor and placed into a recipient to restore a failed organ or tissue.

Type of graft	Description
Allograft (homograft)	A transplant from a genetically nonidentical member of the same species (e.g., heart transplant)
Autograft	A transplant from one part of an individual's body to another location in the same person (e.g., skin)
Heterograft (xenograft)	A transplant between species (e.g., baboon to human)
Isograft (syngraft)	A transplant between genetically identical individuals (e.g., monozygotic twins)
Orthotopic graft	A transplanted organ that is placed in the normal anatomic position (e.g., heart and liver transplants)
Heterotopic graft	A transplanted organ that is placed in a position other than its normal anatomic location (e.g., kidneys usually are placed in the iliac fossa)

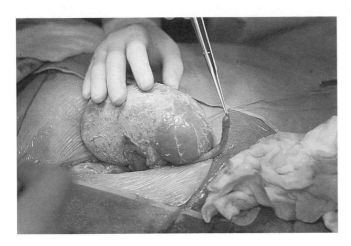

FIGURE 12-3
A donor kidney during the procurement surgery for a living related renal transplant.

determine whether the recipient has preformed antibodies to donor HLA antigens. A positive cross-match indicates the presence of preformed antibodies and is a contraindication for transplantation, because it is associated with early and uncontrolled rejection. The main targets of these preformed antibodies probably are the HLA antigens expressed on the vascular endothelium of capillaries and endothelium.

If a family donor is not available, the individual has the option of a cadaveric renal transplant. The immunologic workup is comparable to that for a living related kidney transplant.

Liver Transplantation

ABO testing is performed on all liver transplant recipients and donors. Although it is preferable that liver transplant recipients receive an ABO-compatible liver, they are not at the same risk of developing a hyperacute rejection as a kidney transplant recipient. However, liver transplant recipients may have antibodies directed against the foreign ABO antigen and may subsequently require retransplantation with an ABO-compatible liver. HLA antigen typing typically is not used to match donors and recipients in liver transplantation; however, the impact of HLA matching and graft survival has not been clarified.

Because hyperacute rejection is uncommon in liver transplantation, cross-matching is not routinely performed before transplantation in most centers; however, it may be performed afterward. The liver's resistance to hyperacute rejection remains unclear.

Pancreas Transplantation

All potential pancreas transplant donors and recipients are typed and matched for ABO and HLA antigens. HLA-DR matching in cadaveric pancreas transplants has proved distinctly beneficial, as demonstrated by prolonged graft survival.

Heart, Lung, and Heart/Lung Transplantation

Pretransplant immunologic screening of heart/lung donors and recipients typically includes HLA typing; however, there rarely is time to identify a matched HLA recipient. Because of this, the impact of HLA typing has not been completely recognized in heart and lung transplantation. The recipient's serum is routinely cross-matched against a panel of lymphocytes from a random donor group. If the reactive antibody level is greater than 15%, a cross-match between the donor and recipient is necessary before transplantation.

PRIMARY HISTOCOMPATIBILITY TESTS PERFORMED IN ORGAN TRANSPLANTATION	
Test	**Reason**
ABO typing	To determine the presence or absence of (1) antigens on donor erythrocytes and (2) specific antibodies in the recipient to the donor antigens
HLA typing	To type class I antigens (HLA-A, HLA-B, and HLA-C) and class II antigen (HLA-DR)
Cross-match (percentage of reactive antibodies [PRA])	To detect preformed circulating cytotoxic antibodies in the recipient
Mixed leukocyte culture	To detect foreign class II antigens and measure donor/recipient compatibility at the HLA-D loci

Table 12-6

TRANSPLANT REJECTION

Type of rejection	Time of onset	Etiology
Hyperacute	Minutes to hours	Humoral response caused by preformed cytotoxic antibodies
Acute	1-3 wk	Cellular immune response caused by trapped antigen that cannot be cleared by the reticuloendothelial system
Accelerated	3-7 days	Cellular immune response
Chronic	3 mo	Cellular and humoral responses

TRANSPLANT REJECTION

Rejection is a phenomenon that is not well understood (Table 12-6). It is a multifactorial immunologic response to foreign donor tissue. It involves recognition of HLA antigens on the donor tissue by receipt lymphocytes or antibodies, which subsequently cause graft damage.

Rejection is classified as hyperacute, accelerated, acute, or chronic. Depending on the organ and the degree of lymphocytic involvement, rejection can also be classified as nonspecific change, minimal, moderate, or severe.

Apheresis

Apheresis is the process of separating whole blood into its various components. It is used to treat a number of diseases, to remove toxins or antibodies, or to harvest specific blood components (e.g., platelets).
Plasmapheresis is a specific type of apheresis in which plasma is removed through the use of a plasma separator or filter or a centrifuge device and replaced with donor plasma or a colloid/crystalloid product.
Leukopheresis is the process of removing plasma enriched with white blood cells and replacing it with donor plasma and/or a plasma substitute.
Platelet pheresis is the removal of plasma enriched with excessive or abnormal platelets.

Apheresis is a Greek word that means "removal" or "to separate." The term "plasmapheresis" refers to the process of removing plasma from whole blood. However, removing large volumes of plasma requires colloidal replacement to maintain oncotic pressure; therefore the term "plasmapheresis" often is used interchangeably with the terms "therapeutic plasmapheresis" and "therapeutic plasma exchange" (TPE).

Apheresis can be performed as a therapeutic procedure to treat such diseases as systemic lupus erythematosus, Goodpasture's syndrome, thrombocytopenic pur-

pura, or Guillain-Barré syndrome (see the following box). However, apheresis may also be performed to obtain plasma and selected blood products from healthy donors, to be administered as replacement therapy for patients.

Plasmapheresis has been therapeutically prescribed for more than 100 different diseases (Table 12-7). The effectiveness of this treatment varies, and several mechanisms of action have been suggested. The proposed actions of plasmapheresis are twofold: (1) removal of autoantibodies, alloantibodies, circulating immune complexes, mixed cryoglobulins, unknown "immune" factors, excess lipoproteins or metabolites, endogenous toxins, monoclonal IgM, and nondialyzable poisons (*Amanita* mushroom poisoning); and (2) replacement of antithrombic factors with fresh frozen plasma (FFP) (Table 14-7).

PROCEDURE FOR PLASMAPHERESIS

The procedure for plasmapheresis must be performed by a nurse trained in apheresis (Figure 12-4). Generally two vascular access sites are established, and peripheral veins are used when possible. A 17-gauge catheter is almost always needed for blood outflow (the bleed line), except in children. An 18-gauge catheter is used for

INDICATIONS FOR THERAPEUTIC APHERESIS

ABO-incompatible bone marrow transplantation
Chronic inflammatory demyelinating polyneuropathy
Coagulation factor inhibitors
Cold agglutinin hemolysis
Cryoglobulinemia
Dermatomyositis/polymyositis
Drug overdose and poisoning
Familial hypercholesterolemia
Goodpasture's syndrome
Guillain-Barré syndrome
Hairy cell leukemia
Hemolytic uremic syndrome (HUS)
Hepatic encephalopathy
Hyperviscosity syndrome (e.g., Waldenström's macroglobulinemia)
Idiopathic inflammatory myopathy
Idiopathic thrombocytopenic purpura (ITP)
Leukemic blast crisis

Multiple sclerosis (MS)
Myasthenia gravis (MG)
Myeloma kidney
Paraproteinemic peripheral neuropathy
Pemphigus
Posttransfusion purpura
Progressive systemic sclerosis
Pure red cell aplasia
Rapid progressive glomerulonephritis (RPGN)
Refsum's disease
Renal graft rejection
Reye's syndrome
Rheumatoid arthritis (RA)
Scleroderma
Sickle cell disease
Systemic lupus erythematosus (SLE)
Systemic vasculitis (e.g., polyarteritis)
Thrombocythemia
Thrombotic thrombocytopenic purpura (TTP)

Table 12-7

DISORDERS AND CONDITIONS TREATED WITH PLASMAPHERESIS

Disorder/condition	Proposed mechanisms of action
Amyloidosis	Removes immunoglobulin
Autoimmune hemolytic anemia	Removes antiplatelet antibodies
Bone marrow transplantation (BMT)	Reduces anti-A or anti-B isoagglutinin titers, or both; prevents transfusion reaction with infusion of BMT
Cardiac transplantation	Used to treat hyperacute rejection (immune [IgG] mediated) in conjunction with steroids
Cold agglutinin hemolysis	Removes pathologic IgM and IgG antibodies (plasmapheresis must be performed at 37° C [98.6° F])
Dermatomyositis/polymyositis	May remove pathologic IgG immunoglobulin
Goodpasture's syndrome	Removes anti–basement membrane antibodies
Guillain-Barré syndrome	May remove pathologic IgG immunoglobulin
Hemolytic uremic syndrome	Replenishes unknown substances (possibly antithrombotic factors) with fresh frozen plasma and liquid plasma
Hepatic failure	Removes endogenous toxins, corrects hepatic coagulopathy, and may improve encephalopathy
Hyperviscosity syndrome (e.g., Waldenström's macroglobulinemia, cryoglobulinemia)	Removes excess antibodies (usually IgM) and improves blood flow
Idiopathic thrombocytopenic purpura	Removes antibodies directed at platelets and improves platelet survival
Multiple sclerosis	Removes putative antimyelin antibodies
Myasthenia gravis	Removes antibodies directed at acetylcholine receptor and improves muscle strength
Polymyositis	Removes unknown immune factors
Refsum's disease	Removes excess metabolites
Rapid progressive glomerulonephritis	Removes circulating immune complexes
Rheumatoid vasculitis	Removes mixed cryoglobulins
Scleroderma	Removes pathologic IgG and circulating immune complexes
Systemic lupus erythematosus	Removes circulating immune complexes or pathologic IgG and triggers endogenous clearance of immune complexes
Thrombotic thrombocytopenic purpura	Replenishes unknown substances (possibly antithrombotic factors) with fresh frozen plasma and liquid plasma

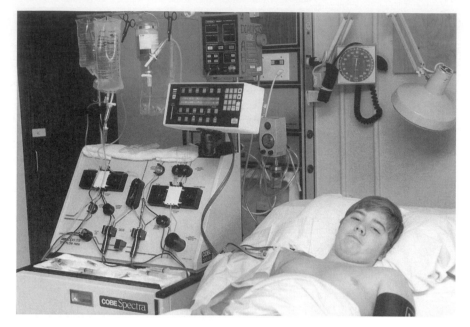

FIGURE 12-4
Patient undergoing plasmapheresis for systemic lupus erythematosus and lupus nephritis.

blood inflow (the return line). When peripheral veins are not adequate, a double-lumen (dialysis) catheter is inserted into a femoral or subclavian vein. Soft catheters (e.g., Hickman or Broviac) cannot be used as outflow lines because they collapse, inhibiting adequate blood flow.

Blood is removed from the patient via the outflow access and anticoagulated with either heparin or, more often, a citrate solution. The blood then enters a centrifuge device (or membrane separator device) and is separated into its cellular components. Plasma, platelets, white blood cells, or red blood cells can be separated and removed selectively. The undesirable components are taken out, and the remaining blood components are returned to the patient along with the prescribed replacement fluid, usually physiologic saline, fresh frozen plasma (FFP), plasma protein fractions, or albumin. Calcium chloride (10% CaCl) may be administered via the return blood line or in conjunc-

tion with the replacement fluid to counteract the effects of the citrate.

The procedure usually takes 2 to 3 hours and consists of six to 12 cycles, or "passes," in an adult. The length of the procedure depends on how much plasma needs to be replaced, the patient's tolerance, and complications. In an adult, the apheresis machine, or cell separator, generally removes blood from the patient at a rate of 40 to 60 ml/minute, a total of 200 to 300 ml per pass, or 2 to 3 L per exchange. No more than 10% to 15% of the patient's total blood volume should be in the machine at any time during the procedure.

COMPLICATIONS

Difficulties with central vascular access
Hypervolemia or hypovolemia
Congestive heart failure
Pulmonary edema
Hypotension
Hemorrhage
Anemia, thrombocytopenia
Air embolism (dyspnea, anxiety, agitation, cyanosis, seizures, respiratory arrest)
Red blood cell lysis
Transfusion reactions
Hepatitis
Infection
Hyperkalemia or hypokalemia
Alteration in pharmacokinetics
Citrate toxicity (if used as an anticoagulant)
Citrate-induced hypocalcemia
Cardiac dysrhythmias

In the event of an air embolism, place the patient in Trendelenburg's position on her **left** side, start oxygen, and initiate CPR if indicated.

Citrate binds calcium and functions as an anticoagulant for apheresis. Calcium chloride is administered to reverse the anticoagulant effects of citrate.

MEDICAL MANAGEMENT

Medical management depends on the specific disorder being treated. Patients undergoing apheresis require meticulous management of their primary disorder and of fluids, electrolytes, and any infections. Cooperation between the apheresis nurse and the primary nurse is crucial. Continual updating about medications, vital signs, fluids, activated clotting times, and changes in the patient's status must be maintained throughout the procedure. Routine orders generally consist of the number of exchanges (e.g., 40-60 ml/kg, or 1 to 1½ plasma volumes), the type of replacement fluid (varies with disorder; e.g., may be one half FFP and one half liquid plasma), the frequency of treatments, the type of anticoagulant (e.g., citrate), replacement of calcium chloride and other electrolytes, blood flow (e.g., 70-90 ml/min with centrifuge), taking vital signs (q 15 min), weighing the patient before and after treatment, laboratory tests, and interventions for complications.

PREPROCEDURAL CARE

1. Review your hospital's policy on apheresis.
2. In collaboration with the apheresis nurse, explain the procedure to the patient and family (i.e., how the machine works, access, how long the procedure will take, any unusual symptoms that may develop; also, answer any questions the patient or family members may have. The pheresis nurse will explain symptoms of hypocalcemia and instruct the patient to tell the nurse if any of these symptoms develop.
3. Make sure that the informed consent form is signed.
4. Record baseline vital signs, neuromuscular status, and level of orientation.
5. CBC, platelet count, fibrinogen, electrolytes, calcium, magnesium, albumin, total protein, activated partial thromboplastin time, and prothrombin time usually are done before apheresis is begun.
6. Ask the physician whether scheduled medications should be delayed until after the procedure to prevent their removal or to prevent hypotension (as with antihypertensive agents).

POSTPROCEDURAL CARE

1. Monitor vital signs.
2. Have laboratory tests done (usually CBC, platelets, electrolytes, calcium, magnesium, and immunoglobulins [e.g., IgG and IgM]). Posttreatment clotting studies are most accurate 24 hours after the procedure, particularly if replacement fluid is crystalloid or albumin.
3. Monitor access site(s) for bleeding, pain, or erythema.
4. Monitor for electrolyte imbalances, hypotension, hypovolemia, and bleeding.

1 ASSESS

ASSESSMENT	OBSERVATIONS
Pulmonary	Dyspnea; orthopnea; rales; pink, frothy sputum; tachypnea; use of accessory muscles
Cardiac	Dysrhythmias secondary to electrolyte imbalances; hypotension
Disequilibrium syndrome	Nausea, vomiting, dizziness, hypotension, diaphoresis, blurred vision
Electrolyte imbalances	Decreased calcium level with numbness, tingling, cramping, muscle fatigue, spasms, positive Trousseau's and Chvostek's signs, malaise, and mental confusion
Hypersensitivity reaction	Dyspnea; hives; diaphoresis; hypotension; weak, thready pulse; low back pain
Bleeding	Petechiae; areas of ecchymosis; decreased platelets, prothrombin time (PT), partial thromboplastin time (PTT), hemoglobin (Hb), and hematocrit (Hct)
Hypothermia	Decreased temperature, chills

→ ❯ ❯

2 DIAGNOSE

NURSING DIAGNOSIS	SUBJECTIVE FINDINGS	OBJECTIVE FINDINGS
High risk for injury related to calcium imbalance	Complains of numbness in fingers and toes, abdominal cramps, leg spasms, circumoral paresthesia, and nausea	Tetany; positive Chvostek's and Trousseau's signs; low calcium level; prolonged QT interval on ECG; disorientation
High risk for injury related to bleeding	Reports bruising easily, oozing of blood from access site, epistaxis, and bleeding gums	Access site bleeding with small hematoma; prolonged PT, PTT; decreased Hb and Hct; old blood in nares
High risk for fluid volume deficit related to rapid fluid shifts during procedure	Complains of lightheadedness, nausea, blurred vision, and dizziness	Hypotension, decreased urine output, tachycardia
High risk for fluid volume excess related to fluid shifts during procedure	Complains of dyspnea, productive cough	Tachypnea; anxiety; breath sounds decreased, with rales; thin, pink, frothy sputum; pale to cyanotic skin; hypertension
High risk for infection related to altered immune response	Complains of tenderness at central line access site, malaise	Fever; access site is erythematous with yellow drainage; increased WBC

Other related nursing diagnoses: Altered thermoregulation related to hypothermia secondary to cool replacement fluid; **High risk for injury** related to hypersensitivity reaction to replacement blood products; **Anxiety** related to a change in health status.

3 PLAN

Patient goals

1. The patient will have no complications related to calcium imbalance.
2. The patient will have no complications related to bleeding.
3. The patient will remain euvolemic with an adequate fluid balance.
4. The patient will have no complications from hypervolemia.
5. The patient will be free of infection.

4 IMPLEMENT

NURSING DIAGNOSIS	NURSING INTERVENTIONS	RATIONALE
High risk for injury related to calcium imbalance	Assess patient for hypocalcemia and citrate toxicity (numbness, tingling, twitching, cramps, spasms, positive Chvostek's and Trousseau's signs, circumoral paresthesia, shivering, nausea, vomiting, cardiac dysrhythmias [prolonged QT interval, ventricular tachycardia]).	To establish baseline and guide therapeutic intervention; citrate acts as an anticoagulant during apheresis by binding calcium.

NURSING DIAGNOSIS	NURSING INTERVENTIONS	RATIONALE
	Administer 1½ - 1 g of calcium chloride (slow IV push) as ordered, and monitor response.	To correct hypocalcemia.
	Add calcium to albumin replacement fluid as ordered.	Because albumin binds calcium, adding calcium prevents double binding of calcium from citrate and albumin.
	Monitor serum calcium levels.	To detect changes and effectiveness of interventions.
High risk for injury related to bleeding	Assess and monitor patient's CBC, PT, PTT, fibrinogen, platelet count, and activated clotting times (ACTs) during the procedure.	These laboratory results are indicators of coagulopathy; hemolysis of RBCs can occur during the procedure; anticoagulation may cause increased bleeding; platelet counts may decrease after treatment; ACTs can change quickly during the procedure and need close monitoring to prevent bleeding complications.
	Monitor for CNS disturbance and evidence of GI bleeding (Hemastix-positive emesis, stool, or aspirate).	To ensure early detection of possible intracranial or GI bleeding.
	Apply pressure dressing to access site after procedure; remove after 3-4 h and replace with plastic bandage strip.	Pressure dressing may prevent bleeding at access sites.
	Observe access site q 15-30 min, then prn for bleeding or development of a hematoma.	To monitor for bleeding at the site.
	Place a sign in patient's room informing other health care providers not to draw blood from antecubitals or central line used for apheresis.	To protect central lines from infection and clotting and antecubital sites from further bruising or trauma so that they may be used repeatedly for apheresis if necessary.
	If patient is severely thrombocytopenic, implement precautions according to hospital policy (e.g., no rectal temperatures, no venous blood work, no razors).	To protect patient from injury and bleeding.
High risk for fluid volume deficit related to fluid shifts during procedure	Assess and monitor vital signs, mental status, and urine output; report change in baseline to physician.	Increased heart rate (HR) and respiratory rate (RR) and decreased BP are indicators of hypovolemia, which can occur at any time during the procedure; a maximum of 10% to 15% of the patient's total blood volume should be extracorporeal at any time during the procedure.
	Monitor weight before and after and, if possible, during the procedure (particularly with children).	To assess and monitor fluid changes during the procedure, to prevent any untoward effects related to fluid imbalances.
	Administer fluids as ordered, and monitor response.	To restore fluid volume.

→ 〉 〉

NURSING DIAGNOSIS	NURSING INTERVENTIONS	RATIONALE
High risk for fluid volume excess related to rapid fluid shifts during procedure	Assess and monitor for volume overload (e.g., hypertension; anxiety; dyspnea; tachypnea; rales; frothy, clear, pink sputum).	To establish baseline values and enhance early intervention to prevent complications of hypervolemia.
	Assess and monitor airway.	To allow early intervention and prevent complications.
	Administer diuretics as ordered, and monitor response.	To remove fluid quickly.
	In collaboration with the apheresis nurse, ascertain the rate of venous/arterial replacement solution and hourly fluid status.	To ensure accurate infusion of replacement fluid and maintenance of fluid balance.
	Administer oxygen as indicated and ordered, and monitor response.	To increase gas exchange, minimize dyspnea, and promote comfort.
	Suction excessive pulmonary secretions as indicated.	To remove excessive secretions, enhance breathing, and maintain airway.
High risk for infection related to altered immune response	Assess and monitor access site and vital signs; notify physician of any changes (increased temperature, HR, and RR, chills, rigors, and purulent drainage from access site are signs of infection that should be addressed).	To establish baseline and to monitor any changes; apheresis depletes the patient of normal immunoglobulins, increasing susceptibility to infection.
	Perform sterile dressing changes per hospital policy for central lines; remember to wash your hands.	To prevent infection.
	Obtain and monitor cultures from site and blood.	To determine exact microorganism.
	Monitor WBC.	Elevations in WBC indicate an infection.
	Administer antibiotics as ordered, and monitor response.	To treat the infection and to determine patient's response to medication.

5   EVALUATE

PATIENT OUTCOME	DATA INDICATING THAT OUTCOME IS REACHED
Patient has no injuries related to calcium imbalance.	Serum calcium levels are normal; patient has no complaints of cramps, spasms, nausea, or vomiting; sinus rhythm is normal.
Patient shows no signs of bleeding.	PT, PTT, Hb, Hct, fibrinogen, and platelet values are all normal; patient has no bleeding from access site and no hematomas, petechiae, or bruising.

PATIENT OUTCOME	DATA INDICATING THAT OUTCOME IS REACHED
Patient is euvolemic, and fluid status is adequate.	BP, HR, and RR are normal; urine output is ≥30 ml/h; patient has no dyspnea or excessive frothy pink sputum; weight is stable.
Complications of hypervolemia have been avoided.	Vital signs normal; anxiety has resolved; breath sounds are clear and there is no sputum; skin is warm, dry, and pink; patient has no complaints of dyspnea or orthopnea.
Patient has no infection.	Patient is afebrile; access site is clear, dry, and without redness, or central line has been removed; WBC is normal.

PATIENT TEACHING

1. Explain the procedure, access, and equipment to the patient and family.
2. Explain how long the procedure will take (2 to 4 hours) and where it will take place.
3. Explain that a number of treatments may be necessary (the number varies with the disorder).
4. Teach the patient and family the signs of bleeding, electrolyte and fluid imbalances, and infection.
5. Instruct the patient to balance activity with rest; encourage scheduled rest periods after treatments to prevent undue fatigue.
6. Instruct the patient to avoid exposure to individuals who are ill or who have recently received immunizations (e.g., oral polio) because of the patient's immunosuppression and increased risk of becoming infected.

Immunoglobulin Therapy

Immunoglobulin is an antibody preparation that contains primarily IgG antibodies.

The extraction of antibody concentrate was achieved successfully in the 1940s through the work of Cohn and Oncley, who developed a process whereby various protein components of human plasma could be precipitated and subsequently purified, allowing removal of the fractions that contained antibodies. This procedure introduced standard immunoglobulin, which could be used intramuscularly (IM) for prophylaxis against infections in individuals with primary immunodeficiency disorders. However, the clinical value of IM immunoglobulin was limited, because the doses that could be given with intramuscular injections were inadequate.

It was not until the mid-1970s that improved fractionation techniques were developed and clinical trials of intravenous (IV) administration of immunoglobulin were begun. This modification of the Cohn-Oncley procedure is known as the Kistler-Nitschmann process. It has demonstrated immunoglobulin preparations safe from viruses and protein aggregates that can cause serious adverse reactions. A variety of processes currently are used to manufacture immunoglobulin derived from human plasma so that it is safe for intravenous administration, and further modification of this technique is continuing today.

IMMUNOGLOBULIN PREPARATION

Immunoglobulin is manufactured by obtaining blood from a large number of donors (more than 1,000), removing the plasma, and purifying and standardizing the immunoglobulin fraction of the serum. Before the single-donor units of plasma are added to the pool of immunoglobulin, they must test negative for hepatitis B surface antigen (HBsAg) and the human immunodeficiency virus (HIV). The purified immunoglobulin contains antibodies (immunoglobulins). Manufactured immunoglobulin contains a wide variety of antibodies, because it is made from a large number of individuals who have developed antibodies to a diverse variety of antigens. Specifically, immunoglobulin preparations contain antibodies that patients with certain immunodeficiency disorders cannot make. Most prepared immunoglobulin has IgG antibodies, with only small amounts of IgM and IgA.

A **specific immunoglobulin** is a preparation obtained from selected donors who process high concentrations of antibodies against a particular illness (e.g., varicella immunoglobulin). Specific immunoglobulin is given to an individual who has not had the disease or vaccine and who has been exposed to the particular disease. The immunoglobulin provides passive immunity to that disease. For example, a child who has undergone transplantation, has never been immunized against chickenpox, and is exposed to chickenpox upon returning to school should receive varicella immunoglobulin.

PROPOSED MECHANISMS OF ACTION

Immunoglobulin contains a broad spectrum of antibody (IgG) specificities against bacterial and viral antigens that are capable of opsonization and neutralization of microbes and toxins. The exact mechanism of action of immunoglobulin is not known, but three types have been suggested: protective, replacement, and immune regulatory. Protective mechanisms are effected through opsonization, which may enhance the nonspecific immune response of phagocytes, may stimulate B cells via the Fc fragment, and may reduce antigenic competition by antibodies directed against dominant antigens. A replacement mechanism would involve the contribution of specific antibodies. Immunoregulatory mechanisms are thought to alter the feedback loop in autoimmune disorders by influencing B-cell proliferation.

INDICATIONS AND CONTRAINDICATIONS FOR USE

Immunoglobulin provides passive prophylactic immunity against bacterial and viral antigens. It is indicated as maintenance treatment for patients with primary immunodeficiency disorders (e.g., CVID, SCID) and primary immune globulin deficiency (X-LA) (see the following box). Although the mechanism is not understood, immunoglobulin has also proved effective in treating chronic and acute idiopathic thrombocytopenic purpura.

Because immunoglobulin generally contains very small amounts of IgA, it is contraindicated in patients with selective IgA deficiency who possess antibody to IgA. Also, because the levels of IgA in immunoglobulin are so small, even those without antibody to IgA would not benefit. Immunoglobulin may also be contraindicated in patients who have had severe systemic reactions to the therapy.

CAUTIONS AND ADVERSE REACTIONS

Rapid infusion of immune globulin (>20 drops [1 ml]/min) may cause an inflammatory reaction in patients with agammaglobulinemia or hypogammaglobulinemia who have never received immunoglobulin, or whose last treatment was more than 2 months ago. These reactions are characterized by fever, chills, nausea, and vomiting.

Because reproductive studies have not been conducted with most immunoglobulins, it is not known whether they can harm a fetus or affect reproductive capacity. Thus immunoglobulin should be given to a pregnant woman only if absolutely indicated.

Symptoms reported in patients receiving immunoglobulin usually occur 30 minutes to 1 hour after administration has been initiated. The severity of the reaction generally is directly related to the rate of infusion. Potential adverse reactions include flushing, chills, fever, dizziness, feeling faint, nausea, chest tightness, diaphoresis, erythema at the site of administration, low back pain, hypotension, abdominal cramps, anxiety, wheezing, myalgia, arthralgia, and rash. Anaphylaxis and hypersensitivity reactions are rare and occur secondary to previous sensitization, most often to

---

INDICATIONS FOR IMMUNOGLOBULIN THERAPY

X-linked agammaglobulinemia (X-LA)	Idiopathic thrombocytopenic purpura (ITP)	Passive immunity to preterm infants
Common variable immunodeficiency (CVID)	Wiskott-Aldrich syndrome (WAS)	Passive immunization
Severe combined immunodeficiency disease (SCID)	CMV prophylaxis or treatment (in conjunction with antibiotics) in transplant recipients	Increased sensitivity to bacterial infections
Hypogammaglobulinemia HIV/AIDS/ARC		Therapy after bone marrow transplantation

IgA. If adverse reactions develop, the infusion should be stopped until the symptoms have subsided; the access is maintained with normal saline.

DOSAGE AND ADMINISTRATION

The dosage of immunoglobulin varies, depending on the company supplying the drug, the disorder, and the patient's response to therapy. It may be given intravenously or intramuscularly. A prophylactic dose generally is 100 mg/kg for weekly treatment and 200 mg/kg for monthly infusions. It may be given in doses as high as 400 mg/kg per treatment if the patient is unresponsive or if the circulating levels of IgG are considered inadequate. The dose for patients with ITP generally is 1 g/kg for 1-3 consecutive days or 400 mg/kg for 5 days. Bone marrow transplant (BMT) patients will receive immunoglobulin therapy at a dosage of 500 mg/kg daily every 7 days while hospitalized. This may vary, depending on the type of BMT and the center's protocols.

Premedication typically includes acetaminophen (10 mg/kg) and diphenhydramine (1 mg/kg). These drugs often are administered 30 minutes before infusion of the immunoglobulin, particularly if the patient has a history of reactions. Children who have a simultaneous infection (e.g., otitis media, viral infection) are at greater risk of having a reaction.

Immunoglobulin generally is reconstituted with sterile water supplied by the manufacturer. When reconstituting, allow the water to wet the dry immunoglobulin by tilting the bottle slowly back and forth. **Do not shake**—excessive shaking will cause the solution to foam, because it is a protein-rich substance. Gently rotate the bottle to prevent foaming. Administration should start within 2 hours of reconstitution, and the solution may be infused through a peripheral or a central line.

Immune globulin should always be hung "piggyback" with normal saline. In the event of an adverse reaction, the immunoglobulin is stopped and the normal saline started. Immunoglobulin infusion rates vary. However, because adverse reactions occur more often at rapid infusion rates, the infusion should start slowly and increase every 15 minutes if tolerated.

Patients must be monitored continuously for adverse effects during the infusion. Vital signs are checked frequently: before the infusion, every 15 minutes for the first hour, then every 30 minutes for 1 hour, and then every hour until the infusion has been completed. Vital signs should be checked again 30 minutes after the infusion. Although anaphylaxis is rare, epinephrine, antihistamines, and oxygen should be readily available.

Before administering immune globulin, read the nursing procedure instructions in your facility.

1 | ASSESS

ASSESSMENT	OBSERVATIONS BEFORE IMMUNOGLOBULIN ADMINISTRATION	OBSERVATIONS DURING IMMUNOGLOBULIN ADMINISTRATION
General	Malaise, fatigue	Arthralgia, myalgia, fever, hypotension
Sinopulmonary	Recurrent infections, bronchitis, sinusitis, rhinitis, pneumonia	Dyspnea, wheezes, chest tightness
Skin	Eczema, rashes, recurrent infections, abscesses (in WAS, petechiae and ecchymosis)	Chills, diaphoresis, sensitivity to touch

→ › ›

ASSESSMENT	OBSERVATIONS BEFORE IMMUNOGLOBULIN ADMINISTRATION	OBSERVATIONS DURING IMMUNOGLOBULIN ADMINISTRATION
Ears	Recurrent episodes of otitis media	Unremarkable change
Eyes	Recurrent conjunctivitis	Unremarkable change
Gastrointestinal	Diarrhea, recurrent infections (e.g., *Giardia lamblia* or *C. difficile*)	Nausea, abdominal cramps

2 DIAGNOSE

NURSING DIAGNOSIS	SUBJECTIVE FINDINGS	OBJECTIVE FINDINGS
High risk for injury related to infusion of immunoglobulin	Complains of dyspnea, headache, myalgia, and arthralgia	Respiratory rate 32-36/min, wheezing on auscultation, patient reluctant to move around due to discomfort
High risk for infection related to inadequate immunity	Reports frequent nasal drainage, frontal headache, and cough	Recurrent episodes of sinusitis and bronchitis, productive cough, yellow-green sputum
Impaired adjustment related to treatment routine and illness	Reports increasing responsibilities at home and inability to prioritize	Consistently late or misses immunoglobulin infusion; unable to recognize change in health status and need for routine infusions

3 PLAN

Patient goals

1. The patient will have no side effects from immunoglobulin infusion or will be able to manage side effects effectively.

2. The patient will show no signs of recurrent sinopulmonary infection.
3. The patient and family will modify their life-style to achieve maximum control and independence within the limits imposed by the patient's altered health status.

4 IMPLEMENT

NURSING DIAGNOSIS	INTERVENTIONS	RATIONALE
High risk for injury related to infusion of immunoglobulin	Before infusion: assess vital signs, obtain nursing history, and perform physical examination.	To record baseline health status and identify changes.
	Explain procedure to patient and family (e.g., immunoglobulin will be given IM or IV and infusion lasts several hours).	To ensure understanding of the process and elicit cooperation.

NURSING DIAGNOSIS	INTERVENTIONS	RATIONALE
	Administer premedications as ordered, and monitor patient's response (usually Tylenol, 10 mg/kg, and Benadryl, 1 mg/kg); repeat as ordered and indicated.	To minimize untoward effects secondary to immunoglobulin administration; repeat dosing may be administered to minimize fever, chills, or sensitivity to touch.
	Normal saline should be hung as backup to the immunoglobulin.	To be readily available if a reaction occurs.
	Immunoglobulin should be administered through a separate line and not in conjunction with other medications.	To prevent precipitation and maintain the access.
	Generally start infusions at 0.5 mg/kg and maintain this rate for 15-30 min (dose varies, depending on drug company used); if tolerated, increase rate gradually no more than every 30 min as tolerated, and document time and rate of increases.	Most reactions are caused by rapid infusion of immunoglobulin.
	Monitor patient's status and vital signs during and after procedure.	To assess for any untoward effects secondary to infusion.
	Have epinephrine, oxygen, and suction readily available.	In the event of an anaphylactic reaction, to prevent aspiration or injury.
	If a reaction occurs: stop the immunoglobulin, start the normal saline, and notify the physician immediately.	To prevent further harm to the patient and recruit other health team members to assist the patient (intubation may be necessary).
High risk for infection related to inadequate immunity	Assess and monitor vital signs and body secretions; monitor exudates for signs of purulent drainage.	To identify early signs of infection, allowing for prompt, aggressive therapy.
	Initiate universal blood and body secretion precautions and other procedures as indicated (e.g., isolation).	To protect patient and staff from infection and observe CDC recommendations.
	Wash hands before and after contact with the patient; use strict aseptic technique when performing invasive procedures (e.g., obtaining central line access for immunoglobulin infusion).	To prevent transmission of microorganisms.
	Perform routine central line care (consult your facility's nursing procedure).	To monitor central line access site and prevent infection.
	Monitor hydration and electrolyte balance.	Adequate fluid status and normal electrolytes are imperative for fighting infection.
	Ensure adequate nutrition; offer meals during infusion.	To support immune functioning.
	Institute chest and/or sinus postural drainage as indicated.	To remove excess secretions, maintain airway patency, and increase patient's breathing comfort.

NURSING DIAGNOSIS	INTERVENTIONS	RATIONALE
	Encourage patient to adhere to recommended routine for immunoglobulin administration.	To prevent recurrent infections.
	Administer antibiotics as ordered, and monitor patient's response.	Antibiotics are use prophylactically and to treat infections.
Impaired adjustment related to treatment routine and illness	Urge patient to discuss impact of change in health status on social life of patient and family; avoid conveying blame; generate hope by helping patient identify previous successful coping behaviors and support systems.	To help patient resolve feelings of loss related to change in health status.
	Assist in actively orienting patient and family to proposed immunoglobulin infusion regimen, and explain why it is necessary.	To help patient modify life-style so as to gain maximum control and independence.
	Investigate home health agencies as appropriate or indicated; collaborate with patient and family in identifying best dates and times for infusion.	To promote coordination between patient's schedule and need for infusion.
	Refer patient and family to other organizations, resources, and self-help groups.	To promote adjustment through support from others and additional information.

5 EVALUATE

PATIENT OUTCOME	DATA INDICATING THAT OUTCOME IS REACHED
Patient is free of injury.	Adverse reactions are avoided during immunoglobulin infusion.
Recurrent infections are minimized.	Patient adheres to antibiotic regimen, shows no signs of sinopulmonary infection, and has no complaints of malaise or fatigue; patient is afebrile, and central line site has no drainage, erythema, or pain.
Patient has adjusted to routine related to immunoglobulin therapy and accompanying disorder.	Patient arrives for treatments on time, attends monthly support group meetings, uses community organizations to assist with child care and respite care, and uses resources to assist with ongoing health management.

PATIENT TEACHING ■

1. Review with the patient and family the effects of the patient's immunodeficiency disorder and routine management.
2. Explain to the patient and family how immunoglobulin is manufactured, to alleviate concern.
3. Discuss with the patient and family routine immunoglobulin therapy, administration, and access.
4. Review the side effects of immunoglobulin therapy.
5. Teach the patient and family techniques for sinus and pulmonary postural drainage as appropriate.
6. Teach central line care if appropriate.
7. Teach patient and family how to monitor for signs and symptoms of infection (e.g., elevated temperatures, decreased appetite, myalgias, arthralgias), and instruct them to notify physician of temperatures $\geq 38°$ C.
8. Provide the patient and family with a list of local and national support organizations.

References

1. Abrams DI: The persistent lymphade-nopathy syndrome and immune thrombocytopenic purpura in HIV-infected individuals. In Levy JA, editor: *AIDS: pathogenesis and treatment*, New York, 1989, Marcel Dekker.
2. Abrams DI: AIDS-related conditions, *Clin Immunol Allergy* 6:581-599, 1986.
3. Abrams DI, Kiprov DD, Goedert JJ, Sarngadharan MG, Gallo RC, and Volberding PA: Antibodies to HTLV-III and development of acquired immunodeficiency syndrome in homosexual men presenting with immune thrombocytopenic purpura, *Ann Intern Med* 104:47-50, 1986.
4. Ammann A: Antibody (B-cell) immunodeficiency disorders. In Stites DP and Terr AI, editors: *Basic and clinical immunology*, ed 7, San Mateo, Calif, 1991, Appleton & Lange.
5. Ammann A and Wara D: Collagen-vascular disease (rheumatic disease). In Rudolf A and Hoffman J, editors: *Pediatrics*, Los Altos, Calif, 1987, Appleton & Lange.
6. Anderson J: Food allergy or sensitivity: terminology, physiologic bases, and scope of the clinical problem. In Perkin JE, editor: *Food allergies and adverse reactions*, Gaithersburg, Md, 1990, Aspen Publishers.
7. Anderson J: Adverse reactions to foods. In Bierman CW and Pearlman DS, editors: *Allergic diseases from infancy to adulthood*, ed 2, Philadelphia, 1988, WB Saunders.
8. Appelbaum R: Bone marrow transplantation. In Wittes R, editor: *Manual of oncologic therapeutic*, Philadelphia, 1989, JB Lippincott.
9. Andreoli T, Carpenter C, Plum F, and Smith L, editors: *Cecil's essentials of medicine*, Philadelphia, 1986, WB Saunders.
10. Appel GP, Silva FG, Pirani CL, Meltzer JI, and Estes D: Renal involvement in systemic lupus erythematosus, *Medicine* 57:371, 1978.
11. Austin KF: Connective tissues diseases other than rheumatoid arthritis. In Beeson P, McDermott W, and Wyngaarden JB, editors: *Cecil's textbook of medicine*, Philadelphia, 1982, WB Saunders.
12. Babior BM: The megaloblastic anemias. In Williams WJ, editor: *Hematology*, New York, 1990, McGraw-Hill.

13. Bach FH and Sachs DH: Current concepts: immunology, *N Engl J Med* 317(8): 1987.
13a. Baker, 1991.
14. Balaban EP, Sheehan RG, Lipsky PE, and Frenkel EP: Treatment of cutaneous sclerosis and aplastic anemia with antilymphocyte globulin, *Ann Intern Med* 106(1):56-58, 1987.
15. Barnes PJ: New concepts in the pathogenesis of bronchiole hyperresponsiveness and asthma, *J Allergy Clin Immunol* 83:1013, 1989.
16. Barrett JT: *Textbook of immunology*, St Louis, 1988, Mosby–Year Book.
17. Bates B: *A guide to physical examination*, ed 3, Philadelphia, 1983, JB Lippincott.
17a. Bell, 1991.
18. Bellanti JA and Rocklin RE: Cell-mediated immune reactions. In Bellanti JA, editor: *Immunology 111*, Philadelphia, WB Saunders.
19. Benjamini E and Leskowitz S: *Immunology: a short course*, New York, 1988, Alan R Liss.
20. Bier OG, Dias da Silva W, Götze D, and Mota I: *Fundamentals of immunology*, ed 2, Berlin, 1968, Springer-Verlag.
21. Bierman CW and Pearlman DS, editors: *Allergic diseases from infancy to adulthood*, ed 2, Philadelphia, 1988, WB Saunders.
22. Blanchette V, Cunningham-Rundles C, Filipovich A, Frenkel L, and Schiff R: *Perspectives on immunotherapy: immune globulin intravenous (human)*, Sandoz Pharmaceutical Corp, 1988.
23. Block G, Nolan W, and Dempsy M: *Health assessment for professional nursing: a developmental approach*, New York, 1981, Appleton & Lange.
24. Blume K, Faiman S, O'Donnell M, et al: Total body irradiation and high-dose etoposide: a new preparatory regimen with bone marrow transplantation in patients with advanced hematologic malignancies, *Blood* 69(4):1015-1020, 1987.
25. Brandt V: Nursing protocol for the patient with neutropenia, *Oncol Nurs Forum* (suppl 17[1]):9-15, 1990.
26. Brannan DP and Guthrie TH Jr: Idio-

pathic thrombocytopenic purpura in adults, *South Med J* 81(1):75-80, 1988.
27. Brenner B and Rector F, editors: *The kidney*, ed 3, Philadelphia, 1986, WB Saunders.
28. Buchanan WW and Kean WF: Sjögren's syndrome. In Katz WA, editor: *Diagnosis and management of rheumatic diseases*, ed 2, Philadelphia, 1988, JB Lippincott.
29. Buckly JM and Pearlman DS: Controlling the environment for allergic diseases. In Bierman CW and Pearlman DS, editors. *Allergic diseases from infancy to adulthood*, ed 2, Philadelphia, 1988, WB Saunders.
30. Bussel JB: Autoimmune thrombocytopenia purpura, *Hematol Oncol Clin North Am* 4(1):179-191, 1990.
31. Calabro JJ: Rheumatoid arthritis: diagnosis and management, *Clin Symp* 38(2): 1986.
32. Carr GS, Newlin B, and Gee G: AIDS-related conditions. In Gee G and Moran TA, editors: *AIDS: concepts in nursing practice*, Baltimore, 1988, Williams & Wilkins.
33. Carson K: Subacute cutaneous lupus, *Bay Area Lupus Foundation Newsletter* 13(2): 1990.
33a. Carter, 1990.
34. Cassidy JT and Nelson AM: The frequency of juvenile rheumatoid arthritis, *J Rheumatol* 15:535-536, 1988.
35. Cassidy JT and Petty RE: *The textbook of pediatric rheumatology*, ed 2, New York, 1990, Churchill Livingstone.
36. Centers for Disease Control: First 100,000 cases of acquired immunodeficiency syndrome—United States, *MMWR* 38:561-562, 1989.
37. Centers for Disease Control: Recommendations for prevention of HIV transmission in health-care settings, *MMWR* 36(2S):3S-18S, 1987.
38. Centers for Disease Control: Revision of the CDC surveillance case definition for acquired immunodeficiency syndrome, *MMWR* 36(1S):3S-15S, 1987.
39. Centers for Disease Control: Classification system for human T-lymphotropic virus type III/lymphadenopathy-associated virus infections, *MMWR* 35:334-339, 1986.
40. Clark C: Nursing care for multiple sclerosis, *Orthop Nurs* 10(1):21-33, 1991.

41. Clark WR: *The experimental foundations of modern immunology*, ed 3, New York, 1986, John Wiley & Sons.

42. Cohen AS, editor: *Laboratory diagnostic procedures in the rheumatic diseases*, Orlando, Fla, 1985, Grune & Stratton.

43. Colletti M, German M, Zeller JM, and Reno-Balkstra C: Immunologic system. In Thompson J et al: *Mosby's manual of clinical nursing*, ed 2, St Louis, 1989, Mosby–Year Book.

44. Corcoran-Buchsel P: Long-term complication of allogeneic bone marrow transplantation: nursing implication, *Oncol Nurs Forum* 13(6):61-70, 1986.

45. Corless IB and Lindeman-Pittman M, editors: *AIDS: principles, practices, and politics*, New York, 1989, Hemisphere Publishing.

46. Damon L, Linker C, and Ries C: Hemolytic reactions after autologous bone marrow infusions (personal communication), 1989.

47. Detels R, Visscher B, Fahey JL, Sever, JL, Gravell M, Madden DL, Schwartz K, Dudley JP, English PA, Powes H, Clark VA, and Gottlieb MS: Predictors of clinical AIDS in young homosexual men in a high-risk area, *Int J Epidemiol* 16:271-276, 1987.

48. Devey ME and Isenberg DA: Immune complex disease: theoretical aspects. In Bird G and Calvert JE, editors: *B lymphocytes in human disease*, Oxford, 1988, Oxford University Press.

49. Devita VT, Hellman S, and Rosenberg SA, editors: *AIDS: etiology, diagnosis, treatment, and prevention*, Philadelphia, 1988, JB Lippincott.

50. Devita VT, Jaffe ES, and Hellman S: Hodgkin's disease and and the non-Hodgkin's lymphomas. In Devita VT, Hellman S, and Rosenberg A, editors: *Cancer: principles and practice of oncology*, Philadelphia, 1988, JB Lippincott.

51. Dietary guidelines for the patient with systemic lupus erythematosus, *Bay Area Lupus Foundation Newsletter* 13(2):7-9, 1990.

52. Dixon FJ and Fisher W, editors: *The biology of immunologic disease*, Sunderland, Mass, 1983, Sinauer.

53. Donham JA and Denning V: Cold agglutinin syndrome: nursing management, *Heart Lung* 17(1):59-67, 1985.

54. Durum SK and Oppenheim JJ: Macrophage-derived mediators: interleukin-1, tumor necrosis factor, interleukin-6, interferon, and related cytokines. In Paul WE, editor: *Fundamental immunology*, ed 2, New York, 1989, Raven Press.

55. Emory D: Juvenile rheumatoid arthritis, Unpublished article, 1990.

55a. Farid and Sternzky, 1988.

56. Fearon DT: Complement. In Wyngaarden JB and Smith LH, editors: *Cecil's textbook of medicine*, Part 21: Diseases of the immune system, Philadelphia, 1985, WB Saunders.

57. Firkin BG, Hunt HA, and Jane SM: Management of refractory idiopathic thrombocytopenia, *Blood Reviews* 2: 149-156, 1988.

57a. Flagg, 1991.

58. Ford R and Ballard B: Acute complications after bone marrow transplantation, *Semin Oncol Nurs* 4(1):15-24, 1988.

59. Foster R, Hunsberger M, and Anderson J: *Family-centered nursing care of children*, London, 1989, WB Saunders.

60. Fries JF and Ehrlich GE: *Prognosis: contemporary outcomes of disease*, Bowie, Md, 1981, The Charles Press Publishers.

61. Fritzler MJ and Tan EM: Antinuclear antibodies and the connective tissue diseases. In Cohen AS, editor: *Laboratory diagnostic procedures in the rheumatic diseases*, Orlando, Fla, 1985, Grune & Stratton.

62. Frober JH: The anemias: causes and courses of action, *RN* 52(5):42-49, 1989.

63. Furukawa T, Takahashi M, Moriyama Y, Koike T, Kurokawa I, and Shibata A: Successful treatment of chronic idiopathic neutropenia using recombinant granulocyte colony-stimulating factor, *Ann Hematol* 62:22-24, 1991.

64. Fye K and Sack K: Rheumatic diseases. In Stites D, Stobo J, and Wells JV, editors: *Basic and clinical immunology*, ed 6, San Mateo, Calif, 1987, Appleton & Lange.

65. Gale R: Management of acute leukemias. I. Bone marrow transplants, *Clin Adv Oncol Nursing* 1(2):1-6, 1989.

66. Gee G and Moran TA, editors: *AIDS: concepts in nursing practice*, Baltimore, 1988, Williams & Wilkins.

66a. George, 1988.

67. Gewanter H: Juvenile arthritis. In Hoekelman R, editor: *Primary pediatric care*, St Louis, 1987, Mosby–Year Book.

68. Giannini AV, Shultz ND, Chang TT, and Wong DC: *Consumers Union edition: the best guide to allergy*, Mt Vernon, New York, 1985, Consumers Union.

69. Gibson J: Autoimmune hemolytic anemia: current concepts, *Aust NZ J Med* 18:625-637, 1988.

70. Glassock R, Cohen AH, Adler S, and Ward HJ: Secondary glomerular diseases. In Brenner B and Rector F, editors: *The kidney*, ed 3, Philadelphia, 1986, WB Saunders.

71. Golub ES and Green DR: *Immunology: a synthesis*, ed 2, 1991, Sinauer.

72. Grady C: Host defense mechanisms: an overview, *Semin Oncol Nurs* 4(2):86-94, 1988.

73. Greenspan JS and Greenspan D: Hairy leukoplakia and other oral features of HIV infection. In Levy JA, editor: *AIDS: pathogenesis and treatment*, New York, 1989, Marcel Dekker.

74. Greenspan D, Greenspan JS, Hearst NG, Li-Zhen P, Conant MA, Abrams DI, Hollander H, and Levy JA: Relation of oral hairy leukoplakia to infection with the human immunodeficiency virus and the risk of developing AIDS, *J Infect Dis* 155:475-481, 1987.

75. Hamilton HK, editor: Nursing clinical library: immune disorders, Springhouse, Pa, 1985, Springhouse.

76. Hansen JH: Current approaches in the treatment of status asthmaticus. Paper presented at Contemporary Forums: Pediatric Critical Care Nursing, San Francisco, Nov 13-16, 1991.

77. Harvey CJ and Verklan T: Systemic lupus erythematosus: obstetric and neonatal implications, *NAACOGS Clinical Issues in Perinatal and Women's Health Nursing* 1(2):177-185, 1990.

78. Henderson CJ and Lovell DJ: Comprehensive nutritional assessment of children and adolescents with juvenile rheumatoid arthritis, *Arthritis Rheum* 30(suppl):202, 1987.

79. Heyward WL and Curran JW: The epidemiology of AIDS in the U.S., *Sci Am* 72-81, 1988.

79a. Hickey, 1991.

79b. Hiller, 1991.

79c. Hillel et al., 1991.

80. Hong R: The DiGeorge anomaly, *Immunodefic Rev* 3(1):1-14, 1991.

81. Huffer T, Kanapa DJ, and Stevenson G: *Introduction to human immunology*, Boston, 1986, Jones & Bartlett.

82. Ishizaka K and Ishizaka T: Allergy. In Paul WE, editor: *Fundamental immunology*, ed 2, New York, 1989, Raven Press.

83. Jacobson MA and Mills J: Serious cytomegalovirus disease in the acquired immunodeficiency syndrome, *Ann Intern Med* 108:585-594, 1988.

84. Jett MF and Lancaster LE: The inflammatory immune response: the body's defense against invasion, *Crit Care Nurse* 64-84, 1983.

85. Kahan A, Amor B, Meckes CJ, and Strauch G: Recombinant interferon-gamma in the treatment of systemic sclerosis, *Am J Med* 87(3):273-277, 1989.

86. Kammer GM: Musculoskeletal and connective tissue diseases. In Andreoli T, Carpenter C, Plum F, and Smith L, editors: *Cecil's essentials of medicine*, Philadelphia, 1986, WB Saunders.

87. Karpatkin S: Immunological platelet disorders. In Samter M, editor: *Immunological diseases*, Boston/Toronto, 1988, Little, Brown & Co.

88. Katz RS: Update: treatment of rheumatoid arthritis, *Compr Ther* 15(5):62-73, 1989.

89. Katz WA: *Diagnosis and management of rheumatic disease*, ed 2, Philadelphia, 1988, JB Lippincott.

90. Kelly B and Mahon S: Nursing care of the patient with multiple sclerosis, *Rehabil Nurs* 13(5):238-243, 1988.

91. Kemp D: Development of the immune system, *Crit Care Q* 9(1):1-6, 1986.

92. Klein RS, Harris CA, Small CB, Moll B, Lesser M, and Friedland GH: Oral candidiasis in high-risk patients as the initial manifestation of the acquired immunodeficiency syndrome, *N Engl J Med* 311:354-358, 1984.

93. Koffler D: Immunology of systemic lupus erythematosus and related rheumatoid diseases, *Clin Symp* 39(2): 1987.

94. Kumagai K, Suzuki S, and Suzuki R: Role of the natural immune system in the antibody response. In Reynolds C and Wiltrout R, editors: *Functions of the natural immune system*, New York, 1989, Plenum Press.

95. Kumararatne DS, Bignall A, Joyce HJ, and Hazlewood M: Antibody deficiency disorders. In Gooi HC, editor: *Clinical immunology: a practical approach*, New York, 1990, Oxford Press.

96. Lancaster L, editor: *American Nephrology Nurses Association core curriculum for nephrology nursing*, ed 2, Pitman, NJ, 1990, The Association.

97. Lancaster L, editor: The patient with end-stage renal disease, New York, 1979, John Wiley & Sons.

98. Lanier R: Discussions in medicine: focus on allergic rhinitis—results of a roundtable discussion, Kenilworth, NJ, 1990, Schering Co.

99. Laubenstein L: Staging and treatment of Kaposi's sarcoma in patients with AIDS. In Friedman-Kien AE and Laubenstein LJ, editors: *AIDS: the epidemic of Kaposi's sarcoma and opportunistic infections*, New York, 1984, Masson.

100. Leach M: Anaemia: nursing care and intervention, *Professional Nurse* 454-456, 1991.

101. Lederle FA: Oral cobalamin for pernicious anemia: medicine's best kept secret? *JAMA* 265(1):94-95, 1991.

102. Legun LA: Systemic lupus during pregnancy, *Patient Care and Teaching* 20(9):86, 1990.

103. Levy JA, editor: *AIDS: pathogenesis and treatment*, New York, 1989, Marcel Dekker.

104. Lewis A, editor: *Nursing care of the person with AIDS/ARC*, Rockville, Md, 1988, Aspen Publishers.

105. Lewis S and Collier I: Medical-surgical nursing, St Louis, 1992, Mosby–Year Book.

106. Lichtenstein L: Insect stings. In Wyngaarden JB and Smith LH, editors: *Cecil's textbook of medicine*, Philadelphia, 1985, WB Saunders.

107. Logue GL, Shastri KA, Laughlin M, Shimm DS, Ziolkowski LM, and Inglehart JL: Idiopathic neutropenia: antineutrophil antibodies and clinical correlations, *Am J Med* 90:211-216, 1991.

108. Lombard CM, Colby TV, and Elliott CG: Surgical pathology of the lung in anti-basement antibody–associated Goodpasture's syndrome, *Hum Pathol* 20(5):445-451, 1989.

109. Malasanos L, Barkauskas V, Moss M, and Stoltenberg-Allen K: *Health assessment*, ed 3, St Louis, 1986, Mosby–Year Book.

110. Male D: *Immunology: an illustrated outline*, New York, 1986, Gower Medical Publishing.

111. Mann JM, Chin J, Piot P, and Quinn T: The international epidemiology of AIDS, *Sci Am* 82-89, 1988.

112. Marieb EN: *Essentials of human anatomy and physiology*, ed 2, Menlo Park, Calif, Benjamin Cummings.

113. Maxfield DL and Boyd WC: Pernicious anemia: a review, an update, and an illustrative case, *J Am Osteopath Assoc* 83(2):133-142, 1983.

113a. McCance and Muether, 1990.

114. McDonald G, Shulman H, et al: Intestinal and hepatic complications of bone marrow transplant. I, *Gastroenterology* 90:460-467, 1986.

115. Medsger TA: Treatment of systemic sclerosis, *Ann Rheum Dis* 4:(suppl 50) 877-886, 1991.

116. Merrill JE: The natural immune system in autoimmune and neurological disease. In Reynolds CW and Wiltrout RH, editors: *Functions of the natural immune system*, New York, 1989, Plenum Press.

117. Michalski JP and Biundo JJ: Histocompatibility antigens. In Katz WA, editor: *Diagnosis and management of rheumatic diseases*, ed 2, Philadelphia, 1988, JB Lippincott.

118. Middleton E, Reed CE, Ellis EF, Adkinson NF, and Yunginger JW, editors: *Allergy: principles and practice*, ed 3, St Louis, 1988, Mosby–Year Book.

119. Mirabelli L: Caring for patients with rheumatoid arthritis, *Nursing 90* 22(9): 67-72, 1990.

120. Morgante LA, Madonna M, and Pokoluk R: Research and treatment in multiple sclerosis: implications for nursing practice, *J Neurosci Nurs* 21(5):285-289, 1989.

121. Muller W, Peter HH, Wilken M, Juppner H, Kallfelz HC, Krohn HP, Miller K, and Rieger CH: The DiGeorge syndrome, *Eur J Pediatr* 147(5):496-502, 1988.

122. Nass T: Helping the patient who has lupus, *RN* 50(10):69-74, 1987.

123. Navia BA, Jordan BD, and Price RW: The AIDS dementia complex. I. Clinical features, *Ann Neurol* 19:517-524, 1986.

124. Navia BA, Cho ES, Petito CK, and Price RW: The AIDS dementia complex. II. Neuropathology, *Ann Neurol* 19:525-535, 1986.

125. Nelson HS: The atopic diseases, *Ann Allergy* 55:441, 1985.

126. Ng SC, Clements PJ, and Paulus HE: *Singapore Med J* 31(3):269-272, 1990.

127. Nickoloff E: Schilling test: physiologic basis for and use as a diagnostic test, *Crit Rev Clin Lab Sci* 26(4):263-276, 1988.

128. Nims J and Strom S: Late complications of bone marrow transplant recipients: nursing care issues, *Semin Oncol Nurs* 4(1):47-54, 1988.

129. Oniboni AC: Infection in the neutropenic patient, *Semin Oncol Nurs* 6(1): 50-60, 1990.

130. Ott MJ, Senner A, and Esker S: Intravenous gammaglobulin: clinical applications in pediatric care, *J Pediatr Nurs* 5(5):307-315, 1990.

131. Page G: Chronic pain and the child with juvenile rheumatoid arthritis, *J Pediatr Health Care* 5(1):18-23, 1991.

132. Page-Goertz S: Even children have arthritis, *Pediatr Nurs* 15(1):1989.

133. Patten E: Immunohematologic diseases, *JAMA* 258(20):2945-2951, 1987.

134. Paul W: Introduction to the immune system. In Wyngaarden JB and Smith LH, editors: *Cecil's textbook of medicine*, Part 21: Diseases of the immune system, Philadelphia, 1985, WB Saunders.

135. Paul WE, editor: *Fundamental immunology*, ed 2, New York, 1989, Raven Press.

136. Perkins JE: Food allergies and adverse reactions, Gaithersburg, Md, Aspen Publishers.

136a. Perlo, 1988.

137. Porth C: Alteration in cardiac function. In Porth C: *Pathophysiology, concepts of altered health states*, Philadelphia, 1986, JB Lippincott.

138. Potter DO and Rose MB: Assessment, patient history, anatomy and physiology, physical examination, nursing diagnosis; Nurse's Reference Library Series, Springhouse, Pa, 1983, Springhouse.

139. Price SA and Wilson LM: Pathophysiology; clinical concepts of disease processes, ed 2, New York, 1982, McGraw-Hill.

140. Queluz TH, Pawlowski I, Brunda MJ, Brentjens JR, Viadutiu AC, and Andres G: Pathogenesis of an experimental model of Goodpasture's hemorrhagic pneumonitis, *J Clin Invest* 85(5):1507-1515, 1990.

141. Reynolds: Functions of the natural immune system, Q Rev 185.2 F86, 1989.

142. Reynolds C and Wiltrout R, editors: *Functions of the natural immune system*, New York, 1989, Plenum Press.

142a. Richards, 1986.

143. Rizzo WB, Dammann AL, Craft DA, Black SH, Tilton AH, Africk D, Chaves-Carballo E, Holmgren G, Jaqell S: Sjögren-Larson syndrome: inherited defect in the fatty alcohol cycle, *J Pediatr* 115(2):223-234, 1989.

144. Roitt I, Brostoff J, and Male D: *Immunology*, London, 1989, Gower Medical Publishing.

145. Roitt I, Brostoff J, and Male D: *Slide*

atlas of immunology, New York, 1985, Gower Medical Publishing.

146. Rosenblum ML, Levy RM, Bredeson DE, So YT, Wara W, and Ziegler JL: Primary central nervous system lymphomas in patients with AIDS, *Ann Neurol* (suppl)23:S13-S16, 1988.

147. Rote NS: Alterations in immunity and inflammation. In McCance K and Huether S, editors: *Pathophysiology: the biologic basis for disease in adults and children*, St Louis, 1990, Mosby–Year Book.

148. Samter M, Talmage DW, Frank MM, Austen KF, and Claman HN, editors: *Immunological diseases*, ed 4, Boston/Toronto, 1988, Little, Brown & Co.

149. Saxona R, Bygren P, Butkowski R, and Wieslander J: Specificity of kidney-bound antibodies in Goodpasture's syndrome, *Clin Exp Immunol* 78(1):31-36, 1988.

150. Scheirberg L: Multiple sclerosis: a guide for patients and their families, ed 4, New York, 1986, Raven Press.

151. Schryber S, Lacasse C, and Barton-Burke M: Autologous bone marrow transplantation, *Oncol Nurs Forum* 14(4):74-80, 1987.

152. Schumacher HR and Gall EP: *Rheumatoid arthritis: an illustrated guide to pathology, diagnosis, and management*, Philadelphia, 1988, JB Lippincott.

153. Schur P, editor: *The clinical management of systemic lupus erythematosus*, New York, 1983, Grune & Stratton.

154. Schwartz R and Datta S: Autoimmunity and autoimmune diseases. In Paul WE, editor: *Fundamental immunology*, ed 2, New York, 1989, Raven Press.

155. Scientific Group on Immunodeficiency sponsored by World Health Organization in *Immunodefic Rev* 1:173-205, 1989.

156. Scoggin C: Pulmonary manifestations. In Katz WA, editor: *Diagnosis and management of rheumatic diseases*, ed 2, Philadelphia, 1988, JB Lippincott.

157. Seidel H, Ball J, Dains J, and Benedict GW: *Mosby's guide to physical examination*, St Louis, 1991, Mosby–Year Book.

158. Selby C and Utsinger PD: Gastrointestinal and abdominal manifestations. In Katz WA, editor: *Diagnosis and management of rheumatic diseases*, ed 2, Philadelphia, 1988, JB Lippincott.

159. Shapiro GG, Virant FS, Furukawa CT, Pierson WE, and Bierman CW: Immunologic defects in patients with refractory sinusitis, *Pediatrics* 87(3):1991.

160. Sheffer A: Guidelines for the diagnosis and management of asthma: National Heart, Lung and Blood Institute National Asthma Education Program expert panel report, Part 2, *J Allergy Clin Immunol* vol 88, no 3.

161. Sheffer AL: Anaphylaxis, *J Clin Immunol* 75:227, 1985.

162. Sienknecht CW: Care of the person with rheumatoid arthritis, *Compr Ther* 16(4):29-35, 1990.

163. Siegel H and Seelenfreund M: Racial and social factors in systemic lupus erythematosus, *JAMA* 191:77, 1965.

164. Smith SL: Physiology of the immune system, *Crit Care Q* 9(1):7-13, 1986.

165. Standen G: Wiskott-Aldrich syndrome: new perspectives in pathogenesis and management, *J R Coll Physicians Lond* 22(2):80-83, 1988.

166. Stevens MB: Sjögren's syndrome. In McGehee A, Johns RJ, McKusick VA, Owens AH, and Ross RS, editors: *The principles and practice of medicine*, ed 21, Norwalk, Conn, 1984, Appleton & Lange.

167. Stevens MB: Systemic lupus. In Harvey AM, Johns RJ, McKusick VA, Owens AH, and Ross RS, editors: *The principles and practice of medicine*, ed 21, Norwalk, Conn, Appleton & Lange.

168. Stevens MB and Halhn BH: Management of systemic lupus erythematosus, *Bull Rheum Dis* 32:35, 1982.

169. Stites DP and Terr AI: *Basic human immunology*, San Mateo, Calif, 1991, Appleton & Lange.

170. Stites DP and Terr AI, editors: *Basic and clinical immunology*, ed 7, San Mateo, Calif, 1991, Appleton & Lange.

171. Storb R: Bone marrow transplantation. In DeVita V, Hellman S, and Rosenberg S, editors: *Cancer: principles and practice of oncology*, Philadelphia, 1989, JB Lippincott.

172. Strand V and Talal N: Advances in the diagnosis and concept of Sjögren's syndrome (autoimmune exocrinopathy), *Bull Rheum Dis* 30:1046, 1979-80.

172a. Swank and Grimsgaard, 1988.

173. Tan EM, Cohen JF, Fries AS, Masi AT, McShane DJ, Rothfield NF, Schaller JG, Talal N, and Winchester RJ: The 1982 revised criteria for the classification of systemic lupus erythematosus, *Arthritis Rheum* 25:1271, 1982.

174. Taylor S: Food allergies and related adverse reactions to foods: a food science perspective. In Perkins JE, editor: *Food allergies and adverse reactions*, Gaithersburg, Md, Aspen Publishers.

175. Taylor J, Passo M, and Champion V: School problems and teacher responsibilities in juvenile rheumatoid arthritis, *J Sch Health* 57(5):186-191, 1987.

176. Terr AI: Allergic diseases. In Stites DP, Stobo JD, and Wells JV, editors: *Basic clinical immunology*, ed 6, Norwalk, Conn, 1987, Appleton & Lange.

177. Tetreault EE: Understanding lupus, *Nursing* 20(9):86, 1990.

178. Thompson J et al: *Clinical nursing*, St Louis, 1989, Mosby–Year Book.

178a. Thompson J et al., 1990.

179. Thorn GW et al: *Harrison's principles of internal medicine*, ed 11, New York, 1986, McGraw-Hill.

180. Ultraviolet light and lupus, *Bay Area Lupus Foundation Newsletter* 13(3):1-5, 1990.

180a. Utiger, 1987.

181. Vanarsdel PP: Drug hypersensitivity. In Bierman CW and Pearlman DS, editors: *Allergic diseases from infancy to adulthood*, ed 2, Philadelphia, 1988, WB Saunders.

182. Virella G, Goust JM, Fudenberg H, and Patrick C: *Introduction to medical immunology*, New York, 1986, Marcel Dekker.

183. Virella G and Spivey MA: Immunohematology, *Immunol Ser* 50:375-394, 1990.

184. Vogelsang G: Bone marrow transplantation, *Mediguide to Oncology* 9(2):1-6, 1989.

185. Volberding PA and Mitsuyasu R: Recombinant interferon-alpha in the treatment of acquired immune deficiency syndrome–related Kaposi's sarcoma, *Semin Oncol* 12(4, suppl 5):2-6, 1985.

186. Wara D: Immunologic disorders. In Rudolph A, editor: *Rudolph's textbook of pediatrics*, ed 19, San Mateo, Calif, 1991, Appleton & Lange.

187. Warkentin TE and Kelton JG: Current concepts in the treatment of immune thrombocytopenia, *Drugs* 40(4):531-542, 1990.

188. Warren RW and Collins ML: Immune hemolytic anemia in children, *Crit Rev Oncol Hematol* 8(1):65-73, 1988.

189. Whaley L and Wong D: *Nursing care of infants and children*, ed 4, St Louis, 1991, Mosby–Year Book.

190. Williams WJ, editor: *Hematology*, New York, McGraw-Hill.

191. Wilson CB and Dixon FJ: The renal response to immunological injury. In Brenner B and Rector F, editors: *The kidney*, ed 3, Philadelphia, 1986, WB Saunders.

192. Wilson CB, Fornasieri A, Moullier P, Tang W, and Ward DW: Renal diseases. In Stites DP and Terr AI, editors: *Basic and clinical immunology*, ed 7, San Mateo, Calif, 1991, Appleton & Lange.

193. Wingard J, Sostrin M, Vriesendorp H, et al: Interstitial pneumonitis following autologous bone marrow transplantation, *Transplantation* 46(1):61-65, 1988.

194. Winston D, Ho W, Lin C, et al: Intravenous immune globulin for prevention of cytomegalovirus infection and interstitial pneumonia after bone marrow transplantation, *Ann Intern Med* 106:12-18, 1987.

195. Wood SF: Lupus: the great imitator, *Nurse Week/North* 3(12):18-20, 1990.

196. Wormser GP, Stahl RE, and Bottone EJ, editors: *AIDS and other manifestations of HIV infection*, Park Ridge, NJ, 1987, Noyes.

197. Yarchoan R, Mitsuya H, and Broder S: AIDS therapies, *Sci Am* 110-119, 1988.

198. Zehr BP and Hunninghake GW: Respiratory diseases. In Stites DP and Terr AI, editors: *Basic and clinical immunology*, ed 7, San Mateo, Calif, 1991, Appleton & Lange.

COMPLETE BLOOD COUNT

Cell type	Purpose	Normal values	Cause for increased value	Cause for decreased value
Red blood cells (RBCs)	To evaluate oxygen-carrying capacity of blood	Men: 4.7-6.1 Women: 4.2-5.4 Children: 3.8-5.5 (100,000/mm^3)	**Polycythemia** Polycythemia vera, chronic anoxia, congenital cardiac disease	**Anemia** Goodpasture's syndrome, SLE, rheumatoid arthritis, aplastic anemia, autoimmune hemolytic anemia, bone marrow failure, hemorrhage, sepsis, dietary deficiency
Hemoglobin (Hb)	To evaluate oxygen-carrying capacity of the blood (part of RBC that carries oxygen [heme] and protein [globulin])	Men: 14-18 Women: 12-16 Children: 11-16 (g/dl)	Severe dehydration increases the percent concentration of RBCs; in normal hydration states, increased Hb indicates increased RBCs	Dilutional overhydration decreases concentration; associated with autoimmune disorders, aplastic anemia, autoimmune hemolytic anemia
Hematocrit (Hct)	To evaluate percent of RBCs and hydration status	Men: 42-52% Women: 37-47% Children: 30-43%	Severe dehydration (same as for increased RBCs)	Aplastic anemia, autoimmune hemolytic anemia
White cell count (WBC) (leukocytes)	To evaluate immune system's response to invading antigens	<4 yr: 5,500-17000/μl ≥4 yr: 3,400-10,000/μd/l	**Leukocytosis** Infection, leukemia, neoplasia, trauma, stress (emotional/physical)	**Leukopenia** Bone marrow failure, overwhelming infection, nutritional insufficiency, autoimmune disorders
Differential WBC Neutrophils (PMNs)	To evaluate percent of neutrophils; may reflect an inflammation	60%-80%	**Neutrophilia** Infection, inflammation, stress (emotional/physical), trauma/hemorrhage, myelocytic leukemia, poisoning, ketoacidosis	**Neutropenia** Overwhelming infection, aplastic anemia, chemotherapy, radiotherapy, vitamin B$_{12}$ or folic acid deficiency
Eosinophils	To evaluate percent of eosinophils and presence as mediator in an inflammation	2%-5%	**Eosinophilia** Parasitic infestation, allergies, asthma, inflammation, eczema, leukemia, autoimmune and inflammatory disorders	**Eosinopenia** Increased adrenal steroid production, stress, SLE, Cushing's syndrome
Basophils	To evaluate percentage (basophils contain vasoactive substances [histamine and serotonin] and are involved in allergic reactions)	0.5%-2%	**Basophilia** Basophilic leukemia, inflammatory and allergic conditions of the skin, small intestine, kidneys, nose, and eyes; graft rejection	**Basophilopenia** Occasionally hyperthyroidism
Lymphocytes	To evaluate percent of lymphocytes and immune response	20%-40%	**Lymphocytosis** Chronic bacterial infection, viral infection, multiple myeloma, infectious mononucleosis, lymphocytic leukemia, Cushing's disease	**Lymphocytopenia** Leukemia, antineoplastic drugs, monoclonal antibodies to treat graft rejection, immunosuppressive medications (e.g., corticosteroids), immunodeficiency diseases, AIDS, sepsis, sometimes in SLE
Monocytes	To evaluate percent of monocytes and potential phagocytic activity	2%-10%	**Monocytosis** Acute HIV mononucleosis, anemia, myelocytic leukemia, cancer, inflammatory disorders	**Monocytopenia** Rarely decreased immunodeficiency disorders

EXAMPLES OF AGGLUTINATION ASSAYS

Assay	Clinical application
Immunologic assays	
Bentonite flocculation	To detect rheumatoid factor, *Trichinella* organisms
Coombs' test	ABO typing before blood transfusions; to evaluate newborns for hemolytic disease and diagnose autoimmune hemolytic anemia
Hemagglutination	To detect antibodies to RBCs (incompatibility, transfusion reactions)
Hemagglutination using nuclear antigens	To detect antinuclear antibodies in various autoimmune disorders (SLE)
Latex fixation	To determine rheumatoid factor (Rh)
Rose-Waaler test	To determine rheumatoid factor (Rh)
Tanned erythrocyte hemagglutination	To detect antithyroid antibodies
Assays for microorganisms	
Antistreptolysin-O (ASO)	To detect antibodies against a single enzyme released early in group A beta-hemolytic streptococcal infections
Cold agglutinins	To detect *Mycoplasma* pneumonia
Febrile agglutinins	To detect agglutinins produced by fever
Hemagglutination inhibition	To detect hepatitis B, rubella, pregnancy
Heterophil antibody titer (HAT)	To detect Epstein-Barr virus (mononucleosis)
Proteus vulgaris test	To detect rickettsial infections (typhus, Rocky Mountain spotted fever)
Rapid plasma reagin (RPR)	To detect syphilis
Widal's reaction	To detect salmonellosis

Index